PRIMO GASTRO
The Pocket GI/Liver Companion

PRIMO GASTRO
The Pocket GI/Liver Companion

Jason M. Guardino, DO, MS Ed.
Cleveland Clinic
Department of Gastroenterology & Hepatology
Cleveland, Ohio

Wolters Kluwer | Lippincott Williams & Wilkins
Health
Philadelphia • Baltimore • New York • London
Buenos Aires • Hong Kong • Sydney • Tokyo

Acquisitions Editor: Charles W. Mitchell
Managing Editor: Sirkka Bertling
Project Manager: Fran Gunning
Manufacturing Coordinator: Kathleen Brown
Marketing Manager: Kimberly Schonberger
Creative Director: Doug Smock
Production Services: International Typesetting and Composition

1st Edition
© 2008 by Lippincott Williams & Wilkins, a Wolters Kluwer business
530 Walnut Street
Philadelphia, PA 19106
LWW.com

All rights reserved. This book is protected by copyright. No part of this book may be reproduced in any form or by any means, including photocopying, or utilizing by any information storage and retrieval system without written permission from the copyright owner, except for brief quotations embodied in critical articles and reviews.

Printed in the USA

Library of Congress Cataloging-in-Publication Data

Guardino, Jason M.
  Primo gastro : the pocket GI/liver companion / Jason M. Guardino.—
1st ed.
    p. ; cm.
  ISBN-13: 978-0-7817-7944-9
  ISBN-10: 0-7817-7944-8
  1. Gastroenterology—Handbooks, manuals, etc. 2. Digestive
organs—Diseases—Handbooks, manuals, etc. 3.
Liver—Diseases—Handbooks, manuals, etc. I. Title.
  [DNLM: 1. Digestive System Diseases—Handbooks. 2. Endoscopy,
Digestive System—methods—Handbooks. WI 39 G914p 2008]
  RC802.G83 2008
  616.3'3—dc22
                               2007029452

  Care has been taken to confirm the accuracy of the information presented and to describe generally accepted practices. However, the authors, editors, and publisher are not responsible for errors or omissions or for any consequences from application of the information in this book and make no warranty, expressed or implied, with respect to the currency, completeness, or accuracy of the contents of the publication. Application of this information in a particular situation remains the professional responsibility of the practitioner.
  The authors, editors, and publisher have exerted every effort to ensure that drug selection and dosage set forth in this text are in accordance with current recommendations and practice at the time of publication. However, in view of ongoing research, changes in government regulations, and the constant flow of information relating to drug therapy and drug reactions, the reader is urged to check the package insert for each drug for any change in indications and dosage and for added warnings and precautions. This is particularly important when the recommended agent is a new or infrequently employed drug.
  Some drugs and medical devices presented in this publication have Food and Drug Administration (FDA) clearance for limited use in restricted research settings. It is the responsibility of health care providers to ascertain the FDA status of each drug or device planned for use in their clinical practice.
  The publishers have made every effort to trace copyright holders for borrowed material. If they have inadvertently overlooked any, they will be pleased to make the necessary arrangements at the first opportunity.
  To purchase additional copies of this book, call our customer service department at (800) 639-3030 or fax orders to (301) 824-7390. International customers should call (301) 714-2324. Lippincott Williams & Wilkins customer service representatives are available from 8:30 am to
6:00 pm, EST, Monday through Friday, for telephone access. Visit Lippincott Williams & Wilkins on the Internet: http://www.lww.com.

10 9 8 7 6 5 4 3 2 1

To Mom & Dad, for giving me roots and wings.
To Gram, for being my confidant.
To Guardino, Corbari & Yee clans, for your unconditional support.
To Stephanie, for being my rock, my best friend, and the love of my life.
To Sofia, for being the one I strive to be like.

Preface

It is with great pleasure that I introduce *Primo Gastro*. The design and ultimate goal of this book is to provide a comprehensive review of several gastroenterology and hepatology topics that are readily available at the reader's fingertips in a pocket-sized handbook.

It is my hope that medical students, residents, fellows, and even staff physicians will find *Primo Gastro* informative and enlightening. While I realize that numerous resources are available at the turn of a page or the click of a mouse, more often than not medical professionals spend much of their time wading through a vast array of information to get answers to a specific question. In an effort to reduce frustration and valuable time spent, *Primo Gastro* includes several unique features. Topics, which are alphabetized, take the practitioner through the digestive, pancreatic, and hepatic systems, as well as incorporate several endoscopy topics. Each topic of the book is arranged to facilitate a rapid but thoughtful initial approach to the diagnosis and treatment of common inpatient and outpatient conditions. Most topics are one or two pages in length with the majority having standardized subtopics and are organized so that pages face each other allowing all related material to be viewed. To provide high-yield information in a concise manner each topic is discussed in bullet format, and several topics include easy-to-understand tables so that the most clinically useful and relevant material is presented. When appropriate, topics are cross-referenced to each other and contain the most recent national guidelines (at the time of publication) at the top of each page. This book would also be a great tool for board review in Gastroenterology/Hepatology, likewise it would be a great tool for board review for the GI/Liver portion of the Internal Medicine and Family Practice boards. Lastly, this pocketbook has been sized to fit into a standard laboratory coat pocket, briefcase, or purse, which allows easy portability during hospital rounds or outpatient visits.

Although the recommendations herein are as evidence-based as possible, one must not forget that medicine is an ever-changing science that must be blended with the art of medical practice. Nothing will replace a clinician's experience and sound medical judgment. I hope you find *Primo Gastro* to be concise, thorough, and most important, clinically useful.

Jason M. Guardino, DO, MS Ed.
www.PrimoGastro.com

Acknowledgments

A special thanks to all my mentors at the Cleveland Clinic who have been inspiring colleagues and friends.

Table of Contents

SECTION I: ESOPHAGUS/GASTRIC

1.01	Achalasia	2
1.02	Barrett's Esophagus (BE)	4
1.03	Diverticula of Esophagus (Zenker's)	8
1.04	Dyspepsia (Indigestion)	10
1.05	Dysphagia/Odynophagia	12
1.06	Eosinophilic Esophagitis	16
1.07	Eosinophilic Gastroenteritis	18
1.08	Esophageal Cancer	20
1.09	Esophageal Infections	22
	Fungal: *Candida albicans*	22
	Viral	22
	Bacterial	22
1.10	Gastric Cancer	24
1.11	Gastric Polyps & Thickened Gastric Folds	28
1.12	Gastroparesis & Dumping Syndrome	30
1.13	Gastropathy/Chronic Gastritis	34
1.14	Gastroesophageal Reflux Disease (GERD)/Nonerosive Reflux Disease (NERD)/Erosive Esophagitis (EE)	36
1.15	Injury (Esophagus): Corrosive	40
1.16	Injury (Esophagus): Pill Induced	42
1.17	Manometry (Esophageal)	44
1.18	Nausea & Vomiting	48
1.19	Non-Cardiac Chest Pain	52
1.20	Percutaneous Endoscopic Gastrostomy (PEG) Tubes	54
1.21	Peptic Ulcer Disease (PUD): *H. Pylori*, NSAIDs	58
1.22	Schatzki's Ring/Esophageal Spasm	62
1.23	Zollinger-Ellison Syndrome (Gastrinoma)	64
1.24	Potpourri	66
	Gastric Physiology (Acid Secretion)	66
	Hiccups	66
	Lichen Planus	67
	Eating Disorders	67
	Bezoars	67

TABLE OF CONTENTS

SECTION II: SMALL BOWEL/COLON/RECTUM

2.01	Abdominal Pain: General	70
2.02	Abdominal Pain: Acute	72
2.03	Abdominal Pain: Chronic	74
2.04	Anorectal Diseases	76
	Hemorrhoids	76
	Solitary Rectal Ulcer Syndrome	77
	Anal Fissures	77
	Pruritus Ani	77
2.05	Appendix Disease & Meckel's Diverticulum	78
2.06	Bacterial Overgrowth	80
2.07	*Clostridium Difficile*	82
2.08	Carcinoid Tumors (Mid-Gut)	84
2.09	Celiac & Tropical Sprue	86
2.10	Colorectal Cancer	90
2.11	Constipation	94
2.12	Diarrhea/Malassimilation	98
2.13	Diarrheal Infections	102
2.14	Diverticulosis & Diverticulitis	106
2.15	Fecal Incontinence	108
2.16	GI Endocrine Tumors	110
	Insulinoma	110
	VIPoma	111
	Glucagonoma	112
	Somatostatinoma	112
	Carcinoid Tumors - See Chapter 2.08/Page 84	
	Zollinger-Ellison Syndrome (Gastrinoma) - See Chapter 1.23/Page 64	
2.17	Irritable Bowel Syndrome (IBS)	114
2.18	Ischemic Colitis	118
2.19	Ischemic Small Bowel	120
2.20	Megacolon (Ogilvie's Syndrome)	122
2.21	Nutrition: Malnutrition & Obesity	124
2.22	Nutrition: Total Parenteral Nutrition (TPN) & Refeeding Syndrome	128
2.23	Short Bowel Syndrome	132
2.24	Small Bowel Tumors	136
2.25	Whipple's Disease	138
2.26	Potpourri	140
	Fecal Fat	140

TABLE OF CONTENTS

SECTION III: INFLAMMATORY BOWEL DISEASE

3.01	Crohn's Disease	142
3.02	Microscopic & Radiation Colitis	146
3.03	Treatment: Crohn's Disease & Ulcerative Colitis	148
3.04	Ulcerative Colitis	152
3.05	Potpourri	156
	IBD Pearls	156
	IBD Mimickers	156
	Small Bowel Resection and Malabsorption	156
	Kidney Stones	156

SECTION IV: LIVER

4.01	α1-Antitrypsin Deficiency	158
4.02	Abscess of Liver	160
4.03	Acute Liver Failure (Fulminant Hepatic Failure)	162
4.04	Alcoholic Liver Disease	166
4.05	Ascites & Portal Hypertension	170
4.06	Autoimmune Hepatitis	174
4.07	Bacterial Peritonitis	178
4.08	Cirrhosis & Encephalopathy	180
4.09	Clots	184
	Budd-Chiari Syndrome	185
	Portal Vein Thrombosis	186
	Veno-Occlusive Disease	186
	Hepatic Artery Thrombosis	187
4.10	Congenital Hepatic Fibrosis	188
4.11	Drug & Toxic Induced Liver Disease	190
4.12	Hemochromatosis & Iron Overload	194
4.13	Hepatitis A, D, E	198
4.14	Hepatitis B	200
4.15	Hepatitis C	204
4.16	Hepatobiliary Cystic Disease	208
	Bile Duct Cysts	208
	Caroli's	209
	Polycystic Liver Disease	209
	Simple Hepatic Cysts	209
	Hydatid Cyst Disease	209
4.17	Hepatocellular Carcinoma	210

xiii

TABLE OF CONTENTS

4.18	Hepatorenal Syndrome	214
4.19	Histopathology of Liver	216
4.20	Liver Function Tests	220
4.21	Mass (Focal Liver) Evaluation	224
4.22	Non-alcoholic Fatty Liver Disease (NAFLD)/Non-alcoholic Steatohepatitis (NASH)/Non-alcoholic Fatty Liver (NAFL)	228
4.23	Primary Biliary Cirrhosis (PBC)	230
4.24	Primary Sclerosing Cholangitis (PSC)	232
4.25	Pregnancy Pearls	234
	Acute Fatty Liver of Pregnancy	234
	Autoimmune Hepatitis	234
	Budd-Chiari Syndrome	235
	Gallstones	235
	Intrahepatic Cholestasis of Pregnancy	235
	Pre-Eclampsia/Eclampsia/HELLP	235
	Viral Hepatitis	236
	Wilson's Disease	236
4.26	Pulmonary Complications	238
	Hepatopulmonary Syndrome	238
	Portopulmonary Hypertension	239
4.27	Transplant Immunosuppression	242
4.28	Transplantation	244
4.29	Wilson's Disease	248

SECTION V: PANCREAS/BILIARY

5.01	Cholangiocarcinoma	252
5.02	Cholecystitis & Cholangitis	256
	Choledochal Cysts, See Hepatobiliary Cystic Disease - Chapter 4.16/Page 208	
5.03	Cholelithiasis & Choledocholithiasis	258
5.04	Cystic Disease of the Pancreas	262
5.05	Pancreatic Carcinoma	266
5.06	Pancreatitis: Acute	270
5.07	Pancreatitis: Chronic	274
5.08	Sphincter of Oddi Dysfunction	278
5.09	Potpourri	280
	Pancreas Anatomy and Physiology	280
	Gallbladder Polyps	280

TABLE OF CONTENTS

SECTION VI: GI BLEED

6.01	Acute GI Bleed Pearls	282
6.02	Diverticular Bleeding	284
6.03	Occult & Obscure Bleeding	286
6.04	Upper & Lower GI Bleeding	288
6.05	Variceal Bleeding	292
6.06	Potpourri	294
	Argon Plasma Coagulation (APC) Therapy	294

SECTION VII: ENDOSCOPY & PROCEDURES

7.01	Anticoagulation & Anti-Inflammatory Management for Endoscopy	296
7.02	Balloon Tamponade	298
7.03	Capsule Endoscopy	300
7.04	Colonoscopy	302
7.05	Esophagogastroduodenoscopy (EGD)	304
7.06	Endoscopic Retrograde Cholangiopancreatography (ERCP)	306
7.07	Endoscopic Ultrasound (EUS)	308
7.08	Foreign Bodies	310
7.09	Gastrointestinal Surgeries	312
	Billroth Type I and II	312
	Roux-en-Y Total Gastrectomy	312
	Whipple's (Pancreatoduodenectomy)	312
	Puestow (Longitudinal Pancreaticojejunostomy)	312
7.10	Infectious Endocarditis Prophylaxis for Endoscopy	314
	Index	316

ABBREVIATIONS

5-ASA:	5-Aminosalycylates
5-HIAA:	5-Hydroxyindolacetic acid
5-HT:	Serotonin
6-MP:	6-Mercaptopurine
α1-AT:	alpha 1 antitrypsin deficiency
Aϕ:	Alkaline phosphatase
AAPC:	Attenuated adenomatous polyposis coli
AC:	Adenocarcinoma
ADPKD:	Autosomal dominant polycystic kidney disease
AFB:	Acid-fast bacilli
AFLP:	Acute fatty liver of pregnancy
AFP:	Alpha fetal protein
AFTP:	Ascites fluid total protein
AGN:	Acute glomerulonephritis
AIH:	Autoimmune hepatitis
AKA:	Also known as
ANA:	Antinuclear antibody
APC:	Argon plasma coagulation
ARDS:	Acute respiratory distress syndrome
ASA:	Aspirin
ASD:	Atrial septal defect
ASMA:	Anti-smooth muscle antibody
ATN:	Acute tubular necrosis
BB:	Beta blocker
BCS:	Budd-Chiari syndrome
BE:	Barrett's esophagus
BM:	Bowel movement
BMI:	Body mass index
BO:	Bacterial overgrowth
BRAVO:	Wireless gastric pH monitoring system
BRBPR:	Bright red blood per rectum
CA:	Cancer
CBD:	Common bile duct
CCB:	Calcium channel blocker
CCK:	Cholecystokinin
CD:	Crohn's disease
CDC:	Center for Disease Control
CEA:	Carcinoembryonic antigen
CHO:	Carbohydrate
CIS:	Carcinoma in situ
CK:	Creatinine kinase
CLO:	Campylobacter-like organism
CMP:	Complete metabolic panel
CMV:	Cytomegalovirus
CNS:	Central nervous system
CPP:	Cerebral perfusion pressure
CRC:	Colorectal cancer
CREST:	Calcinosis, Reynaud's phenomenon, sclerodactyly, esophageal dysmotility, telangiectasia
CRF:	Chronic renal failure
CTP:	Child-Turcotte-Pugh class
CVA:	Cerebral vascular accident
CVVHD:	Continuous veno-venous hemodialysis
DCT:	Distal convoluted tubule
DDX:	Differential Diagnosis
DES:	Diffuse esophageal spasm
DIC:	Disseminated intravascular coagulation
DKA:	Diabetic ketoacidosis
DM:	Diabetes mellitus
DU:	Duodenal ulcer
EBL:	Esophageal band ligation
EBV:	Epstein-Barr virus
ELISA:	Enzyme linked immunosorbent assay
EMR:	Endoscopic mucosal resection
EN:	Erythema nodosum
ENT:	Ear, nose, throat
ESR:	Erythrocyte sedimentation rate
ETOH:	Alcohol
EUS:	Endoscopic ultrasound

ABBREVIATIONS

FAP:	Familial adenomatous polyposis	HIDA:	Hepatobiliary iminodiacetic acid
FFP:	Fresh frozen plasma	HIV:	Human immunodeficiency virus
FHF:	Fulminant hepatic failure	HLA:	Human leukocyte antigen
FNA:	Fine needle aspiration	HNPCC:	Hereditary nonpolyposis colorectal cancer
FNH:	Focal nodular hyperplasia	HPS:	Hepatopulmonary syndrome
FOBT:	Fecal occult blood test	HPV:	Human papilloma virus
GAVE:	Gastric antral vascular ectasia	HR:	Heart rate
GB:	Gallbladder	HRS:	Hepatorenal syndrome
GDM:	Gastroduodenal manometry	HSM.	Hepatosplenomegaly
GE:	Gastroesophageal	HSV:	Herpes simplex virus
GEJ:	Gastroesophageal junction	HTN:	Hypertension
GERD:	Gastroesophageal reflux disease	HVWPG:	Hepatic venous wedge pressure gradient
GES:	Gastric emptying study	IBD:	Inflammatory bowel disease
GFR:	Glomerular filtration rate	IBS:	Irritable bowel syndrome
GIB:	Gastrointestinal bleed	IC:	Ileocecal
GIST:	Gastrointestinal stromal tumors	ICP:	Intracranial pressure
GN:	Glomerulonephritis	IDA:	Iron deficiency anemia
GNB:	Gram negative bacilli	IHCP:	Intrahepatic cholestasis of pregnancy
GNR:	Gram negative rod	IHSS:	Idiopathic hypertrophic subaortic stenosis (term replaced with HCM)
GPC:	Gram positive cocci		
GU:	Gastric ulcer		
GVHD:	Graft-versus-host disease		
HAV:	Hepatitis A Virus	IL:	Interleukin
HBIG:	Hepatitis B Immune Globulin	IM:	Intestinal metaplasia
		INH:	Isoniazid
HBV:	Hepatitis B Virus	INR:	International normalized ratio
HCC:	Hepatocellular carcinoma		
HCG:	Human chorionic gonadotropin	IPMN:	Intraductal papillary mucinous neoplasm
HCL:	Hydrochloric acid	IVC:	Inferior vena cava
HCM:	Hypertrophic cardiomyopathy	IVIG:	Intravenous immune globulin
HCV:	Hepatitis C Virus	JET:	Jejunal extension tube
HDV:	Hepatitis D Virus	LAN:	Lymphadenopathy
HELLP:	Hemolysis, elevated liver enzymes, low platelets	LDH:	Lactic dehydrogenase
		LES:	Lower esophageal sphincter
HEV:	Hepatitis E Virus	LFT:	Liver function test
HGD:	High-grade dysplasia	LGD:	Low-grade dysplasia
HH:	Hereditary hemochromatosis	LGIB:	Lower gastrointestinal bleed

ABBREVIATIONS

LMWH:	Low molecular weight heparin	PAP:	Pulmonary arterial pressure
LPR:	Laryngopharyngeal reflux	PAS:	Periodic Acid Shiff
MAC:	*Mycobacterium avium* complex	PBC:	Primary biliary cirrhosis
		PCP:	*Pneumocystis carinii* pneumonia
MALT:	Mucosal associated lymphoid tumors	PCR:	Polymerase chain reaction
MAP:	Mean arterial pressure	PCWP:	Pulmonary capillary wedge pressure
MCN:	Mucinous cystic neoplasm	PD:	Pancreatic duct
MCTD:	Mixed connective tissue disease	PDA:	Patent ductus arteriosus
		PEEP:	Positive end expiratory pressure
MELD:	Model for end stage liver disease	PEG:	Percutaneous endoscopic gastrostomy
MEN:	Multiple endocrine neoplasia	PEJ:	Percutaneous endoscopic jejunostomy
MOA:	Mechanism of action		
MPGN:	Membranoproliferative glomerulonephritis	PET:	Positron emission tomography
MRA:	Magnetic resonance angiogram	PG:	Prostaglandin
		PG:	Pyoderma gangrenosum
MRCP:	Magnetic resonance cholangiopancreatography	PHG:	Portal hypertensive gastropathy
MS:	Multiple sclerosis	PHTN:	Portal hypertension
MWT:	Mallory-Weiss tear	PID:	Pelvic inflammatory disease
N/V/D:	Nausea/vomiting/diarrhea	PLD:	Polycystic liver disease
N/V:	Nausea/vomiting	PMN:	Polymorphonuclear leukocyte
NA:	Nucleoside analogues (i.e. Lamivudine)	PPHTN:	Portopulmonary hypertension
NAC:	N-acetylcysteine		
NAFL:	Non-alcoholic fatty liver	PPI:	Proton pump inhibitor
NAFLD:	Non-alcoholic fatty liver disease	PPN:	Peripheral parenteral nutrition
NASH:	Non-alcoholic steatohepatitis	PRO:	Protein
		PSC:	Primary sclerosing cholangitis
NERD:	Nonerosive reflux disease		
NO:	Nitric oxide	PSE:	Portosystemic encephalopathy
NPO:	Nothing by mouth		
NSAID:	Nonsteroidal anti-inflammatory drug	PTLD:	Post-transplant lympho-proliferative disorder
NUD:	Non-ulcer dyspepsia	PUD:	Peptic ulcer disease
O&P:	Ova and parasite	PVR:	Pulmonary vascular resistance
OCP:	Oral contraceptive pill		
OLT:	Orthotropic liver transplantation	PVT:	Portal vein thrombosis
		RA:	Rheumatoid arthritis
OTC:	Over the counter	RBV:	Ribavirin
PAN:	Polyarteritis nodosa	S/E:	Side Effect(s)

ABBREVIATIONS

SAAG:	Serum-ascites albumin gradient	TMP-SMX:	Trimethoprim/Sulfamethoxazole
SB:	Small bowel	TNF:	Tumor necrosis factor
SBP:	Spontaneous bacterial peritonitis	TPMT:	Thiopurine s-methyltransferase
SBS:	Small bowel series	TPN:	Total parenteral nutrition
SCJ:	Squamocolumnar junction	TSH:	Thyroid stimulating hormone
SCN:	Serous cystic neoplasm		
SLE:	Systemic lupus Erythematosus	UC:	Ulcerative colitis
		UDCA:	Ursodeoxycholic acid
SMA:	Superior mesenteric artery	UES:	Upper esophageal sphincter
SOD:	Sphincter of Oddi dysfunction	UGIB:	Upper gastrointestinal bleed
SPEP:	Serum protein electrophoresis	UGIS:	Upper gastrointestinal series
SSCY:	*Salmonella, Shigella, Campylobacter, Yersinia*	ULN:	Upper limit of normal
		VIP:	Vasoactive intestinal peptide
SSRI:	Selective serotonin reuptake inhibitor	VL:	Viral load
		VOD:	Veno-occlusive disease
STD:	Sexually-transmitted disease	VSD:	Ventricular septal defect
TCA:	Tricyclic antidepressant	VZV:	Varicella zoster virus
TEE:	Transesophageal echocardiogram	WHO:	World Health Organization
TG:	Triglyceride	XO:	Xanthine oxidase
TI:	Terminal Ileum	XRT:	Radiation therapy
TIPS:	Transjugular Intrahepatic Portosystemic Shunt	ZES:	Zollinger-Ellison syndrome

ESOPHAGUS/GASTRIC

1.01 ACHALASIA

(Am J Gastroenterol. 1999;94:3406-12. Gastroenterology. 1999;117:229-32 & 233-54)

DEFINITION:
- Achalasia = "lack of relaxation"; The hallmark is the failure of the lower esophageal sphincter (LES) to relax
  - Secondary features include aperistalsis of the body of the esophagus
- Vigorous Achalasia = prominent contractions can be noticed in body of esophagus (radiographic/manometry)
  - These contractions are simultaneous and therefore fulfill manometric definition of aperistalsis
- Secondary Achalasia = associated with various diseases: cancer, Chagas' disease, amyloid, mixed connective tissue disease
- Pseudoachalasia = achalasia-like symptoms produced by infiltrating cancer at the GE junction; Consider with ↓ symptom duration & wt loss
- Diffuse esophageal spasm vs. Achalasia: at least some normal peristalsis in DES and LES dysfunction to a lesser degree

EPIDEMIOLOGY:
- Relatively uncommon: Prevalence 10/10,000; Incidence 0.5 cases/year/100,000 population
- Thought to be acquired disorder affecting any age group, however uncommon before the age of 25 (most common 30-60 years old)
- ♂ = ♀; All races equally affected

ETIOLOGIES:
- Remains a mystery; Thought to be associated with a viral infection, particularly Herpes, but no concrete evidence
  - Other theories include the possibility of autoimmune disorders
- Chagas' disease has a similarly pathological condition which is due to an infection by *Trypanosoma cruzi*
  - This parasitic antigen has a protein similar to that of myenteric neurons and produces an immunologic attack against the plexus
- **Pseudoachalasia** DDX: cancer of GE junction (most common), amyloidosis, sarcoidosis, postvagotomy, chronic intestinal pseudoobstruction

PATHOPHYSIOLOGY:
- Myenteric plexus: loss of ganglion cells (inhibitory function); Relative sparing of cholinergic (stimulatory function); Therefore persistent LES constriction

CLINICAL MANIFESTATIONS/PHYSICAL EXAM:
- Dysphagia to solids and liquids (motor disorder); However, most may only complain of solid food dysphagia; Isolated liquid dysphagia is rare
- Regurgitation in 60-90% with bending or recumbent position; Awakening with previous night's supper in their mouth
- Heartburn is common not only from acid reflux but also from fermentation of food in the aperistaltic esophagus
- Weight loss is common, but not invariable
- Chest pain can often be confused with GERD for years
- Pseudoachalasia is suggested by older age, short duration of symptoms and rapid weight loss

LABORATORY STUDIES:
- Not helpful

DIAGNOSTIC STUDIES:
- Barium swallow: atonic and dilated esophageal body, narrowing of the GE junction "bird's beak"
  - Excellent screening test, if diagnosis is relatively certain (i.e. birds beak, dilated esophagus) still need to exclude pseudoachalasia
- Manometry: *See also Esophagus/Gastric- Manometry (Chapter 1.17)*
  - Absent distal peristalsis in body (smooth muscle); Incomplete LES relaxation (residual >8 mmHg); High resting LES (> 45 mmHg)

- EGD: rule out pseudoachalasia; May observe retained food, esophageal dilation, feel a 'pop' at the GE junction
  - EUS if strongly suspected and biopsies negative

TREATMENTS:
- All treatment is considered palliative and directed at removing the functional obstruction at the LES
  - Therefore allowing gravity to compensate for lack of esophageal pumping
- Pharmacologic:
  - Nitrates (Isosorbide dinitrate 5-10 mg SL 30 minutes AC), acts in 15 min, last 90 min
  - CCB (Nifedipine 10-20 mg po, poor SL absorption), acts 30 min, last 60 min
  - Botox: blocks the excitatory neural input to the LES by inhibiting the release of acetylcholine; Success 60-75%
    - Usually lasts 3-12 months, leading to repeated injections; Ideal for frail elderly who are not surgical candidates
- Endoscopic:
  - Pneumatic balloon dilation with Rigiflex balloon, beginning with 3 cm diameter at 7-10 psi for 60 seconds; Success 75-85%
    - Post procedure give water-soluble contrast and observation 6 hours
      - Small contained perforations can be observed with NPO/Antibiotics with a surgical colleague observation
    - Risk of perforation 3% and require thoracotomy repair
- Surgical: Heller Myotomy:
  - Success 90%; Side effect: long term GERD and PPI need; Need highly experienced surgeon

COMPLICATIONS:
- Esophageal cancer risk 2-7%; Pathogenesis unknown, but chronic stasis is thought to play a role
  - Mean interval between diagnosis and cancer: 17 yrs; Most are squamous cell type; 5-year survival <5%
  - There is a nationally recognized endoscopic surveillance program; Suggested: 15 yrs after initial symptoms, 10 yrs after surgery

PROGNOSIS:
- Depends on Treatment modality as above

1.02 BARRETT'S ESOPHAGUS (BE)

(Gastroenterol 2006;131:1392-99 & 2005;128:1468-70. Am J. Gastroenterol 2002;97:1888-95)

DEFINITION:
- Barrett's esophagus (BE) is displacement of the squamocolumnar junction (SCJ) proximally to the gastroesophageal junction (GEJ) ***and*** intestinal metaplasia (IM)
  - Intestinal metaplasia is histologically characterized by acid mucin-containing **goblet cells** using H & E alcian blue (pH 2.5) stain
- Short and Long segment BE: Short segment BE <3 cm, Long Segment BE ≥3 cm
- BE is of little importance if not for the well established association with adenocarcinoma (AC) of the esophagus (BE is a premalignant condition)
- Note: The endoscopic Prague C & M Criteria (first presented in Prague in 9/2004) has recently been proposed as a standard way of accurately recognizing and grading BE
  - This classification may likely replace the standard 'Short' or 'Long' segment terminology

EPIDEMIOLOGY:
- Short segment BE is found 10-15% and Long segment BE is found in 3-7% of symptomatic GERD patients undergoing endoscopy
- IM of cardia (not BE) can be found in as much as 6-35% of patients undergoing endoscopy for any reason
  - Prevalence increases with age, suggesting an acquired condition; Unlike BE it is found equally in ♂ & ♀ and whites & blacks
- Reports of up to 25% of BE patients are under the age of 50 – not just an "old person's disease" (Am J Gastroenterol 2006;101:2187-93)

ETIOLOGIES:
- Risk factors:
  - Acquired disorder: Age and Duration of reflux (<1 year of symptoms: 4% prevalence; >10 years of symptoms: 21% prevalence)
  - Men > Women; Ethnicity (Caucasian > African American); Obesity; Average age at diagnosis: 63

PATHOPHYSIOLOGY:
- Acquired condition resulting from severe esophageal mucosal injury; Unclear why some GERD patients get BE and others do not
- Most BE patients have larger hiatal hernias and lower basal LES pressures (as compared to those with esophagitis or those without reflux)
- Cyclooxygenase (COX)-2 is involved in chronic inflammation and may be increased by exposure to acid; Possible chemoprevention role in future
- **Evolution of BE [Intestinal metaplasia (IM)] to cancer:**
  Negative for dysplasia » Indefinite for dysplasia » Low-grade dysplasia (LGD) » High-grade dysplasia (HGD) » Adenocarcinoma (AC)
  - Time course variable and most never progress to dysplasia
  - Progression not preordained (i.e. some can go from HGD back to intestinal metaplasia)

CLINICAL MANIFESTATIONS/PHYSICAL EXAM:
- ± long standing symptoms of GERD

LABORATORY STUDIES:
- None

CHAPTER 1.02 BARRETT'S ESOPHAGUS (BE)

DIAGNOSTIC STUDIES:
- EGD: presence of intestinal metaplasia anywhere in the tubular esophagus (salmon colored tongues of tissue extending proximally from GEJ)
  - Find landmarks:
    - Diaphragmatic hiatus
    - GEJ (Anatomical junction where distal end of the esophagus is defined by the most proximal margins of the gastric folds)
    - SCJ or Z line (Mucosal junction formed by the juxtaposition of squamous and columnar epithelia)
  - If SCJ above the GEJ then biopsy (i.e. 1 of 2 criteria for BE, other is IM)
    - Should *NOT* routinely biopsy SCJ if at the level of GEJ (that is the normal position)
  - Biopsies should be 4 quadrant with jumbo forceps every 1-2 cm
    - Inflammation related to GERD should be controlled (with PPI) before biopsies
  - If intestinal metaplasia (goblet cells) present: BE diagnosed, patient needs surveillance
- Note: difficult to distinguish short segment BE due to precise junction of stomach/esophagus
  - Biopsies from normal GEJ may reveal columnar epithelium with pseudogoblets, which is **gastric fundic/cardia epithelium** (not BE)
  - Biopsies from normal GEJ may also reveal intestinal metaplasia, presumably representing **intestinal metaplasia of cardia** (not BE)
    - Intestinal metaplasia of cardia does not (yet) require surveillance because cancer risk much less than short segment BE
- As noted above under Definitions, the Prague C & M Criteria are defined *endoscopically* by C = circumferential extent and M = maximum extent of the Barrett's esophagus (Note: still need histological conferment of intestinal metaplasia)
  - Example:
    - True GEJ at 40 cm from gums: Call this origin = 0.0 cm
    - The circumferential extent of the BE (i.e. SCJ) is at 38 cm: call this C = 2.0 cm
    - The maximal extent of any metaplastic tongue of BE is at 35 cm: call this M = 5.0 cm
    - So this would be classified as Prague C2M5
- Pathology: Many pathologists continue to classify gastric (cardia or fundic) epithelium or metaplasia without intestinal metaplasia as BE
  - Thereby increasing patient alarm and subjecting many to unnecessary surveillance endoscopy
  - A reliable biomarker to distinguish between intestinal metaplasia of cardia versus that of the esophagus would be beneficial

TREATMENTS:
- Goals: control reflux symptoms: PPI (heal erosive esophagitis), surgery (laparoscopic fundoplication), prevent adenocarcinoma (surveillance)
  - PPI/surgery (acid normalization) and decreased cancer risk: unproven to date; However, use of aggressive PPI is still standard to prevent esophagitis
  - Chemoprevention (NSAIDs/aspirin) may be protective (suggested by observational studies); premature to suggest regular usage
  - Mucosal ablation (thermal, photodynamic, endoscopic mucosal resection): regeneration of squamous mucosa in low acidity (theory)
    - Problem: residual intestinal metaplasia and even cancer development underlying new squamous epithelium
    - Use: for those non-surgical candidates with HGD or AC; Not indicated for those with IM or no dysplasia
- Screening:
  - Any patient of any age (especially white ♂) with a chronic history of GERD
  - Smoking and Obesity are other considerations to keep in mind
  - No proof if widespread screening will alter survival of AC

SECTION I ESOPHAGUS/GASTRIC

- Surveillance: intervals based on detection of dysplasia with the goal of early intervention to improve survival associated with cancer
  Note: Best if done on PPI (↓ erosions/ulcerations and ↓ inflammation on biopsy)
  - No Barrett's:
    - No further EGD screening for Barrett's; Additional EGD only to investigate new symptoms
  - No dysplasia:
    - Repeat biopsies × 2 (confirm, as with *all* BE biopsies, with expert pathologist); then if no dysplasia, EGD every 3 years
  - Low-grade dysplasia (LGD): 10-25% will progress to HGD or AC, and up to 65% will regress to no dysplasia
    - EGD every 6 months to 1 year until no dysplasia, then every 1-2 years
    - Indefinite for dysplasia usually handled like LGD
  - High-grade dysplasia (HGD): Confirm with expert pathology peer review and repeat biopsy within 1 month to confirm no AC
    - See treatment below; Some are considered for continued surveillance every 3 months: 4 quadrant 1 cm intervals ("Seattle protocol" biopsy method) until cancer
- Treatment of HGD: controversial; Range of unexpected cancer in those with HGD is 0-73%
  - Esophagectomy, but most patients will be elderly and poor surgical candidates; Key is a center performing a high volume
    - Complications: 30-50%; Mortality 3-20%; Long-term morbidity is frequent
  - Mucosal ablation (thermal/cryo, photodynamic, endoscopic mucosal resection)
    - Use: for those non-surgical candidates with HGD or AC; Not indicated for those with IM or no dysplasia
  - Others advocate continued surveillance and surgery only for those with intramucosal or submucosal carcinoma
  - Natural history suggests that 14-56% of HGD patients go on to develop cancer over the course of 3 years
  - Ultimate approach: consider factors such as surgical/endoscopic expertise, age, BE length requiring surveillance, compliance

COMPLICATIONS:
- Patients have 30-125% higher risk of developing AC; However, a 50 y/o man with BE and otherwise normal lifespan: 3-10% risk of developing AC
  - Esophageal cancer develops in 0.5% of patients with BE (i.e. very low risk)

PROGNOSIS:
- Risk of developing cancer from BE is approximately 0.5% per year (or an incidence of 1 in 52-175 patient years): Most never get cancer!
- Adenocarcinoma is the cancer with the most rapidly rising incidence in the U.S. (but not from BE); *See also Esophagus/Gastric- Esophageal Cancer (Chapter 1.08)*

NOTES

1.03 DIVERTICULA OF ESOPHAGUS (ZENKER'S)

DEFINITION:
- Zenker's Diverticula: upper esophageal diverticula
- Traction Diverticula: midesophageal diverticula
- Epiphrenic Diverticula: distal esophageal diverticula

PATHOPHYSIOLOGY:
- Zenker's: Impaired cricopharyngeal compliance, usually due to fibrotic changes, causes increased intrabolus pressure with swallowing
  - Relaxation of UES is usually normal
  - The result is increased hypopharyngeal pressure with herniation at a weak point just above the cricopharyngeus
- Traction: thought to result from esophageal motility disorders

CLINICAL MANIFESTATIONS/PHYSICAL EXAM:
- Zenker's: regurgitation of undigested food, bad breath, visible lump on side of neck, dysphagia in lower neck area

DIAGNOSTIC STUDIES:
- Barium Swallow
- EGD

TREATMENTS:
- Symptomatic Zenker's requires surgery; Should also have cricopharyngeal myotomy, otherwise the recurrence rate is high
- Traction: Few cause symptoms and need treatment
- Epiphrenic: usually no surgery needed unless large diverticula or producing symptoms such as regurgitation or aspiration
  - Manometry should be done, as the results can change the surgical approach to include long myotomy or LES myotomy

ESOPHAGEAL INTRAMURAL PSEUDODIVERTICULOSIS (EIPD)

Definition:
- Benign, multiple tiny flask-shaped out-pouching in esophagus; Formed by dilation of submucosal esophageal glands

Epidemiology:
- Uncommon (200 cases reported in the literature)

Etiologies:
- Candidiasis (50% of cases), Reflux esophagitis, Esophageal malignancy

Pathophysiology:
- Benign, multiple tiny flask-shaped out-pouching in esophagus; Stricture (upper/middle esophagus)
- Dilated submucosal glands, chronic inflammatory infiltrate, smooth muscle fibrosis (stricture)

Clinical Manifestations/Physical Exam:
- Intermittent solid food dysphagia (esophageal motor disorders and esophageal strictures)

Diagnostic Studies:
- EGD
- Barium Esophagram: pseudodiverticula, stricture
- Abd CT: non-diagnostic, may show esophageal wall thickening

Treatments:
- Esophageal dilation of symptomatic strictures
- Treatment of candidiasis
- PPI acid suppression
- Biopsy to rule out malignancy of adjacent mucosa

Complications:
- ? increased risk of esophageal cancer

CHAPTER 1.03 DIVERTICULA OF ESOPHAGUS (ZENKER'S)

NOTES

1.04 DYSPEPSIA (INDIGESTION)

(Am J Gastroenterol. 2005;100:2324-37; Gastroenterology. 1998;114:579-81 & 582-95)

DEFINITION:
- Chronic or recurrent pain or discomfort centered in upper abdomen
  - Patients with predominant or frequent (>once/week) heartburn should be considered to have GERD until proven otherwise
- Functional Dyspepsia:
  - Chronic or recurrent pain or discomfort centered in upper abdomen without endoscopic or other test evidence of disease

EPIDEMIOLOGY:
- Prevalence of the population: 25% (excluding those who have typical GERD symptoms)
- Incidence: 9% per year (however may be an overestimate due to those with past history of dyspepsia and PUD)

ETIOLOGIES:
- GERD (characteristic heartburn)
- Organic: PUD (15-20%), gastric cancer (<3%)
  - Other: lactose intolerance, biliary (cholelithiasis, cholecystitis, colic), mesenteric ischemia, chronic pancreatitis
- Functional ('non-ulcer dyspepsia' or NUD, ~60%):
  - ? delayed gastric emptying, ↓ fundic accommodation, gastric dysrythmias, visceral (afferent) hypersensitivity, IBS, Brain/Gut (psych)
- Complete DDX:
  - Abdominal wall pain, Biliary pain/Liver disease, Chronic pancreatitis, Small bowel pathology (chronic mesenteric ischemia), Colonic (transverse) pathology, Diabetic radiculopathy, Thyroid, Electrolyte abnormalities (calcium, heavy metal), Porphyria, Familial Mediterranean Fever, Eosinophilic gastritis, Connective tissue disease
- **Criteria suggesting organic disease and warrant an EGD: Age older than 55 years (However, no age threshold is absolute) or Alarm Features (any age):**
  - Weight loss, Persistent Anorexia/Vomiting, Dysphagia/Odynophagia/Early Satiety, Anemia, Bleeding/+FOBT
  - Positive Family History (GI cancer), Previous documented PUD, Palpable Mass/Adenopathy

CLINICAL MANIFESTATIONS/PHYSICAL EXAM:
- Chronic or recurrent pain or discomfort centered in upper abdomen
  - Discomfort defined as subjective negative feeling that is non-painful and can incorporate a variety of symptoms

LABORATORY STUDIES:
- Depends on DDX as listed above (i.e. amylase/lipase for suspected pancreatitis)

CHAPTER 1.04 DYSPEPSIA (INDIGESTION)

DIAGNOSTIC STUDIES:
- Age >55 years or Alarm Features (any age) present?
    Weight loss, Persistent Anorexia/Vomiting, Dysphagia/Odynophagia/Early Satiety, Anemia, Bleeding/+FOBT, Positive Family History (GI cancer), Previous documented PUD, Palpable Mass/Adenopathy

    - No: Stop NSAIDs, Test for *H. Pylori* (especially with high prevalence area/population)
      See also Esophagus/Gastric- Peptic Ulcer Disease (Chapter 1.21)
        - Pos: Treat with antibiotics »
            Asymptomatic: cured
            Symptomatic: PPI; If symptoms persist or poor response to therapy » EGD

        - Neg: Empiric therapy with PPI for 4-8 weeks (can use this strategy first if in area with low prevalence of *H. Pylori*) »
            Asymptomatic: stop therapy after 4-8 weeks; If reoccurs, repeat course
            Symptomatic after 2-4 weeks: Step up therapy (based on expert opinion only): change drug class/dosing
    - Yes: Endoscopy
        - Ulcer: Biopsy and treat for *H. Pylori*
        - Normal/No Ulcer: Functional Dyspepsia

TREATMENTS:
- Empirical therapy is NOT currently recommended in individuals over 55 yrs who develop new dyspeptic symptoms:
    - Risk of malignancy increases with age
- *H. Pylori* eradication useful for PUD » therefore empiric Rx reasonable if + serology; minimal data that eradication useful without PUD
- Functional dyspepsia: Patients who fail to respond to simple measures need to have their diagnosis reconsidered first; See Complete DDX under Etiologies above
    - Delayed gastric emptying in 40%
    - Consider first: education and reassurance; Avoid fatty meals or aggravating foods, consider frequent small meals
    - Consider trial: Acid suppression with PPI ± H2 blockers, Prokinetic agents (not first-line drug for dyspepsia), TCAs (i.e. Nortriptyline)
- Young patients with no alarm symptoms:
    - Wait-and-see strategy with reassurance and education, OTC preparations, Re-evaluation
    - Test and treat for *H. Pylori* as above or go straight to Empiric therapy with PPI (ACP guidelines for primary care)

1.05 DYSPHAGIA/ODYNOPHAGIA

(Gastroenterology. 1999;117:229-32 & 233-54)

DEFINITION:
- Difficulty swallowing and passing food from the mouth or esophagus to the stomach
  - Divided into: Oropharyngeal or Esophageal (See Etiologies below)
- Globus (hystericus): feeling of lump in throat; Not to be confused with dysphagia
  - Not related to swallowing, present continually and may be temporarily alleviated during swallowing
- Dysphagia Lusoria (Lusoria = trick of nature): impingement of aberrant vasculature on proximal esophagus
  - Most common type involves an aberrant right subclavian artery and compresses the esophagus
  - Diagnosis: MRI is believed to be most accurate in defining lesion; Also should have manometry and barium swallow to confirm

ETIOLOGIES:
- **Causes of Esophageal Dysphagia:**
  Solids (Mechanical Obstruction): **RPC**
  - INTERMITTENT » **R**ing *See also Esophagus/Gastric- Schatzki's Ring (Chapter 1.22)*
  - PROGRESSIVE/GERD » **P**eptic stricture (Simple: <2 cm, focal, nonangulated)
                       (Complex >2 cm, angulated, severe narrowing)
  - PROGRESSIVE » **C**ancer (pseudoachalasia)

  Solids & Liquids (Motility): **SSA**
  - INTERMITTENT » **S**pasm
  - PROGRESSIVE/GERD » **S**cleroderma
  - PROGRESSIVE » **A**chalasia

- **Causes of Oropharyngeal Dysphagia:** problems with initiating swallowing (Gastroenterology 1999; 116:452-54 & 455-78)
  Propulsive:
  - Neurologic (CVA, Parkinson's, ALS, Multiple Sclerosis, Brain cancer)
  - Muscular (Muscular Dystrophy, Dermatomyositis, Poliomyelitis, Myasthenia gravis): ↑ Creatine Kinase/Aldolase
  - Autoimmune (SLE, Sarcoid, Amyloid)
  - (Note: Stroke patients usually take 2 weeks to improve, if none after that time, then swallowing function should be evaluated)

  Structural: Neoplasm, Cricopharyngeal bars, Zenker's, Lymphadenopathy, Cervical osteophytes, Infections, Oral CD, Behçet's, Dentition
  - Cricopharyngeal bar: indentation of the cricopharyngeal muscle seen as barium passes by slowly and the muscle poorly relaxes
    - Can be the sole cause of oropharyngeal dysphagia but other neuromuscular diseases should be excluded

  Iatrogenic: Oropharyngeal resections, Mucositis due to chemo, Radiation-induced, Neck stabilizations (hardware, halo), Dental prostheses

- **Other:**
  - Zenker's (diverticula that can occur throughout hypopharynx); *See also Esophagus/Gastric- Diverticula of Esophagus (Chapter 1.03)*
    - Caused by constrictive myopathy of the cricopharyngeus = relative obstruction
    - Increased resistance with intrabolus pressures above this relative obstruction: muscle stress and herniation with diverticula formation
    - Halitosis, regurgitation/choking
  - Pill-induced: i.e. Bisphosphonates, Potassium
  - Globus causes: GERD > Anxiety > Early hypopharyngeal cancer > Goiter; Consider CT neck; Symptomatic treatment with TCAs
  - Odynophagia: herpes (multinucleated giant cells, ground glass), CMV (inclusion bodies), candida (pseudohyphae), reflux

CHAPTER 1.05 DYSPHAGIA/ODYNOPHAGIA

PATHOPHYSIOLOGY:
- Swallowing is a complex neuromuscular process that depends on intact motor and sensory innervation
  - Oropharyngeal phase is under voluntary control; however once bolus moved into pharynx the process becomes involuntary
- Sensory cues: swallowing requires afferent signal from both peripheral (input via oropharyngeal afferents) and central nervous system
  - Therefore swallowing can't be initiated during sleep (high centers turned off) or deep anesthesia (oral peripheral afferents turned off)
- Swallowing center in the brainstem; Therefore brainstem strokes are more likely to cause most severe impairment
- Compare:

Oropharynx	Esophagus
Striated muscle	Striated and smooth muscle proximally, and smooth muscle mid to distally (approximately 25 cm long)
Direct nicotinic innervation	Myenteric plexus with longitudinal and circular smooth muscles
Cholinergic	Cholinergic/nitric oxide, vasoactive intestinal peptide

- Compare:
  - UES (striated muscle that depends on tonic excitation to maintain contractility), if innervation lost = flaccid
  - LES in achalasia results in a loss of *inhibitory* myenteric plexus neurons = contraction
- Most difficult substance to swallow (Oropharyngeal)? Water
  - Normally: Preparatory phase (chewing, sizing, shaping, position with tongue); Oral phase (bolus propelled while airway protected)
  - Water is difficult to shape, size, hardest to control for propulsion; Therefore, more viscous foods used to feed patients with oropharyngeal dysphagia
- GERD association with dysphagia: Inflammation, Stricture, Peristaltic dysfunction, Hiatal hernia

CLINICAL MANIFESTATIONS/PHYSICAL EXAM:
- Oropharyngeal dysphagia: patients can accurately recognize problem: food accumulation, can't initiate pharyngeal swallow, aspiration
  - Symptoms: nasopharyngeal regurgitation, coughing, choking (aspiration), can't initiate swallow, change in speech, ptosis
- Esophageal dysphagia: patients identification of localizing obstruction is ~60% accurate; 40% mistakenly localizing the problem proximally

LABORATORY STUDIES:
- As above for oropharyngeal dysphagia, most likely TSH, aldolase, CK

SECTION I ESOPHAGUS/GASTRIC

DIAGNOSTIC STUDIES:
- EGD, Esophagram or Video-swallow; ± Manometry; Rarely esophageal pH monitoring
  Which first?
    - EGD first if you suspect esophageal structural/mechanical diagnosis
        - Abnormal: Endoscopic dilation/biopsy
        - Normal: Manometry
    - Esophagram first if you suspect esophageal dysmotility or ring
        - Probably dysmotility: Manometry
        - Ring: Endoscopic dilation/biopsy
        - Normal: Endoscopy; If normal, consider Manometry
    - Video-swallow first if you suspect oropharyngeal disorder or malignancy or no apparent cause
        - Abnormal: Endoscopy
            - Normal endoscopy (i.e. motor disorder): ENT consult with laryngoscopy and/or Speech pathology consult
            - Abnormal Endoscopy (i.e. cancer, web, stricture, pouch): Surgical consultation
        - Normal: Follow Esophagram algorithm
    Note: Esophagram and Video swallow often done simultaneously at many centers
- If suspected Zenker's, there is increased risk of perforation with EGD, so important to intubate under direct visualization if history suggests oropharyngeal dysphagia; Another reason to get video-swallow first if history suggestive of oropharyngeal dysphagia
- CT of neck and/or ENT may be helpful to detect cervical osteophytes and/or occult malignancy for suspected oropharyngeal dysphagia

TREATMENTS:
- Oropharyngeal Dysphagia:
    - Treat any underlying neuromuscular disorder; Speech therapy: learning new swallowing maneuvers
    - PEG tube may be needed for malnutrition
    - Indications for Cricopharyngeal myotomy: Zenker's, Cricopharyngeal bar with symptoms, Parkinson's?
        - Risks: aspiration in patients with GERD; worsening of swallow function
- Esophageal Dysphagia:
  Dilation (selection based on stricture configuration, comfort of endoscopist, availability of equipment)
  Rule of 3's: dilate a total of three times in one session (first dilation is the one with mild resistance)
  End point is a lumen diameter of >14 mm, followed by control of reflux (PPI) if any
    - Mercury-filled tapered bougies (Maloney): axial shearing and radial forces; best for simple symmetric strictures <10 mm
    - Guidewire placed tapered polyvinyl dilators (Savary): axial shearing and radial forces; best for <10 mm, long, tortuous, post-op strictures
    - Through-the-scope (TTS) balloons: only radial force; best for <10 mm, long, tortuous, post-op strictures
  Note: French sizes are circumferences sizes, divided by 3 they give the diameter in mm; So 30 Fr is 10 mm in diameter

COMPLICATIONS:
- Suspected failed Nissen workup: Barium swallow, manometry, pH test off medications, EGD ± GES
    - Thorough and proper evaluation needs to be done before considering re-operation

NOTES

1.06 EOSINOPHILIC ESOPHAGITIS

DEFINITION:
- Characterized by eosinophilic infiltration of the esophagus presumably due to allergic or idiopathic causes

EPIDEMIOLOGY:
- Not well studied, but reported in several countries in the world
  - Majority of case reports are men in their 20-30's and among children with the majority being boys
- Case reports in families demonstrate a possible genetic link

ETIOLOGIES:
- Has been described in association with eosinophilic gastroenteritis, *See also Esophagus/Gastric-Eosinophilic Gastroenteritis (Chapter 1.07)*
  - However most reports are isolated esophageal involvement
- DDX:
  - GERD, infections (parasitic/fungal), Crohn's, drug injury, allergic vasculitis, connective tissue diseases, carcinoma, periarteritis

PATHOPHYSIOLOGY:
- The normal esophagus is devoid of eosinophils, but like the colon is capable of recruiting eosinophils to a variety of stimuli (i.e. GERD)
- The pathophysiology of Eosinophilic Esophagitis is unknown
  - The recruitment of eosinophils is observed in a variety of inflammatory or infectious disorders such as IBD, GERD, food allergy
  - Association with allergies is common suggesting that there may be a response to environmental antigens
  - Eotaxin, Interleukin 5 (IL-5) and STAT6 may play important roles
  - Some patients have at least partially improved with antisecretory therapy, suggesting that acid reflux may be a contributor
- Several morphologic features have been described:
  - Strictures (especially proximally); Mucosal rings; Linear furrowing; Ulceration/Corrugation; **"Feline esophagus"; "Trachea-like esophagus"**
  - Multiple whitish papules that may be confused with candida represent small eosinophilic abscesses
- Dysphagia likely caused by ongoing inflammatory response via local eosinophilic infiltration
- Rings are caused by lamina propria and dermal papillary fibrosis due to mediators that stimulate eosinophils or from eosinophils themselves

CLINICAL MANIFESTATIONS/PHYSICAL EXAM:
- General:
  - Has been described in children and adults with **dysphagia** either alone or as a manifestation of eosinophilic gastroenteritis
  - In its isolated form, it is recognized to cause dysphagia and possibly **heartburn unresponsive to therapy**
  - A history of **esophageal perforation** or **severe pain after dilation** of strictures should make one think about this disease
- Adults usually present with dysphagia; **A history of food impaction is common**
  - Esophageal dysmotility may be observed suggesting deeper muscular layer involvement
- Children's symptoms vary with age:
  - Feeding disorders (median age 2); vomiting (median age 8); abdominal pain (median age 12); food impaction (median age 16)
- A history of allergies has been described (i.e. asthma, allergic rhinitis, urticaria, hay fever, atopic dermatitis, food/medicine allergy)

LABORATORY STUDIES:
- Peripheral eosinophilia has been described, but appears to be less common in adults
- Serum IgE may be elevated

DIAGNOSTIC STUDIES:
- Consensus not uniform on diagnostic criteria
  - Based on characteristic clinical features, presents of eosinophils in esophagus and exclusion of other causes
- EGD:
  - An association with Schatzki ring has been described, but association is unclear
  - Biopsy is key, and they should be performed not only in esophagus, but also stomach and duodenum for eosinophilic gastroenteritis
  - **More than 20 eosinophils per high power field** likely to be associated with non acid-related causes (Am J Gastroenterol 2004;99:801-05)
- Barium swallow and pH study can help define esophageal anatomy and evaluate for reflux, but shouldn't be routinely obtained

TREATMENTS:
- Optimal treatment consensus has not been defined
- Acid suppression:
  - Usually not successful or only achieves partial response; however a subset of patients appear to have coexisting reflux
  - An empiric trial of acid suppression may be warranted
- Esophageal dilation:
  - Should be performed carefully since it has been associated with *deep mucosal tears and esophageal perforation*
  - Not unreasonable to inspect the esophagus after each dilation
  - Generally reserve for patients with strictures/rings refractory to therapy
- Elimination diets:
  - Rational that there is a component of allergic reaction to a food antigen; Efficacy is variable, and practicality is unclear
- Systemic corticosteroids:
  - May be helpful but relapse seen with withdrawal; Role as long-term management is unclear
- Topical corticosteroids:
  - Patients instructed to swallow, rather than inhale followed by rinsing mouth with water
  - Relief often within several days and lasting effect for months
  - Long-term safety has not been established and likely relapse is common
- Antihistamines and Cromolyn
  - Occasional patients are reported to respond to medications aimed at controlling allergies (i.e. Doxepin, Cromolyn sodium)
- Montelukast (Singulair)
  - Symptomatic improvement observed (unlike eosinophilic gastroenteritis with esophageal involvement)
  - High doses used: begin at 10 mg/day and titrated to as high as 100 mg/day, then a slow taper to effective dose
- A good game plan:
  - Refer to Allergist with expertise in the evaluation of food allergies with a discussion of pros/cons of elimination diet
    - Likely to work best in children
  - Treatment with swallowed Fluticasone: Adults: 220 mcg/puff; Two puffs BID for 6-8 weeks (repeat for 4-6 weeks if symptoms recur)
    - Do not use spacer as would be used for asthma therapy
    - Small amount of water should be sipped and swallowed immediately after actuation to help carry medicine into esophagus
    - Do not eat/drink 30 minutes following administration
    - Patients who will respond tend to do so quickly (within days to one week); Repeat courses may be necessary
  - Trial of PPI except in patients who have already tried and not responded
  - Repeat EGD in patients whose symptoms have changed or who require esophageal dilation

COMPLICATIONS:
- Perforation and mucosal tears with EGD can occur even just from the passage of the scope without noting any resistance

PROGNOSIS:
- Long term prognosis is unknown
  - Untreated patients may remain asymptomatic or have episodic symptoms
  - Whether or not a child's symptoms will persist in adulthood is unknown
  - Malignant potential has not been reported

1.07 EOSINOPHILIC GASTROENTERITIS

DEFINITION:
- A rare, nonparasitic inflammatory disease of the GI tract with various degrees of eosinophilic infiltration anywhere in the tubular intestinal tract and biliary tree in the absence of vasculitis

ETIOLOGIES:
- DDX (must exclude):

Syndromes and Disorders	Systemic Vasculitis	Parasitic
IBS	Churg-Strauss	*Ancylostoma* spp. (hookworm)
Reflux esophagitis	Polyarteritis nodosa	*Anisakis* spp.
IBD (CD, UC, Collagenous)	Dermatomyositis/	*Ascaris* spp.
Idiopathic hypereosinophilic syndrome	Polymyositis	*Capillaria* spp
Eosinophilic granuloma (Histiocytosis X)	Scleroderma	*Strongyloides* spp.
Lymphoma	Eosinophilic fasciitis	*Isospora belli* (immunocompromised)

PATHOPHYSIOLOGY:
- Immune-mediated; Most likely result of several different factors affecting immunologic regulation (i.e. allergic, autoimmune)
- Although it is associated with allergic illnesses in almost half of patients, a specific allergic stimulus has not been identified
  - Food Allergy: (Gastroenterology 2001;120:1023–25 & 1026–40)
  - Less than 50% of cases have an identifiable precipitant
- Note: the affected organs and depth of inflammatory infiltration of intestinal wall layers determine the clinical manifestations
  - **Mucosal, without muscular involvement:** Mucositis has symptoms of abdominal pain, N/V/D; May have malabsorption, protein losing enteropathy, iron deficiency anemia
  - **Muscular (Submucosal) involvement:** Muscularis propria, rigid gut with symptoms of dysmotility i.e. dysphagia, gastric outlet obstruction, small/large intestinal obstruction, bacterial overgrowth, ampullary stenosis and cholangitis or pancreatitis
  - **Subserosal/Serosal inflammation:** peritonitis, ascites, pleural effusions; Ascitic eosinophils >80%; Often with muscular involvement as well
- Eosinophils in extra-intestinal organs is suggestive of Hyper-Eosinophilic Syndrome or Loeffler's Syndrome
  - This may be present with GI eosinophilia, but is distinct from Eosinophilic Gastritis

CLINICAL MANIFESTATIONS/PHYSICAL EXAM:
- Note: the affected organs and depth of inflammatory infiltration of intestinal wall layers determine the clinical manifestations as above under Pathophysiology
  - Abdominal pain, diarrhea, nausea, vomiting, dysphagia, gastric outlet obstruction
  - May have weight loss and malabsorption (protein-losing enteropathy)

LABORATORY STUDIES:
- Peripheral blood eosinophilia is present 80% of cases, but not necessary for diagnosis

DIAGNOSTIC STUDIES:
- Upper GI Series: gastric retention or small intestinal hypomotility
- Barium enema: mucosal thickening with cobble-stoned or saw-tooth silhouette, nodular filling defects; Can mimic Crohn's disease
- CT: duodenal wall thickening, inflammatory tumors, ascites
- Diagnosis:
  - Check history for atopic disease (present in 50% of patients)
  - Exclude parasitic intestinal disease by history and stool samples
  - Eosinophilic counts, supporting the diagnosis:
    - Peripheral smear: 5–35% (normal peripheral blood counts can be found in 20% of patients)
    - Stool: >5% of eosinophils in differential counts of leukocytes
    - Deep mucosal biopsy: 20 eosinophils/high-powered field; Biopsy should be from 10 sites (deep muscular or peritoneal disease may require full-thickness biopsy)

CHAPTER 1.07 EOSINOPHILIC GASTROENTERITIS

TREATMENTS:
- Oral prednisone 0.5 mg/kg per day for 2 weeks; Often induces remission, regardless of the layer of the gut involved
- If severe disease, may need IV therapy followed by 2 week taper
- A few patients need long-term steroid therapy (several months)
- Nonsteroid, immune-modulatory therapies may be alternative in future: Montelukast, Cromolyn
- Rarely, suspected food allergy; May need trial of elimination diets to resolve disease
- Symptomatic: loperamide for diarrhea, supplementation for electrolyte deficiencies
- Recurrence can be treated with repeat short courses of prednisone

1.08 ESOPHAGEAL CANCER

(Gastroenterology 2005;128:1468-70. Am J Gastroenterol 1999;94:20-29)

DEFINITION:
- Cancer of the esophagus

EPIDEMIOLOGY:
- Incidence <10/100,000
  - However, the incidence of esophageal adenocarcinoma has increased sharply in U.S.
  - The incidence of esophageal squamous cell cancer has decreased in U.S.

ETIOLOGIES:
- Squamous cell cancer: smoking and alcohol; More common in African Americans
  - World wide, squamous cell is the most common cancer of the esophagus and is related to tobacco/alcohol
- Adenocarcinoma (AC): GERD, Barrett's esophagus; More common in White Americans
  - AC is the most common type of esophageal cancer in the U.S.; Incidence of cancer with BE is low (0.5% per patient year)
- Obesity as an independent risk factor is quite possible
- Diet: some research suggest that low intake of fresh fruits and vegetables may be risk; Fiber is protective
- Tylosis: uncommon genetic disorder characterized by hyperkeratosis of the palms and soles; Autosomal dominant
  - Predisposition to develop squamous esophageal cancer (prevalence can be >90% by age 65; death reported in young as 30 years)
  - Surveillance endoscopy begins early; Swallowing symptoms should be evaluated promptly

CLINICAL MANIFESTATIONS/PHYSICAL EXAM:
- Dysphagia 90% of patients; Odynophagia in 50% of patients
  - Unfortunately, dysphagia associated with esophageal cancer usually signals an advanced stage, typically T3
- Pseudoachalasia = achalasia-like symptoms produced by infiltrating cancer at the GE junction; Consider with ↓ symptom duration & weight loss

LABORATORY STUDIES:
- Not helpful

DIAGNOSTIC STUDIES:
- EGD and Biopsy
  - Location: Upper to middle one-third are mostly squamous cell and those in the distal third are generally AC
  - Most rare tumors (sarcoma, melanoma, choriocarcinoma) tend to occur in the distal esophagus
- CT for staging distant metastases (60% accuracy for T score)
- EUS for staging; Better than CT for staging the depth (T) of invasion (90% accuracy) and lymph node (N) involvement (80% accuracy)
  - Muscularis propria is seen as the hypoechoic layer most distal from the esophageal lumen
    - Critical area: extension to this level is T2 (↑ risk of nodal metastases), T1 lesions do not extend to this region
- PET Scan, unlike CT/EUS, is a functional test that does not demonstrate anatomical changes
  - IV contrast concentrates rapidly in metabolizing cells; Used primarily to detect metastatic disease (more value in nodal metastases)
- Screening:
  - Currently no acceptable screening method for esophageal cancer
- Surveillance:
  - Recommended in patients with Barrett's esophagus; *See also Esophagus/Gastric- Barrett's Esophagus (Chapter 1.02)*

CHAPTER 1.08 ESOPHAGEAL CANCER

Staging:	Primary Tumor	Regional LN	Distant Mets	Stages:	
	Tx: Tumor can't be assessed	Nx: LN can't be assessed	Mx: Mets can't be assessed	0:	Tis, N0, M0
	T0: No evidence of tumor	N0: No LN metastases	M0: No distant metastases	1:	T1, N0, M0
	Tis: Carcinoma in situ	N1: LN metastasis	M1: Distant metastases	2A:	T2 _or_ T3, N0, M0
	T1: Invades lamina propria/submucosa		M1a: In celiac region for AC	2B:	T1 _or_ T2, N1, M0
	T2: Invades muscularis propria		M1b: Other distant mets	3:	T3 _or_ T4, N1, M0
	T3: Invades adventitia (outside wall)			4:	Any T, Any N, M1
	T4: Invades adjacent structures (i.e. pleura, aorta)				

TREATMENTS:

- Stage 0, 1, 2A: curative surgery (occurs in only 50% of patients due to metastases at diagnosis): resection (esophagectomy) with gastric pull up
  - Mortality is 10% (5% with specialized centers having more experience)
  - Morbidity is primarily related to leakage from anastomosis (10% of cases) or pulmonary complications (40% of cases)
  - No study has found that the addition of adjuvant therapy before or after surgery affects outcome in this group
- Stage 0 and 1: Endoscopic Mucosal Resection (EMR) may be curative
- Stage 2B, 3: Triple therapy: surgery, chemotherapy, radiation; If poor patient functional ability may pursue palliative therapy
- Stage 4: Palliation
- Endoscopic Mucosal Resection (EMR): can remove pieces of mucosa at least 1cm in diameter down to the level of the deep submucosa
  - Can eliminate superficial cancer in about 94% of patients
- Endoscopic palliation options: esophageal dilation, self expanding metal stenting, PEG placement; Radiation
  - Stent complications: poor position/migration, perforation, pain, bleeding, compression of bronchi/trachea; Mortality rate 1-2%
    - If dyspnea occurs in relation to large midesophageal lesion, bronchoscopy may be indicated before stent placement

PROGNOSIS:

- Squamous cell: with either surgery or chemoradiation: 5 year survival: 20-30%
- Adenocarcinoma: Surgery alone: 3 year survival: 6-20%; Chemoradiation then surgery: 3 year survival: 30%
- Metastatic disease for either: 5 year survival: <5%

1.09 ESOPHAGEAL INFECTIONS

- Odynophagia, and to a lesser degree, dysphagia are most common symptoms
- Others: Nausea, dysgeusia, heartburn, chest pain, fever, bleeding, hiccups

FUNGAL: *CANDIDA ALBICANS*
- Most common cause of infectious esophagitis; Ubiquitous yeast found in normal oral flora
  - First step: colonization with mucosal adherence and proliferation; 20% of asymptomatic persons
  - Second step: impaired host defense; Creamy white plaques or exudates seen endoscopically
- 75% of patients with candidal esophagitis have coincident oral infections; However, the absence of thrush does not exclude the diagnosis
- Predisposing medications: corticosteroids, antibiotics affecting normal flora, acid suppression
- Predisposing conditions: impaired immunity: HIV, hematologic malignancies, DM, Cushings, ETOH, disease of peristalsis (achalasia)
- In immunocompromised population, trial of fluconazole 100-200 mg/day for 10-14 days; If no resolution in 5-7 days: EGD
  - Nystatin is effective at a swish-and-swallow 500,000 units 5/day; However oral imidazoles are preferred
  - Prophylaxis with fluconazole 150 mg/week can be recommended
  - If patient is granulocytopenic, should receive amphotericin B because of high risk of fungal dissemination

VIRAL
HERPES SIMPLEX VIRUS (HSV):
- Most common cause of viral esophagitis; Typically seen in conjunction with orolabial infection
- EGD: small vesicles, may progress forming circumscribed ulcers up to 2 cm in diameter with raised yellow edges: volcano ulcers
- Microscopic: infects squamous epithelium, multinucleated giant cells with ballooning and degeneration of squamous cells
  - Cowdry type A intranuclear inclusions are pathognomonic for HSV
- Severely symptomatic or immunocompromised: acyclovir IV

CYTOMEGALOVIRUS (CMV):
- Most common cause of viral esophagitis in the immunocompromised; Usually widespread infection, not just limited to esophagus
- EGD: linear, serpiginous ulcers in mid-distal esophagus and may coalesce to form giant ulcers
- Microscopic: infects submucosal fibroblasts and vascular epithelium, which require deep biopsies from ulcer crater
  - Large cells with both intracytoplasmic inclusions and amphophilic intranuclear inclusions
- Treatment is ganciclovir IV (most common side effect is granulocytopenia) and relapse is common

OTHER:
Epstein-Barr (EBV): reported in patients with AIDS and immunocompetent patients with infectious mononucleosis; Therapy: acyclovir
Varicella zoster (VZV): immunocompromised hosts; May have skin manifestations
Human papilloma virus (HPV): both normal and immunocompromised hosts; Seldom symptomatic

BACTERIAL
- *H. Pylori* is the most common cause of bacterial gastritis, ***See also Esophagus/Gastric- Gastropathy & Peptic Ulcer Disease (Chapter 1.13 & 1.21)***
- Most significant risk factor is granulocytopenia
- Most polymicrobial:
  - G+ found in normal flora
  - G− can be seen
- Diagnose with tissue gram stain of mucosal biopsies
- Risk of overwhelming sepsis is high, due to granulocytopenia; Aggressive treatment with beta-lactam and aminoglycoside

NOTES

1.10 GASTRIC CANCER

(N Engl J Med 1995;333:32-41)

DEFINITION:
- Cancer of the stomach; Adenocarcinoma is classified, via Lauren in 1965, into:
  - Intestinal variant: arise from gastric mucus cells that have undergone intestinal metaplasia in setting of chronic gastritis
    - Microscopically resembles colonic adenocarcinoma; may be polypoid or ulcerated or both
    - Better differentiated; becoming less prevalent in the U.S.
    - Risk factors: Diet (nitrates, smoked foods, ↓ vegetable/fruits), *H. Pylori*, Pernicious anemia (Type A gastritis), Billroth I & II
  - Diffuse variant: arise directly from native gastric mucus cells, is not associated with chronic gastritis
    - Poorly differentiated and infiltrating; accounts for half of all gastric cancers in U.S.; Poorer prognosis
    - Risk factors: *H. Pylori,*? association with blood group A
    - Can infiltrate the stomach extensively given thickened appearance: *Linitis Plastica* ("leather bottle stomach")

EPIDEMIOLOGY:
- World wide: second most common cancer with 750,000 new cases per year; Second most deadly cancer behind lung cancer
  - In U.S.: 22,000 new cases per year, 8th most deadly cancer for men, 10th for women; Incidence increases dramatically >50 yrs old
- **Over 80% are adenocarcinomas**
  - Less common: gastric lymphomas, gastric stromal tumors, leiomyosarcomas, carcinoid, metastatic (i.e. melanoma, breast)
  - *H. Pylori* causes *more* adenocarcinoma than MALTs
- Mucosal Associated Lymphoid Tumors (MALT): often low grade **B-cell** lymphomas (non-Hodgkin's), but may be high grade aggressive tumors
  - Cause: association (90%) with infection by *H. Pylori* (seems to drive lymphoid proliferation in the lamina propria and tumor development)
- Gastric Lymphoma (non-MALT)
  - Primary gastric lymphoma is rare and accounts for less than 5% of gastric malignancies
  - Immunoperoxidase staining or lymphoma markers increase diagnostic accuracy
  - Non-Hodgkin's is much more common than Hodgkin's lymphoma
- Gastric Carcinoid (neuroendocrine cell growths): benign or malignant, stain for chromogranin; *See also Bowel- Carcinoid Tumors (Chapter 2.08)*
  - Cause: de novo malignant transformation or loss of normal growth regulation in response to chronic elevation of serum gastrin levels
- Gastritis Type A (Pernicious anemia) has gastric cancer incidence of 2-10% (i.e. elevation in serum gastrin levels) *See also Esophagus/Gastric- Gastropathy (Chapter 1.13)*
- There is a risk of gastric cancer in the gastric remnant after gastrectomy (Gastric stump carcinoma): 2-4 fold increase 15 years after surgery
  - Initiate surveillance endoscopy 15 years after surgery with biopsies
- Gastrointestinal Stromal Tumors (GISTs); occur most commonly stomach (50%) > small intestine (25%); *See also Bowel- Small Bowel Tumors (Chapter 2.24)*

ETIOLOGIES:
- Genetics: evidence supports genetic factors; Gastric cancers common in families with Lynch Syndrome
  - First-degree relatives of patients with gastric cancer have a twofold to threefold greater incidence of gastric cancer
- *H. Pylori* is a well established risk factor: 2-6 fold increase in gastric cancer; In 1994, the WHO classified *H. Pylori* as a group I carcinogen
- Achlorhydria (generally caused by immune destruction of parietal cells, Type A Chronic Gastritis): 4-6 fold increase in gastric cancer
- Gastric Stump Cancer: after partial gastric resection, 2 fold increase in gastric cancer after 15 yrs post surgery; Initial 5 years is protective

CHAPTER 1.10 GASTRIC CANCER

- Diet may play a role; In general, higher incidence of gastric cancer with diet high in salted, smoked, preserved meats/fish (i.e. nitrates, nitrites)
  - Fruit/Vegetables appear to be protective (? If direct effect of vitamins or if these vitamins act through effects such as antioxidants)
- Smoking appears to increase the risk of gastric cancer
- Cancers that metastasize *to* stomach: Colon, Liver, Lung, Breast, Ovary/Testes, Melanoma, Kaposi sarcoma, Parotid (not thyroid)

PATHOPHYSIOLOGY:
- Presentation is in two major sites: Proximally (Barrett's, reflux related) and Distally in antrum (more common worldwide, less common in U.S.)
- Probable sequence of developing gastric carcinoma
  - Normal gastric mucus with an insult from a diet high in salt, low in vitamins, *H. Pylori* colonization, mucosa then goes through:
    - Chronic superficial gastritis » Atrophic gastritis » Intestinal metaplasia » Dysplasia » Gastric cancer
- Adenocarcinoma Staging TNM; T: relation to muscularis propria; N: number and location of lymph nodes; M: metastases

CLINICAL MANIFESTATIONS/PHYSICAL EXAM:
- Most clinical features are vague and nonspecific and therefore rarely lead to an early diagnosis
  - Epigastric pain, early satiety, abdominal bloating, meal-induced dyspepsia, gastric outlet obstruction with distal cancers
  - Weight loss, nausea, anorexia or bleeding malignant ulcer disease in advanced cases
- Virchow's (supraclavicular) or Sister Mary Joseph's (umbilical) lymph nodes:
  - Both intestinal and diffuse types can penetrate gastric wall to involve serosal surface and spread via lymph
- Trousseau's syndrome: a paraneoplastic syndrome that includes acanthosis nigricans or venous thrombi (rare)

LABORATORY STUDIES:
- *H. Pylori* testing, ***See also Esophagus/Gastric- Peptic Ulcer Disease (Chapter 1.21)***
- Nonspecific: anemia, hypoproteinemia, abnormal LFTs if metastases

DIAGNOSTIC STUDIES:
- EGD
  - If ulcer suspicious of cancer (i.e. in Fundus): 8 biopsies (base and margin) and Brush cytology = 98% accuracy
    - Need follow up EGD to confirm healing if negative biopsies
- CT abdomen
  - Tends to understage gastric cancer, but useful for identifying those not suitable for curative surgical resection
- EUS
  - More accurate for staging gastric cancer, but not suitable for assessing metastases

TREATMENTS:
- Adenocarcinoma:
  - Surgery: potentially curative for localized cancers
    - Occasionally palliative surgery is considered for tumor obstruction, perforation or bleeding
  - Chemotherapy: metastatic disease
    - Neoadjuvant: given prior to surgery
    - Adjuvant: given after attempted curative surgery without evidence of residual cancer
    - Conflicting results on survival benefit
  - Radiation:
    - Gastric carcinoma is relatively radiation resistant and is usually administered only to palliate symptoms

SECTION I ESOPHAGUS/GASTRIC

- MALT: Low grade tumors usually lead to regression with treatment for *H. Pylori* (50-90% of patients have complete regression)
  - Need EGD biopsy, abdominal CT, and EUS to adequately stage
  - For those with normal appearing mucosa/CT/EUS, one theory suggests two 21-day antibiotic courses at baseline and at 8 weeks
  - Others should be considered for initial treatment with traditional forms of therapy for gastric lymphoma via Oncology colleagues
  - Frequent follow-up is required after the initial therapy to verify treatment response
- Gastric Lymphoma (non-MALT): If Ann Arbor stage I or II: surgery can be curative; However ? if chemo ± radiation is equally efficacious
- Gastric Carcinoid: gastrectomy or endoscopic removal (smaller tumors)

COMPLICATIONS:
- Metastases of gastric carcinoma (hematogenous) to: liver, lung, bone, brain; Metastases to ovaries in women

PROGNOSIS:
- Primarily related to depth of tumor penetration through the gastric wall (irrespective of the extent of nodal involvement)
- In the U.S. Adenocarcinoma 5-year survival is 28% and 10-year survival is 20% (i.e. most are diagnosed at an advanced stage)
- Gastric lymphoma 5-year survival is 50% (80% for stage I & II with tumor <5 cm)

NOTES

1.11 GASTRIC POLYPS & THICKENED GASTRIC FOLDS

DEFINITIONS:
- Gastric Polyp: any abnormal growth or epithelial tissue arising from the otherwise smooth surface of the stomach
  Sessile or pedunculated polyps:
  - Hyperplastic: **70–90%** of gastric polyps, hyperplastic, elongated glands with abundant edematous stroma; Benign
  - Adenomatous: neoplastic growths composed of dysplastic epithelium, not normally present in stomach; Pre-malignant
  - Fundic gland: hypertrophied fundic gland mucosa, normal variant; found throughout fundus and body, Benign
  - Hamartomatous: branching bands of smooth muscle surrounded by glandular epithelium, Benign
  - Early gastric cancer
- Thickened Gastric Folds: folds appearing larger than normal and do not flatten with insufflation of air during endoscopy
  - (Radiographically, folds >10 mm in width after distention of the stomach with contrast during UGIS)

EPIDEMIOLOGY: GASTRIC POLYPS
- Risk of cancer (*malignant transformation*) with gastric polyps:
  - Hyperplastic (70–90% of polyps): very low 0.6–4.5% transformation; Most common gastric polyp seen in FAP, Gardner's syndrome
  - Adenomas: true neoplasms, as high as 75% malignant transformation, >2 cm is critically significant and need removal
  - Fundic gland: generally benign, rare cases of malignant transformation reported in large polyps associated with FAP syndromes
  - Hamartomas: thought to have no malignant potential; Most common polyp seen in Peutz-Jeghers, Juvenile polyposis syndromes

ETIOLOGIES: GASTRIC POLYPS
- Gastric adenomatous and hyperplastic polyps: commonly appear in background of chronic gastritis Type A and *H. Pylori*
  - Adenomatous polyps need removal, usually accomplished endoscopically but >2 cm may need surgical resection

ETIOLOGIES:
- **DDX of thickened gastric folds:**

Lymphoma	Lymphocytic gastritis	Eosinophilic gastritis	Mucosa-associated lymphoid tissue (MALT)
Linitis plastica	Gastritis cystica profunda	Menetrier's disease	
Kaposi's sarcoma	Gastric adenocarcinoma	Gastric anisikiasis	Gastric antral vascular ectasia (GAVE)
Gastric varices	*H. Pylori* gastritis (acute)	Sentinel fold	Zollinger-Ellison syndrome
			Infection: TB, Syphilis

  DDX of systemic diseases associated with thickened gastric folds:
  - Gastric Crohn's disease, Sarcoid (most common granulomatous gastropathies)
  - Others: Histoplasmosis, Candida infections, Blastomycoses, Secondary syphilis, Disseminated TB, Systemic mastocytosis

- **DDX of submucosal mass seen on endoscopy:**
  - Common: leiomyoma, lipoma, aberrant pancreas, gastric varices, external compression by liver or spleen
  - Less Common: carcinoid, leiomyosarcoma, granular cell tumor, lymphoma, splenic remnant, submucosal cyst, splenic artery aneurysm
  - Rare: leiomyoblastoma, liposarcoma, schwannoma

- **High-grade non-Hodgkin lymphoma** account for only 3% of gastric cancers, but makes up largest group secondary to adenocarcinoma
  - Endoscopically may present as discrete lesion, ulcerated mass, diffuse submucosal infiltration with enlarged rugal folds
  - When suspected, large-particle or snare biopsy or needle aspiration should be attempted; EUS is useful for visualization, nodes, etc

CHAPTER 1.11 GASTRIC POLYPS & THICKENED GASTRIC FOLDS

- **MALT:** classified as extranodal marginal zone lymphoma; Histologically, large lymphoid follicles and dense B-cell lymphocytic infiltrate
  - Majority associated with *H. Pylori* infection; Most common in 5th decade, but can occur in any age; Most are low grade, indolent course
  - If diagnosed, should have gastric mapping and EUS to assess the depth of wall layer involvement
  - Therapy options: surgery, radiation, chemotherapy, *H. Pylori* eradication (low-grade diseased limited to submucosa) ***See also Esophagus/Gastric- Gastric Cancer (Chapter 1.10)***
- **Menetrier's Disease:** rare condition with giant gastric rugal folds that often spare the antrum; Gastric cancer in 10% (premalignant condition?)
  - Typically men over age 50; Characterized by rugal fold hypertrophy, hypochlorhydria, and protein-losing enteropathy (low albumin/protein)
  - Histologically marked foveolar hyperplasia with cystic dilations penetrating submucosa; Cause is unclear
  - May be confirmed with EUS findings of thickening of deep mucosal layer; Therapy with H2 or PPI is successful in some patients

DIAGNOSTIC STUDIES:
- EGD with Biopsy: must confirm histology; Polyps with diameter 3-5 mm removed entirely by forceps, >5 mm excised by snare
- EUS: most accurate diagnostic imaging study for thickened gastric folds (can't tell if malignant, but is discriminatory in the DDX)

TREATMENTS:
- See Etiologies, above

PROGNOSIS:
- Surveillance for Gastric Polyps (recurrence rate for gastric adenomas is 16%):
  - Begin surveillance endoscopy at 1 year after removal looking for recurrence and new or missed polyps
    - If this is negative, endoscopy should be performed no more frequently than 3-5 years for patients with adenomas
    - If intestinal metaplasia (no dysplasia) found in polyp, surveillance should be performed no less than every 2-3 years

1.12 GASTROPARESIS & DUMPING SYNDROME

(Gastroenterology 2004;127:1589-91 & 1592-1622. Neurogastroenterol Motil 2006;18:263-83)

GASTROPARESIS
Definition:
- Motility disorder of the stomach, often associated with other intestinal motility disorders; Results from impairment of normal gastric emptying
- Factors of gastric motility and emptying:
    1. Composition of the meal: liquids/solids empty at different rates, content influence (i.e. fat empties slow)
    2. Neuroregulators: Neural innervation is complex but largely involves the vagus (innervates stomach to right colon)
    3. Hormonal regulators: Motilin/Neurotensin accelerate, Secretin/cholecystokinin delay gastric emptying
    4. Gastric pacemaker: on greater curve of stomach, oscillates at 3 cycles/min

Etiologies:
- **Idiopathic: most common cause;** May be sudden or insidious development of symptoms; ? viral association
- **Gastrointestinal:**
    - Paraneoplastic: gastric cancer, pancreatic cancer, metastatic disease: breast, small cell lung
    - Atrophic gastritis (Type A): most commonly with solid food delayed emptying
    - Chronic intestinal pseudoobstruction
    - Radiation-induced: any abdominal radiation
    - Anorexia nervosa, Obesity
- **Endocrine:**
    - Diabetic: Well established; Gastroparesis does not necessarily correlate with symptoms; some asymptomatic patients have abnormal GES
    - Hypo/Hyperthyroidism, Hypoparathyroidism
- **Surgical:**
    - Post-op complications: Vagotomy, Roux-en-Y gastrojejunostomy, Fundoplication, Gastric bypass, Esophagectomy, etc
- **Rheumatological**
    - Scleroderma, polymyositis, dermatomyositis, SLE
- **Infectious disorders:**
    - Chagas' disease (Trypanosoma Cruzi), VZV, CMV, EBV, Clostridium Botulinum, HIV
- **Neurologic:**
    - Porphyria, Brainstem tumor, Parkinson's disease, Multiple sclerosis, Spinal cord injury, Heavy-metal poisoning
- **Other:**
    - Stress from pain or anxiety
    - Myotonic dystrophy, Muscular dystrophy, Amyloid, Idiopathic constipation

- Drugs that *delay* gastric emptying:

Alcohol	Aluminum antacids	Anticholinergics	Atropine	Beta agonists
Calcitonin	CCB	Diphenhydramine	Glucagon	IL-1
L-dopa	Lithium	Ondansetron	Opiates	PPIs
Phenothiazine	Progesterone	Sulcrafate	Tobacco	TCAs

- Drugs that *accelerate* gastric emptying:

BB	Cisapride	Diazepam	Domperidone	Erythromycin
H2s	Metoclopramide	Naloxone	PG-E	

Clinical Manifestations/Physical Exam:
- Chronic nausea, vomiting, early satiety, abdominal discomfort - bloating, distention, anorexia/weight loss
- Succussion splash is usually indicative of a region of stasis, typically in the stomach
- Disturbances of bowel movements (i.e. diarrhea and constipation) indicate that the motility disorder is more extensive than gastroparesis
- Neurological exam may be helpful (papillary response, ocular movements, etc)
- Confirm rumination is not playing a role, *See also Esophagus/Gastric- Nausea & Vomiting (Chapter 1.18)*

CHAPTER 1.12 GASTROPARESIS & DUMPING SYNDROME

Laboratory Studies:
- Routine laboratory testing is not useful, although it may help identify diseases that are associated with gastroparesis
  - Hb, fasting plasma glucose, serum total protein, albumin, TSH, cortisol stimulation test, HCG
  - Most of these tests help assess the nutritional state of the patient

Diagnostic Studies:
- Thorough history is critical, including medication use, underlying collagen vascular disease, neurological symptoms (orthostatic dizziness)
- Ask the following:
  - Are the symptoms acute or chronic?
  - Is the disease due to a neuropathy or myopathy?
  - What is the status of hydration and nutrition?
  - What regions of the digestive tract are affected?
- Proposed sequence of investigation
  - Suspect and exclude mechanical obstruction
    - Abd X-ray: show dilated loops of small bowel with air-fluid levels (taken at time of symptoms); CXR for paraneoplastic considerations
    - EGD or Barium study (Small bowel series)
  - Assess gastric and small bowel motility
    - Gastric emptying study (solid phase; off narcotics and promotility drugs) or EGD demonstrating a bezoar
    - If cause is unclear, gastroduodenal manometry may distinguish neuropathic from myopathic processes
  - Identify the pathogenesis (See Etiologies above)
    - May be necessary to purse paraneoplastic workup, autonomic testing for orthostatic hypotension, brain imaging
    - Other tests: thyroid, ANA, CK, Aldolase, Scl-70 for scleroderma, Porphyrins, Serology for Chagas' disease
    - Rarely small bowel full-thickness biopsy
  - Identify complications
    - Bacterial overgrowth, dehydration, malnutrition
- Work-up and DDX as outlined in *See also Esophagus/Gastric- Nausea & Vomiting (Chapter 1.18)* may be appropriate; Rule out pregnancy, Addison's disease, Hyperthyroid

Treatments:
- Treatment ultimately designed for each patient, depending on findings of the investigation
- Correct electrolytes, stop offending medications (including all narcotics)
- Correct constipation (i.e. Miralax); may be related to a functional bowel problem
- CT needed to rule out malignancy/paraneoplastic? (i.e. alarm signs present)
- **Dietary** (rate of emptying inversely proportional to fat & calorie content); recommendations:
  - Small but frequent meals (6/day), reduced fat (<40 gm/day), Soups/crackers/noodles/potatoes
  - Reduced fiber helps avoid bezoars, liquid caloric supplementation (e.g. BOOST)
- **Prokinetic medications:**
  - Metoclopramide (Reglan): Elixir is best; Dopamine antagonist with potent cholinergic effects mainly on proximal GI tract (stomach)
    - Dose: 40–80 mg/day and/or 10 mg sq 2–4 times daily
    - Side effects: dystonic reactions can be permanent (Parkinson-type syndrome, tardive dyskinesia), drowsiness, tolerance
  - Erythromycin: Motilin agonist (stimulates antral contractions); No known antiemetic effect; Effect diminishes after several weeks
    - Dose: 3 mg/kg IV q 8 hours, alternative is elixir 40–80 mg TID ac or pills 125–250 mg BID ac (efficacy: IV >> po)
  - Tegaserod: 6mg BID or TID (if diarrhea is not a prominent symptom) (FDA restricted 2007)
  - Domperidone: similar effects of metoclopramide; 40–80 mg/day in QID doses; Not available in U.S.
  - Cisapride (Propulsid): facilitates acetylcholine release at myenteric plexus; 40–80 mg/day; Taken off market due to arrhythmias
  - Bethanechol (Urecholine): cholinergic drug stimulating muscarinic receptors; Limited use
- **Antiemetic medications:** *See also Esophagus/Gastric- Nausea & Vomiting (Chapter 1.18)*
- Antibiotics for bacterial overgrowth, *See also Bowel- Bacterial Overgrowth (Chapter 2.06)*
- JET with venting PEG (especially if enteral supplementation is required for more than 3 months)
- Gastric pacing is only considered if the above fails while off all narcotics for 6 months

SECTION I ESOPHAGUS/GASTRIC

Complications:
- If N/V severe, can lead to weight loss and malnutrition, GI hemorrhage due to Mallory-Weiss tears, aspiration pneumonia

DUMPING SYNDROME:

Definition:
- Accelerated gastric emptying typically occurring after truncal vagotomy and gastric drainage procedures (i.e. Roux-en-Y gastric bypass)

Epidemiology:
- Prevalence decreasing due to high selective vagotomy and effective anti-acid secretory therapy

Pathophysiology:
- Thought to result from impaired gastric accommodation after the ingestion of a meal and the presence of the drainage procedure
- A high caloric content of the liquid phase of the meal evokes a rapid insulin response with secondary hypoglycemia
- Impaired antral contractility and gastric stasis of solids has a paradoxical result with clinical features of both gastroparesis for solids and dumping for liquids

Clinical Manifestations/Physical Exam:
- Nausea, shaking, diaphoresis and diarrhea immediately after eating foods containing high amounts of refined sugars

Diagnostic Studies:
- Dual-phase (liquid and solid) gastric emptying study

Treatments:
- Dietary: avoid high-nutrient hyperosmolar liquid drinks
- Rarely octreotide (50-100 mcg subcutaneously before meals) is needed
  - Retards intestinal transit and inhibits the hormonal responses that lead to hypoglycemia

Complications:
- Rarely sever enough to cause significant nutritional problems

NOTES

1.13 GASTROPATHY/CHRONIC GASTRITIS

GASTROPATHY

Definition:
- Any disease or inflammation of the stomach

Etiologies:
- Increased frequency with age; Approximately 60% of adults have histological evidence of nonspecific gastritis

In general, chronic dyspepsia » EGD with inspection and biopsy:
(See corresponding chapter of each topic for more detail)

- Gastric Carcinoma » Surgery/Chemotherapy
- Gastric Lymphoma » Chemo/Debulking surgery
- Hypertrophic Folds
  - Menetrier's Disease » PPI, Prokinetics; Rarely surgery
  - ZES » Fasting gastrin, gastric acid analysis, secretin stimulation test; Surgery for localized tumor; PPI/Chemo for metastatic disease
  - Gastric pseudolymphoma » Normal variant (1%)
- Specific Gastritis
  - Eosinophilic gastritis » Corticosteroids
  - Alkaline/Bile gastritis occurs with surgery (i.e. Billroth I or II) » Bile acid binders (cholestyramine), Bile analog (ursodiol), Prokinetics, Surgery (Roux-en-Y)
  - Granulomatous gastritis » Crohn's disease, Sarcoid, TB, Syphilis, Histoplasmosis, Parasites; Treat specifically
  - Portal HTN gastropathy » If blood loss, then BB, Nitrates, PPI
  - Collagenous gastritis » No known effective therapy
- Nonspecific Gastritis
  - Nonerosive gastritis: Type A, Type B; See Chronic Antral & Fundal Gastritis on page 35
  - Erosive gastritis:
    - *H. Pylori:* treat appropriately
    - Crohn's disease: treat appropriately
    - Idiopathic/?Allergic: Trial of acid suppression; If continued symptoms: trial of oral cromolyn or steroids

Pathophysiology:
- Acute/Stress Gastropathy:
  - NSAIDs, Alcohol, corticosteroids
  - Stress Gastritis:
    - Any critical illness resulting in stress-related mucosal disease from under perfusion
    - Respiratory failure, liver or renal disease with coagulopathy, sepsis, surgery or trauma, burns, CNS insult
    - Can develop within 24 hrs; GIB in up to 30%
    - Unique lesions: Curling's (or Stress) ulcers (i.e. ulcer develops in a patient in a burn unit), Cushing's ulcers (eponym for ulcer developing after head injury/trauma/surgery)
- Chronic Gastritis (Type A and B):
  - See Chronic Antral & Fundal Gastritis on page 35
- Congestive Gastropathy:
  - Cirrhosis and portal HTN; Acute treatment: octreotide, PPI; Chronic treatment: Beta blocker, TIPS

Clinical Manifestations/Physical Exam:
- Many asymptomatic
- Dyspepsia (epigastric discomfort), N/V, Postprandial fullness, bloating, occasionally GI bleeding

Diagnostic Studies:
- EGD: scattered mucosal erosions or foci of intramucosal hemorrhage

Treatments:
- Goal is increase stomach pH >4.0 (pepsin is inactivated and blood coagulation is enhanced): PPIs and supportive measures
- **ICU acid suppression indications:** Coagulopathy, Mechanical ventilation (possible ↑ nosocomial pneumonia 2° to micro aspiration of bacteria via ↓ gastric acid)

CHAPTER 1.13 GASTROPATHY/CHRONIC GASTRITIS

CHRONIC ANTRAL GASTRITIS (*TYPE B*, NON-ATROPHIC)
Definition:
- Chronic inflammation of the stomach, especially mucosal (Gastritis is a histological diagnosis)

Etiologies:
- ***H. Pylori*** infection (80% of cases)
  - Characterized by: surface degeneration, foveolar hyperplasia, hyperemia with lamina propria edema, neutrophilic infiltration

Clinical Manifestations/Physical Exam:
- Most asymptomatic
- Most patients who have non-ulcer dyspepsia (NUD) do not have *H. Pylori* gastritis as a cause

Laboratory Studies:
- *See also Esophagus/Gastric- Peptic Ulcer Disease (Chapter 1.21)* For *H. Pylori* testing

Diagnostic Studies:
- EGD: more intense inflammation located in antrum (termed: gastropathy)

Treatments:
- *H. Pylori* treatment
- PPI, H2 blocker

Complications:
- Can progress to atrophic gastritis with ↑ risk of gastric adenocarcinoma

CHRONIC FUNDAL GASTRITIS (*TYPE A*, ATROPHIC):
Definition: Type A = Anemia, Antibodies, Atrophic
- Chronic inflammation of the stomach, especially mucosal (Gastritis is a histological diagnosis)

Etiologies:
- **Autoantibodies** against intrinsic factor and parietal cells, leading to loss of intrinsic factor and achlorhydria

Clinical Manifestations/Physical Exam:
- Atrophic gastritis, **achlorhydria, hypergastrinemia;** pernicious anemia
- Often associated with other autoimmune diseases:
  - Hashimoto's thyroiditis, Thyrotoxicosis, Myxedema, Addison's disease, Diabetes mellitus, Sjogren's syndrome, Vitiligo
- **Pernicious anemia (B12 deficiency/malabsorption):**
  - DDX of low B12:
    - Gastric: pernicious anemia, gastrectomy; Pancreases (insufficiency); Diet: vegan
    - Small Bowel: ileal resection, Crohn's, blind loop, malabsorption states; Meds: neomycin, metformin, PPI

Laboratory Studies:
- Low B12 and Iron
- Autoantibodies against intrinsic factor are more sensitive/specific than antibodies to parietal cells (anti-parietal cell antibodies)
- Schilling's test (labeled B12 and follow urinary excretion)–rarely used in clinical practice

Diagnostic Studies:
- EGD: chronic inflammation located in corpus-fundal mucosa (termed: gastropathy)
- Colonoscopy (with TI intubation)

Treatments:
- B12 injections 1-3 times/month, ? PPI for reflux (but they are already achlorhydria), ? regular screening for gastric cancer
- Associated carcinoids are generally benign and can be removed endoscopically, whereas adenocarcinomas are malignant

Complications:
- Associated ↑ risk of gastric cancers: **gastric carcinoid tumors,** adenocarcinoma, lymphoma
  - Gastrin may be the link between the increased risk of carcinoids with Chronic Type A Gastritis and ZES
  - Most gastric carcinoids (75%) associated with females with Chronic Type A Gastritis: <1 cm endoscopically remove, >1 cm surgery
  - Most sporadic gastric carcinoids (25%) associated with males without chronic gastritis: typically require aggressive surgery
- Also associated with hyperplastic and adenomatous polyps of the stomach

1.14 GASTROESOPHAGEAL REFLUX DISEASE (GERD)/NONEROSIVE REFLUX DISEASE (NERD)/EROSIVE ESOPHAGITIS (EE)

(Am J Gastroenterol 2005;100:190-200)

DEFINITION:
- GERD: Pathologic condition of chronic symptoms or histopathologic injury via percolation of gastroduodenal contents into the esophagus
  - NERD: typical symptoms of GERD caused by intraesophageal acid in the absence of visible mucosal injury at endoscopy
  - EE (or sometimes referred to as Reflux Esophagitis): patients with histopathologically demonstrated changes in esophageal mucosa

EPIDEMIOLOGY:
- Symptoms. 7% daily, 14% weekly, 15-40% monthly
  - Note that the prevalence varies markedly from country to country due to physicians' awareness and understanding the condition
- ♂ = ♀, but ♂ experience more complications: esophagitis 2:1, Barrett's 10:1
- GERD becomes more common with increasing age (incidence increases markedly after age 40)
- Actual organ damage is less frequent as <50% of patients who present with reflux symptoms have esophagitis

ETIOLOGIES:
- There is a potential genetic contribution to GERD; A gene for severe pediatric GERD has been mapped to chromosome 13q14

PATHOPHYSIOLOGY:
- Excessive transient LES relaxations (tLES) or incompetent LES (normal pressure: 10-30 mmHg) or ↑ abdominal pressure
  - ↑ LES pressure: cholinergic agonist, protein, gastrin, motilin, antacids, metoclopramide, domperidone
  - ↓ LES pressure: cholinergic antagonist, fatty food, peppermint, chocolate, ETOH, tobacco, secretin, glucagon, OCPs, CCB, morphine, obesity
- Hiatal hernia: contributes to ↓ LES tone; acts as reservoir for refluxed gastric contents; may widen diaphragmatic hiatus
  - Size may be the best predictor of the severity of esophagitis
- Esophageal mucosal damage (esophagitis) due to prolonged contact with gastric contents: acid, pepsin and duodenal contents: bile salts
- Protective: Swallowing; Reflux can trigger salivary production; Saliva has neutral pH, can clear reflux, and contains healing growth factors
  - Swallowing #/hr: awake/upright: 70/hr; meals 200/hr; sleep <10/hr; Reduced with sedatives/alcohol
    - Scleroderma/CREST and Sjogren's syndrome have reduced amounts of saliva production
    - Saliva is naturally decreased at night, hence nighttime reflux has less saliva and gravity clearance = more injury

CLINICAL MANIFESTATIONS/PHYSICAL EXAM:
- **Heartburn,** retrosternal burning discomfort and regurgitation of stomach contents; atypical "angina"; dysphagia as a complication
  - Waterbrash (foam at mouth as salivary glands produce up to 10 ml of saliva/min as an esophagosalivary response to acid reflux)
- Extraesophageal manifestations (most patients lack classic GERD symptoms and there is no gold standard for diagnosing GERD):
  - Pulmonary: asthma, chronic bronchitis, aspiration pneumonitis, sleep apnea, atelectasis, interstitial pulmonary fibrosis
  - ENT: cough (chronic nocturnal aspiration), hoarseness (vocal cord inflammation), sore throat, posterior laryngitis, sinusitis,
    - Laryngealpharyngeal Reflux: hoarseness, contact ulcers/granulomas, vocal cord nodules, globus, arytenoid fixation
  - Other: dental erosions, globus, scleroderma/mixed connective tissue disease (MCTD)

An empiric trial of PPI bid for 3 months is preferred diagnostic and treatment approach; If symptoms persist than a pH study on therapy can prove one way or the other if acid reflux playing a role

CHAPTER 1.14 GERD/NONEROSIVE REFLUX/EROSIVE ESOPHAGITIS

- Asthma and GERD or ENT symptoms and GERD: Possible mechanisms: Reflex vs. Reflux
  - Reflex: esophagus, bronchial tree and ENT share innervations via vagus; acid infusion of esophagus/ENT can irritate vagus
  - Reflux: microaspiration of acid into bronchial tree/ENT irritates the respiratory epithelium, stimulating inflammatory mediators
    - Clues GERD (rather than asthma): adult onset, nonallergic, poor response to asthma medications, nocturnal cough, related to meals
    - Clues GERD related cough: normal CXR, non smoker/exposure to irritants, no use of ACE-I, negative methacholine challenge
    - Diagnostic trial of PPI bid for 3 months; If no response then pH study on therapy to prove acid related or not
- Chest pain, may be indistinguishable from cardiac pain and cardiac evaluation should precede esophageal evaluation
  See also Esophagus/Gastric- Non-Cardiac Chest Pain (Chapter 1.19)
- Can be associated with: Cerebral palsy, Down syndrome, Mental retardation
- Precipitants: large meals, supine position, fatty foods, peppermint, ETOH, tobacco, caffeine, CCB, obesity, progesterone (pregnancy)
  - Aerophagia (unknowingly swallowing air) triggers burps, belch, and heartburn cycle

LABORATORY STUDIES:
- Not helpful

DIAGNOSTIC STUDIES:
- Diagnosis often based on history, trial of PPI; No diagnostic gold standard
  - If resolution of symptoms and relapse when treatment is stopped the diagnosis is confirmed and suggest need for long-term PPI
- Further testing based on: failure to respond to PPI, alarm signs suggesting complications (dysphagia, odynophagia, risk for Barrett's, etc)
- EGD to detect esophagitis, ulcer, BE, or stricture; EE grading scheme (LA Classification):
    A = One or more mucosal breaks <5 mm and not contiguous with adjacent mucosal fold tops
    B = One or more mucosal breaks >5 mm and not contiguous with adjacent mucosal fold tops
    C = Mucosal breaks contiguous between tops of two or more folds, but involving <75% of esophageal circumference
    D = Mucosal breaks contiguous between tops of two or more folds, but involving $\geq$75% of esophageal circumference
- **Laryngopharyngeal reflux (LPR):** Prescribe BID PPI for 3 months
  - Symptoms improved: Stop PPI » Symptoms recur, maintain PPI; Symptoms do not recur, observe
  - Symptoms not improved: pH testing on PPI » Acid normalized, consider alternative diagnosis; Acid persists with pH testing, change PPI, $\uparrow$ dose
- 24-hr ambulatory esophageal pH monitoring via nasal catheter or BRAVO (normal in 25% of EE, 33% of NERD) (Gastro 1996;110:1981–96)
  -Most important parameter is percent time that pH < 4
  -Indications: Patient refractory to therapy with negative EGD; Prior to any consideration of surgery; Diagnosis is uncertain/atypical symptoms
  - Normal % time pH < 4: Total time 5.5%, Upright 8.2%, Recumbent 3.0%
  - Symptom Index: # of symptoms during acid reflux / total # of symptoms during pH monitoring; >50% is considered positive
    - I.e. 2 symptoms occurred during acid reflux/4 symptoms total during study = 50%
  - Limitations: may give false-negative results in 17% of those with EE (may reflect day-to-day variations of reflux)
    - Some have physiologic degree of acid but have symptoms, may be due to hypersensitivity ("Functional heartburn")
  - Ideally performed off of PPIs; Indications to test on PPI: reflux symptoms refractory to what should be adequate acid-suppression
- Barium esophagram: no role for routine evaluation of GERD, demonstrates reflux only 25–75% of symptomatic patients, false positive: 20%
  - Useful prior to antireflux surgery to asses the size and reducibility of a hiatal hernia and the presence of strictures
- Esophageal manometry: no role for routine evaluation of GERD; essential for accurate transnasal 24-hour pH probe placement
  - Useful prior to antireflux surgery to exclude achalasia
- Impedance: permits the detection of both liquid and gas flow through esophagus independent of pH; role outside of research is currently unclear

SECTION I ESOPHAGUS/GASTRIC

TREATMENTS:
- Conservative measures: avoid precipitants (noted above, i.e. stop tobacco, weight loss, etc), elevate head of bed, avoid late/fatty meal
- Graded approach: (1): life style modification (works in 25%), antacids, prokinetics (2): H2s, reinforced need for lifestyle modification (3): PPI, reinforced lifestyle modification (4): Consider antireflux surgery (only if response to PPI)
- Life style: Elevate head of bed, Weight loss, Avoid: recumbency after meals, bedtime snacks, tobacco/alcohol, reflux promoting foods
- Medical (most effective with EE, and less effective with NERD):
  - Antacids: 1-2 ac & hs (diarrhea: magnesium containing; constipation: aluminum and calcium containing)
  - Sucralfate: 1 gm 4/day
  - H2 blockers: Ranitidine 150-300 mg 2-4/qd, Famotidine 20-40 mg 1-2/qd (tolerance likely develops to H2 blockers within days)
    - Works by blocking histamine induced stimulation of gastric parietal cells, Caution with renal impairment
  - PPI: Omeprazole, Lansoprazole, Rabeprazole, Pantoprazole, Esomeprazole; Never administer on 'as needed' basis
    - Long-term therapy does not result in gastric carcinoids or cancer; although mucosal atrophy with *H. Pylori* can occur
    - Esophagitis: 80% healing in 4 weeks, 100% healing in 8 weeks; However rate of symptom relief is less than healing rate
    - Give 30 min before meals (i.e. pumps need to be working to inactivate); Takes 3-5 days to reach steady state acid inhibition; No need to lower dose with renal insufficiency (primary liver metabolism)
    - Work by an irreversible complex to H+/K+ ATPase pump, which is the final step in acid production
    - To produce acid, parietal cells must form new pumps which can take many hours
  - Prokinetic: Metoclopramide 5-10 mg TID (S/E: extrapyramidal dysfunction, Parkinsonian-like reaction, irreversible tardive dyskinesia)
    - Not a good idea to use for GERD unless associated with gastroparesis; Caution with renal impairment
  - Avoid meds if possible: Theophiline, Anticholinergics, CCB, Diazepam, Morphine, Barbiturates, Alpha-adrenergic antagonists
- Surgical: an option for carefully selected patients with well-documented GERD that responds completely to PPI therapy
  - Laparoscopic (preferred): restoration of intra-abd esophagus, reconstruction of diaphragmatic hiatus, reinforcement of LES by fundoplication; Success >90% (in experienced surgical hands)
  - Failures of wrap: disruption, improper placement, too long/short
  - Note: surgery offers no clear advantage to medication with respect to healing EE, preventing strictures or BE or cancer
- Endoscopic therapy to LES: suture fundoplication, radiofrequency ablation, injection of bulking agent or implantation of bioprosthesis
  - No indications for these techniques in clinical practice at this time; Enteryx withdrawn from market due to complications (2005)
- **GERD despite BID PPI Therapy:** **Incorrect diagnosis** (Non-reflux esophagitis: pill, skin disease, infection, eosinophilic); **Additional diagnosis** (Dyspepsia- gastroparesis, PUD, NERD, NUD); **Inadequate acid suppression** (noncompliance, rapid metabolizer, dose timing, too low dose); **Dysmotility** (achalasia, spasm, nutcracker, gastroparesis); **Functional** (hypersensitivity, brain/gut or psychiatric depression)
  - Consider: EGD, pH Testing off meds (BRAVO), Gastric emptying study, Barium swallow, Motility study
  - Consider adding pain modulator (once all else is excluded): TCA, Trazodone, SSRI

COMPLICATIONS:
- Esophagitis, Peptic strictures, Ulcers, Barrett's esophagus
  - Strictures: develops 1–23% of GERD patients;
    Treatment is dilation (selection based on stricture configuration, comfort of endoscopist, availability of equipment)

    Rule of 3's: dilate a total of three times in one session (first dilation is the one with mild resistance) End point is a lumen diameter of >14 mm, followed by control of reflux (PPI) if any
  - Mercury-filled tapered bougies (Maloney): axial shearing and radial forces; best for simple symmetric strictures <10 mm
  - Guidewire placed tapered polyvinyl dilators (Savary): axial shearing and radial forces; best for <10 mm, long, tortuous, post-op strictures
  - Through-the-scope (TTS) balloons: only radial force; best for <10 mm, long, tortuous, post-op strictures

  Note: French sizes are circumferences sizes, divided by 3 they give the diameter in mm; So 30 Fr is 10 mm in diameter

  - If BE: endoscopic surveillance for dysplasia is warranted; ***See also Esophagus/Gastric- Barrett's Esophagus (Chapter 1.02)***
- Note: Cimetadine (Tagamet) can cause confusion in elderly, and increase PT/INR with coumadin
- Cough (rule out non-GERD causes too): ACE-I, environmental, smoking, parenchymal lung disease, allergic rhinitis, sinusitis, asthma
- Non-Cardiac Chest Pain (cardiac excluded); ***See also Esophagus/Gastric- Non-Cardiac Chest Pain (Chapter 1.19)***

PROGNOSIS:
- Likelihood of stopping meds: 50% stay on PPI lifelong, 30% can be weaned to H2s, 20% can get off all meds (i.e. GERD can be a lifelong disease)
- *H. Pylori* and GERD: Those with *H. Pylori* have no different or less severe reflux; Controversial whether *H. Pylori* is protective or not
  - In patients with GERD, eradication of *H. Pylori* does not effect the relapse rate of either symptoms or erosive esophagitis

1.15 INJURY (ESOPHAGUS): CORROSIVE

DEFINITION:
- Injury of the esophagus caused by any number of caustic agents

EPIDEMIOLOGY:
- Approximately 26,000 caustic ingestions occur per year; suicidal gesture is most common and most injurious compared to accidental ingestion
- Approximately 80% of caustic ingestions occur accidentally in children less than 5 y/o, who most often consume household cleaners

ETIOLOGIES:
- Severity of damage depends on corrosive properties and concentration of ingested agents
- **Alkaline cleaning products = most severe injury**
- Alkali esophagitis (i.e. Lye): upon exposure to esophagus, result in liquefactive necrosis: complete destruction of entire cells and membranes; Phases of injury:
  - Acute (day 1-4): Liquefactive necrosis: sloughing or ulcer not apparent <24 hr, vascular thrombosis, inflammation
  - Subacute (day 5-14): Sloughing of casts: esophageal wall is thinnest, granulation, fibroblast/collagen deposition
  - Cicatrization (day 15-3 mon): Fibroblast proliferate, further collagen deposition, stricture formation, epithelialization
- Acid esophagitis: coagulation necrosis with clumping and opacification of cellular cytoplasm, retained cell boundaries, unlike alkali injury

Class	Caustic Agent	Product
Strong Alkalis	Ammonia	Cleaning products
	Lye (Sodium hydroxide, Potassium hydroxide)	Disc batteries, drain cleaners, nonphosphate detergents, paint removers, washing powders
Strong Acids	Hydrochloric acid	Muriatic acid, soldering fluxes, swimming pool cleaners, toilet bowel cleaners
	Nitric acid	Gun barrel cleaners
	Oxalic acid	Antirust compounds
	Phosphoric acid	Toilet bowel cleaners
	Sulfuric acid	Battery acid, Toilet bowel cleaners
Miscellaneous	Sodium hypochlorite	Liquid bleach

Reprinted with permission from McNally P: GI/Liver Secrets 3rd ed. Elsevier/Mosby, 2006:60.

PATHOPHYSIOLOGY:
- See Phases of injury under Etiologies, above

CLINICAL MANIFESTATIONS/PHYSICAL EXAM:
- Early signs and symptoms are not reliable indicators of the severity of caustic injury; Can be easily fooled either way of the severity

LABORATORY STUDIES:
- Not helpful

DIAGNOSTIC STUDIES:
- Ng lavage is controversial: potential risks include inducing vomiting, perforation; Consider fluoro; If Ng placed, aspirate before cold lavage
- Endoscopy: may help guide surgery; The risk is acceptable once decision to operate has been made
  - If no surgery, endoscopy still should be performed to triage severity and patients hospital stay; Timing is based on clinical judgment
  - Classification of injury by endoscopy:

CHAPTER 1.15 INJURY (ESOPHAGUS): CORROSIVE

Endoscopic Findings	Hospital Stay	Risk of Stricture	Treatment
No injury	None	None	Discharge
Gastric only	Observe 24–48 hrs	None	Liquid diet
Linear esophageal injury	Observe 24–48 hrs	Low	Liquid diet
Circumferential injury	Observe at least 48 hrs	High	NPO, Ng Tube

Reprinted with permission from McNally P. GI/Liver Secrets. 3rd ed. New York: Elsevier/Mosby; 2006:60.

TREATMENTS:
- Emergency treatment always begins with ABCs; ? need for intubation, ? obvious signs of mediastinitis/peritonitis requiring surgery
- Determine the quantity and type of caustic agent and time of ingestion; Is the container available?
- Poison control center should be contacted
- Emesis should not be induced, because it will re-expose the esophagus and perhaps the larynx
- If known acid and within minutes of injury, large volumes of water/milk may dilute and neutralize the acid; Otherwise NPO
- Steroids: thought to reduce the potential for strictures in high risk lesions; However, no consensus on their use
  - If used, should only be with circumferential injury: prednisone 1.5 mg/kg/day and tapered over 2 months
  - Probably a better use is in those patients with airway compromise and bronchospasm
- Antibiotics: role has never been established
- In acute setting, get CXR or CT to rule out perforation *before* endoscopy:
  - Prophylactic dilation: once acute injury has resolved, strictures are likely with circumferential burns; First dilation about 3rd week
    - ? role for removable stents while healing

COMPLICATIONS:
- Strictures: threshold for evaluating swallowing problems in these patients should be low
- Esophageal Cancer: 1000× fold risk of developing esophageal cancer compared to general population
  - Begin endoscopic surveillance 15 years after ingestion (generally not performed more than every 1-3 years)

PROGNOSIS:
- Mortality has decreased markedly over that last several decades from 20% to 1-3%
  - Due to improvements of supportive care, change in products
- Association between esophageal cancer and caustic lye ingestion is strong
  - Approx 1-7% of patients with esophageal cancer have a history of caustic ingestion; Latent period can be long, up to 40+ years

1.16 INJURY (ESOPHAGUS): PILL INDUCED

DEFINITION:
- Injury of the esophagus caused by a any of a number of pills/medications

EPIDEMIOLOGY:
- Anyone who can ingest caustic pills is susceptible to pill-induced injury
- Esophageal dysmotility or structural abnormalities, such as rings or strictures, are clearly not required for pill-induced injury

ETIOLOGIES:
- Antibiotics: more than one-half of all reported causes: Doxycycline, Tetracycline, Clindamycin, Erythromycin, Penicillin
- Cardiac meds: antihypertensives, antiarrhythmics, Quinidine
- NSAIDs: 30 million people use every day, 16% have GI side effects; NSAIDs inhibit the protective prostaglandins
- Other: Potassium chloride, Ascorbic Acid, Ferrous sulfate, Theophylline, Antiretroviral drugs Fosamax and other bisphosphonates; Manufacturer recommends 8oz water and sitting upright 30 min after ingestion

PATHOPHYSIOLOGY:
- Upright posture and increased volume of water ingested with pills improves the clearance of pills
  - Taking the pill with inadequate fluid and lying down immediately afterwards are often the only identifiable risk factors (most common)
- Patients at particular risk: structural abnormalities of the esophagus:
  - Pathologic (stricture, tumor, esophageal ring)
  - Physiologic narrowing areas: Sphincters, Cervical spine degenerative arthritis, Aortic arch, Left atrium, Left main stem bronchus
  - GERD: can cause more acidic environment, and since many pills are weak acids, their absorption into tissues is increased
- Synergistic role with Alcohol; May decrease the primary and secondary contractions of the esophagus

CLINICAL MANIFESTATIONS/PHYSICAL EXAM:
- Typical patient:
  No history of esophageal disease, chest pain awakening from sleep (recent pill ingestion with little fluid), exacerbated by swallowing
- Odynophagia, dysphagia, chest pain (rarely upper GI bleeding or perforation)

LABORATORY STUDIES:
- Not helpful

DIAGNOSTIC STUDIES:
- Suspected on basis of history when typical symptoms suddenly appear soon after ingestion of a pill
- EGD required if symptoms are severe, persist longer than 3-4 days, have atypical features, or suggest complication (stricture/bleed)
  - EGD shows one or more discrete ulcers with normal surrounding mucosa; Pill fragments may be seen

TREATMENTS:
- Most heal without intervention
- Avoid initial drug responsible for injury; If avoidance not possible, effort must be made to decrease potential: elixir, sitting upright, fluids

COMPLICATIONS:
- Ulcers typically involve only mucosa, but deeper lesions can occur: erosions into vascular structures
- Strictures that may require dilation

NOTES

1.17 MANOMETRY (ESOPHAGEAL)

(Gastroenterology. 2005;128:207-08 & 209-24. Gut 2001;49:145-51)

INDICATIONS:
- Dysphagia not explained by stenosis or inflammation, Chest pain not explained by heart disease, Before fundoplication to exclude achalasia *See also Esophagus/Gastric- Schatzki's Ring (Chapter 1.22)*

GENERAL/NORMAL: (Fig. 1.17.1A)
- The **Basal LES** (tonically closed) at rest with a normal mean pressure of 20 mmHg (range 10-45 mmHg)
  - A wet swallow can alter subsequent swallows for up to 20-30 seconds, so it is important to note time intervals between swallows
- After a wet swallow, **Peristaltic wave progression** occurs at a rate of 2-8 cm per second
  - Following peristalsis there is complete **LES relaxation** to allow bolus to pass (pressure drops to <8 mmHg above gastric pressure)
- The normal **Distal wave amplitude** is 30-180 mmHg
- Asymptomatic esophageal manometric findings should be ignored; Symptoms may not respond to therapies that correct abnormalities

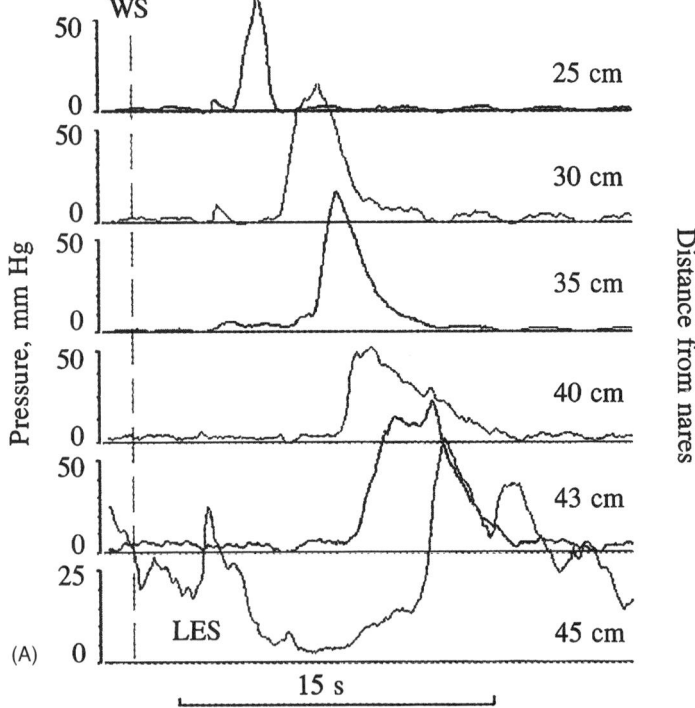

Figure 1.17.1 A. Normal esophageal motility.
Reprinted from Talley NJ. Normal and abnormal esophageal motility. In: Hauser SC Ed. Mayo Clinic Gastroenterology and Hepatology Board Review 2nd ed. Mayo Clinic Scientific Press. 2006:37,38,40 with permission.

CHAPTER 1.17 MANOMETRY (ESOPHAGEAL)

ACHALASIA (Fig. 1.17.1B)

Basal LES: Usually high/>45 mmHg (may be normal)
Peristaltic wave progression: Absent or simultaneous with identical configurations

LES relaxation: Incomplete (residual >8 mmHg)
Distal wave amplitude: Low or low-normal (<40 mmHg)

- Intraesophageal pressure can be increased because the esophagus is accommodating and behaving as a common cavity
- Manometry can not distinguish between Achalasia and pseudoachalasia, the clue to either is aperistalsis
- Vigorous achalasia is a combination of diffuse esophageal spasm and failure of the LES to relax
- Note: Chagas' Disease is identical to Achalasia

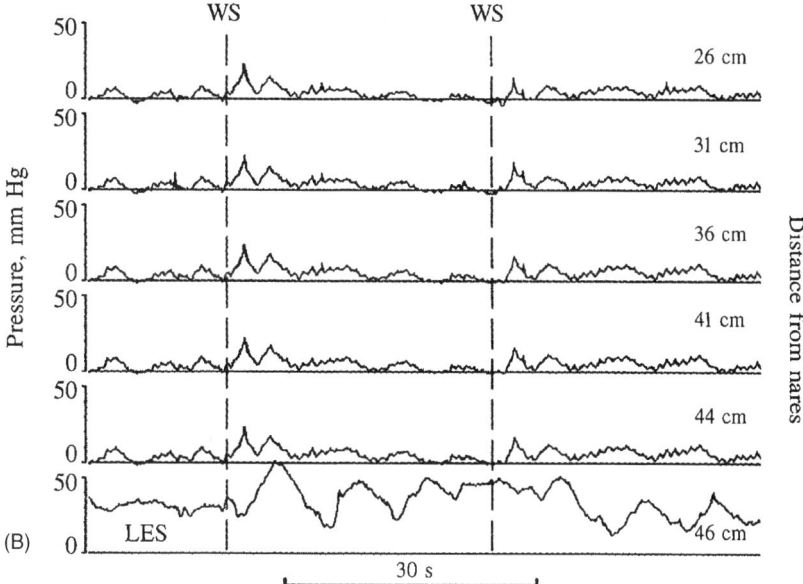

Figure 1.17.1 B. Achalasia.
Reprinted from Talley NJ. Normal and abnormal esophageal motility. In: Hauser SC Ed. Mayo Clinic Gastroenterology and Hepatology Board Review 2nd ed. Mayo Clinic Scientific Press. 2006:37,38,40 with permission.

SECTION I ESOPHAGUS/GASTRIC

DIFFUSE ESOPHAGEAL SPASM: (Fig. 1.17.1C)

<u>Basal LES:</u> Low, normal or high

<u>Peristaltic wave progression:</u> Simultaneous contractions in >20-30% of wet swallows

<u>LES relaxation:</u> Complete relaxation supports the diagnosis

<u>Distal wave amplitude:</u> Normal or high (>30 mmHg)

- Peristaltic wave progression may display >3 repetitive contractions (i.e. >8 cm/sec) & prolonged contractions (>6 seconds in duration)
  - i.e. normal pressures, but the contractions land on top of one another

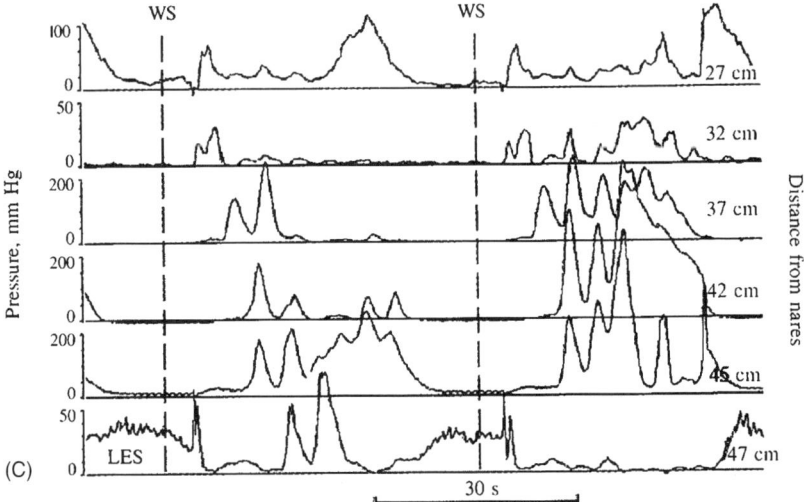

Figure 1.17.1 C. Diffuse esophageal spasm.
Reprinted from Talley NJ. Normal and abnormal esophageal motility. In: Hauser SC Ed. Mayo Clinic Gastroenterology and Hepatology Board Review 2nd ed. Mayo Clinic Scientific Press. 2006:37,38,40 with permission.

SCLERODERMA/INEFFECTIVE ESOPHAGEAL MOTILITY: (Fig. 1.17.1D)

Basal LES: Low (<10 mmHg) or rarely normal
Peristaltic wave progression: Normal, simultaneous, or absent

LES relaxation: Complete
Distal wave amplitude: Low (<30 mmHg) in >30% wet swallows

- Low amplitude or absent peristaltic waves progression in the smooth muscle of esophagus (i.e. loss of distal smooth muscle peristalsis)
- Clue: Normal striated UES, hence the proximal pressures are normal

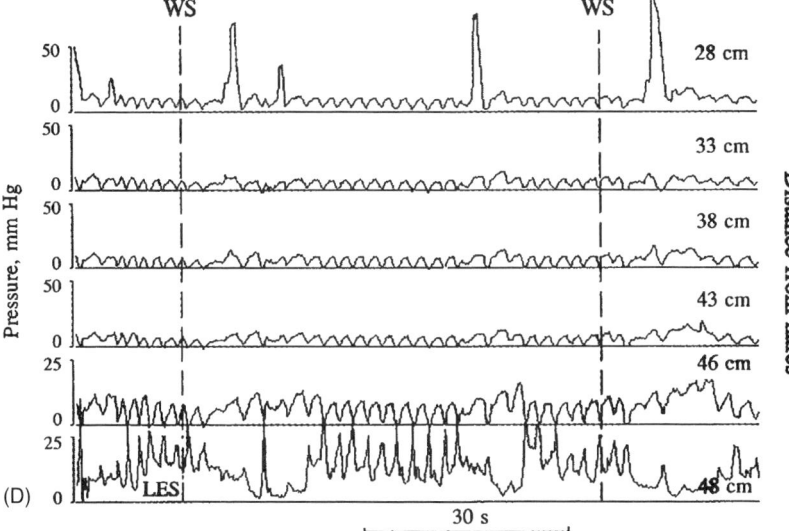

Figure 1.17.1 D. Scleroderma/Ineffective esophageal motility.
Reprinted from Talley NJ. Normal and abnormal esophageal motility. In: Hauser SC Ed. Mayo Clinic Gastroenterology and Hepatology Board Review 2nd ed. Mayo Clinic Scientific Press. 2006:37,38,40 with permission.

HYPERTENSIVE PERISTALSIS/NUTCRACKER

Basal LES: Low, normal or high
Peristaltic wave progression: Normal

LES relaxation: Complete
Distal wave amplitude: High (total amplitude >180 mmHg)

- High mid/distal wave amplitude with a total amplitude >180 mmHg and ↑ distal peristaltic duration (>6 sec)
- Clue: the peristaltic wave progressions propagate normally in the esophagus and the LES relaxes normally
  - i.e. looks exactly like a normal swallow except the mid and distal pressures add to an average of >180 mmHg (very high)

ISOLATED HYPERTENSIVE LES

Basal LES: High (>45 mmHg)
Peristaltic wave progression: Normal

LES relaxation: Usually complete
Distal wave amplitude: Normal

- High basal LES (>45 mmHg); May be incomplete relaxation (residual pressure >8 mmHg)

1.18 NAUSEA & VOMITING

(Gastroenterology. 2001;120:261-62 & 263-86)

DEFINITION:
- Vomiting: forceful expulsion of gastric contents associated with contraction of abdominal and chest wall musculature
- Nausea: unpleasant sensation of the imminent need to vomit (above); a sensation that may or may not ultimately lead to the act of vomiting
- Regurgitation: act by which food is brought back into the mouth without the abdominal and diaphragmatic muscular activity of vomiting
- Anorexia: loss of desire to eat (true loss of appetite)
- Sitophobia: fear of eating because of subsequent or associated discomfort
- Retching: spasmodic respiratory movements against closed glottis with contraction of abdominal muscles without expulsion of gastric contents (dry heaves)
- Rumination: chewing & swallowing of regurgitated food that came back into mouth within minutes of eating without an organic cause (See end of chapter)

PATHOPHYSIOLOGY: GM_3PIC_2 (mnemonic to help remember categories)
Medications & Toxic:
- Chemo: cisplatinum, methotrexate, vinblastine, tamoxifen
- Analgesics: asa, NSAIDs, Antigout
- CV Meds: digoxin, Anti-HTN, Anti-arrhythmics, BB, CCB
- Hormonal: OCP
- Abx: tetracycline, sulfonamides, acyclovir
- GI: sulfasalazine, azathioprine
- Nicotine: Narcotics, Anti-parkinsonian, Anti-convulsants
- ETOH
- Misc: Radiation, Hypervitaminosis, Theophylline

Infectious:
- Gastroenteritis (Viral, Bacterial)
- Non-GI: otitis media

Gut Disorders:
- Mechanical: gastric outlet obstruction, small bowel obstruction, pyloric stenosis, SMA syndrome, volvulus, Zenker's diverticulum
- Functional: gastroparesis, chronic intestinal pseudo-obstruction, nonulcer dyspepsia, IBS
- Organic: pancreatic adenocarcinoma, intraperitoneal disease, PUD, cholecystitis, pancreatitis, hepatitis, CD, mesenteric ischemia, retroperitoneal fibrosis

CNS:
- Migraine
- Increased intracranial pressure: hemorrhage, infarctions, abscess, meningitis, hydrocephalus, pseudo-tumor cerebri
- Cancer (glioblastoma), can also increase ICP: think about it with sudden early am vomiting and no nausea
- Seizure, Demyelinating disorders
- Emotional
- Psychiatric: psychogenic vomiting, anxiety, depression, pain, anorexia, bulimia
- Labyrinthine: motion sickness, labyrinthitis, tumors, meniere's disease

Metabolic/Endocrine
- Pregnancy, Uremia, DKA, Hyper/Hypoparathyroidism, Hyperthyroidism, Addison's (abrupt steroid withdrawal), Acute intermittent porphyria

Postoperative Nausea and Vomiting
Cyclic Vomiting Syndrome
Miscellaneous: Cardiac (MI, CHF), Starvation, Paraneoplastic

CLINICAL MANIFESTATIONS/PHYSICAL EXAM:
- See Definitions above

LABORATORY STUDIES:
- Alkalosis (loss of hydrogen ions in vomitus); Potassium deficiency common due to loss in vomitus and kidney wasting

CHAPTER 1.18 NAUSEA & VOMITING

DIAGNOSTIC STUDIES:
Initial evaluation with H & P Labs: Electrolytes, Albumin, CortStim (Addison's), Eosinophiles, ?ABG
Restoration of fluid/electrolytes; Empiric antiemetic therapy

Underlying disorder » Known: treatment
Unknown:

Abdominal X-rays (KUB/SBS) » Bowel obstruction: Surgical consult
No bowel obstruction:

Endoscopy ± Barium studies (UGIS/SBS/CT enterography) » Lesion identified: Medical or Surgical treatment
No lesion identified:

Radionuclide gastric emptying study » Abnormal: prokinetic drugs, further evaluation with **manometry and electrogastrography**
?GDM (gastroduodenal manometry): If normal, think outside the GI tract
Normal:

Further evaluation »
CT/MRI scan (Brain/Abdomen) ± angiography (if indicated); Vestibular Battery Testing with ENT
Many need psychiatric consult (if indicated) with antiemetic & nonpharmacological approaches

TREATMENTS:
- General: NPO, Ng tube, treat underlying disease
- Diet: low fat, small portions, etc
- Gastroparesis: diet, prokinetic/anti-emetic, botox of pylorus, PEG/PEJ
- Antiemetics: act primarily within CNS to suppress nausea and vomiting; Prokinetics: stimulate GI motility

Class/Drug	Dose	Indications
5-HT$_3$ Antagonists		
Ondansetron (Zofran)	8 mg IVP, then 9 mg q 8 hr	Chemo-induced
Dolasetron (Anzemet)	1.8 mg/kg IV (max 100/dose)	
Corticosteroid		
Dexamethasone	10 mg IV q 6 hr	Chemo-induced
Dopamine Antagonists		
Prochlorperazine (Compazine)	10 mg po/IM/IV q 6 hr	All; Not helpful in motion sickness and vertigo; S/E: sedation, parkinsonism
Metoclopramide (Reglan)	1–3 mg/kg q ac/hs	Use elixir in refractory cases; Can cause permanent dystonia in patients
Domperidone	Not available in U.S.	
Antihistamine (H$_1$ antagonist)		
Diphenhydramine (Benadryl)	25–50 mg po/IV q 4–6 hr	Motion sickness/inner ear-vestibular, pregnancy, uremia, post op
Promethazine (Phenergan)	25 mg po/IM/IV q 8 hr	
Dimenhydrinate (Dramamine)	50–100 mg po q 6 hr	
Benzodiazepines		
Lorazepam	0.5–2.0 mg po/IV q 4–6 hr	Psychogenic or anticipatory
Alprazolam	0.25–0.5 mg po/IV q 8 hr	
Anticholinergics		
Scopolamine	1.5 mg patch q 3 days	Motion sickness/inner ear-vestibular
Meclizine (Antivert)	25–100 mg po qd (divided TID)	
Other		
Erythromycin	250 mg po/IV q 8 hr	Acts on motilin receptors in smooth muscle, independent of antibiotic effect
Haloperidol (Haldol)	0.5 mg IV q 6 hr	Psychogenic or anticipatory
Octreotide	50–500 mcg sq QD-TID	May be beneficial for small bowel motility in scleroderma

COMPLICATIONS:
- Mallory Weiss Tear (or Boerhaave's syndrome: transmural tear of esophagus), Aspiration, Electrolyte disturbance

RUMINATION:
- Typical history of a person is early (0-30 minutes) postprandial, effortless regurgitation of undigested food that happens with most meals
- Patients (mostly males) do not describe it as distressful and are often embarrassed and attempt to hide the symptom
  - Often occurs in mentally challenged children (i.e. Down syndrome) as well
- Most people have abdominal and thoracic movements that precede and accompany the process; There is a voluntary component
  - Eating large meals with a lot of liquids facilitates rumination; Usually rumination begins 15-20 minutes following a meal
- Behavioral therapy is treatment of choice:
  - Biofeedback directed against the increased intra-abdominal pressure
  - Teaching diaphragmatic breathing techniques (Am J Gastroenterol 2006;101:2449-52)
  - Changing composition of food, slowing the speed of eating, and giving less water with meals have been effective approaches

NOTES

1.19 NON-CARDIAC CHEST PAIN

(Neurogastroenterol Motil 2006;18:408-17)

DEFINITION:
- Chest pains of non-cardiac origin
- Initial approach is to exclude coronary artery disease (CAD); Cardiac causes other than CAD: Mitral valve prolapse
- *See also Esophagus/Gastric- GERD (Chapter 1.14)*

ETIOLOGIES:
- **Non Cardiac Chest Pain (cardiac excluded)**
  - **DDX:** GERD, Esophageal dysmotility, Musculoskeletal, Brain/Gut, Gallstones (rarely)
- GERD: most frequent cause, up to 50% of unexplained chest pains
- Esophageal dysmotility: up to 25-30% of unexplained chest pains (See below in order of frequency: highest to lowest)
  - Hypertensive peristalsis/Nutcracker: most common manometric abnormality, high pressures during esophageal peristalsis
  - Ineffective esophageal motility/Nonspecific esophageal dysmotility: weak or poor conducted waves
  - Diffuse esophageal spasm
  - Achalasia
- Musculoskeletal (chostochondritis): remaining 20-30%
- Psychological (Brain-gut) i.e. panic disorder, acting either independently or cofactors are responsible for many of these pain syndromes
- More rare: biliary tract disease (gallstones)

PATHOPHYSIOLOGY:
- The mechanism whereby GERD causes chest pain remains obscure
  - Possible that intraepithelial free nerve endings act as acid sensitive nociceptors
  - Patients can also develop hypersensitivity to physiologic amounts of intraesophageal acid
- Predisposition to GERD:
  - Drugs commonly used to treat coronary disease (nitrates, CCB) can ↓ LES pressure and distal esophageal contraction amplitudes

CLINICAL MANIFESTATIONS/PHYSICAL EXAM:
- Chest discomfort/pains

LABORATORY STUDIES:
- Often not helpful

DIAGNOSTIC STUDIES:
- Exclude cardiac disease
  - Alarm Symptoms? (Dysphagia, Odynophagia, Weight loss, Anorexia, etc.)
    - No: PPI trial BID for 2-3 months (relatively inexpensive, noninvasive, easy to perform)
      - Relief: taper down to lowest effective dose
      - No relief: Manometry (see below)
    - Yes: EGD
      - Negative: PPI trial (see above)
      - Findings: treat accordingly

      Manometry *See also Esophagus/Gastric- Manometry (Chapter 1.17)*
      - Achalasia *See also Esophagus/Gastric- Achalasia (Chapter 1.01)*
      - Spastic motility disorder *See also Esophagus/Gastric- Schatzki's Ring (Chapter 1.22)*
      - Negative: treat with pain modulator (i.e. TCA, SSRI)

- pH monitoring (i.e. 24 hr nasal or BRAVO); best done off therapy
  - Normal: pH <4; Total time 5.5%, Upright 8.2%, Recumbent 3.0%
  - Symptom Index: # of symptoms during acid reflux/total # of symptoms during pH monitoring; >50% is considered positive
    - I.e. 2 symptoms occurred during acid reflux/4 symptoms total during study = 50%
- ? RUQ U/S if history warrants it

TREATMENTS:
- PPI Trial: BID for 8-12 weeks
- Treatment of reflux-induced chest pain is no different from normal management of GERD
- Esophageal dysmotility:
  - CCB, nitrates, anticholinergics

PROGNOSIS:
- Generally poor functional outcome; Morbidity and mortality is the same as for the general population

1.20 PERCUTANEOUS ENDOSCOPIC GASTROSTOMY (PEG) TUBES

(Am J Gastroenterol 2003;98:272-7. Endoscopy 1998;30:781-89. Gastroenterology 1995;108:1282-1301)

INDICATIONS: In general, patients should have a functional GI tract and anticipated life expectancy >30 days
- Malnutrition/poor volitional intake (BMI <18.5, Wt.loss >10%, Starvation >7-10 days); Oropharyngeal dysphagia (i.e. throat cancer)
- Malabsorption, Short Gut Syndrome; Need for gastric decompression; Major trauma/burns
- Permanent neurological impairment: CVA, MS, Parkinson's, Dementia

PRE-PEG CHECKLIST:
- Obtain consent from the patient or healthcare power of attorney
- Check vitals: any recent fevers, homodynamic/respiratory instability?
- Check basic labs: CBC, PT/PTT
- Does this patient have any contraindications (see below)
- Adjust any anticoagulation/anti-platelet agents (see page 58)
- NPO/stop enteral feeds after midnight
- Antibiotic prophylaxis needed? See below and *See also Endoscopy & Procedures- Infectious Endocarditis Prophylaxis (Chapter 7.10)*

POST-PROCEDURE CARE:
- Clean area with soap and water
- Dressing: cut drain sponge placed over the external bumper to avoid unnecessary tension at the site

CONTRAINDICATIONS:
General:
- Cannot pass endoscope (i.e. obstructing esophageal malignancy) » Consider percutaneous radiological or surgical gastrostomy
- Inability to transluminate abdominal wall; Inability to appose the anterior gastric wall (peritoneal carcinomatosis, ascites)
- Gastric outlet obstruction (unless PEG is for venting reasons) or Severe malabsorption
- Others: Severe diarrhea or vomiting, SBO or severe intestinal dysmotility (Ileus/pseudo-obstruction), Peritonitis, High-output fistula

Relative:
- Coagulopathy, Gastric varices, Morbid obesity, Prior abdominal/gastric surgery, Ascites, Peritoneal dialysis, Gastric/abdominal wall neoplasm
- Technically difficult, but not contraindication: Pregnancy, Liver disease, Obesity, and Prior abdominal/gastric surgery

COMPLICATIONS: (TOTAL 4–23%)
Minor: 7-20%: ileus, peristomal infection, stomal leak, buried bumper, gastric ulcer, fistulous tracts, inadvertent removal
Major: 3-4%: peritoneal leak/peritonitis, hemorrhage, aspiration (higher risk as patient left decub position); these may require surgery
Death: 0-2%

- Bleeding:
  - Check post-procedure hemoglobin and inspect site for hematoma
- Perforation/Peritonitis:
  - Think about peritonitis if patient has abdominal pain, high WBC, ileus, fever (Transient subclinical pneumoperitoneum occurs in 56% of PEGs; It is usually of no clinical significance but may persist making use of post-procedure X-ray very limited; A better evaluation post-PEG in a patient with suspected peritonitis would be a gastrografin injection)
- Ileus:
  - Most post-procedure related ileus are managed conservatively; If concern for acute gastric distention, uncap and decompress; Also consider if the bumper of the PEG tube could have migrated and be causing gastric outlet obstruction
- Excessive granulation tissue (at PEG site):
  - Apply topical silver nitrate to reduce irritation and decrease drainage

CHAPTER 1.20 PERCUTANEOUS ENDOSCOPIC GASTROSTOMY (PEG) TUBES

- Infections:
  - 30% of PEGs may have peristomal infections at some time but 70% are minor
  - Decrease risk: limit tension between bumpers; Pre-PEG antibiotics 30 min prior to procedure (Cefazolin 1 gm IV); small skin incision
  - Early diagnosis: po antibiotics for 5-7 days; More severe infection: may require IV antibiotics
- Site Irritation/Leak:
  - Identify cause: Infection/ulceration at site; High gastric acid secretion (Tx: PPI); Patient cleaning excessively with hydrogen peroxide; Buried bumper; Torsion of PEG (consider clamping device to stabilize tube or replace with low-profile); No external bumper to stabilize tube
  - Prevent local skin irritation: Zinc oxide applied topically as a barrier to irritation; Use foam dressing rather than gauze (foam will help lift away drainage from skin); Topical antifungal if suspicion for local fungal infection
  - Refractory leakage/irritation: may need to relocate PEG site
- Buried Bumper:
  - Partial or complete growth of gastric mucosa over the internal bumper
  - The bumper may migrate through the gastric wall and lodge anywhere along PEG tract
  - Can present as: peritubal leakage or infection, immobile catheter, abdominal pain, resistance to infusions of feeds, bleeding
  - Increased risk: PEG with high tension between bumpers; malnutrition; poor wound healing; significant weight gain after placement
  - Diagnosis: gastrografin study with patient prone (supine may appear that contrast is entering into gastric lumen)
- Bleeding:
  - May be caused by PUD, ulceration of gastric wall opposite bumper, ulceration under the internal bumper
  - May need EGD to evaluate PEG site with external manipulation of PEG to look 'under' internal bumper
  - Avoid excessive lateral traction on PEG tube
- Gastrocolocutaneous Fistula:
  - If caused by placement of PEG through colon, patients usually have symptoms of colonic perforation/obstruction
  - Due to erosion of the tube into the colon: usually have stool seepage and diarrhea that looks like formula
- Inadvertent removal of PEG:
  - PEG tract matures within first 7-10 days, but can take up to 4 weeks in the setting of malnutrition or chronic steroid use; If assessed acutely, can temporarily place foley in PEG site
  - Treatment: Ng suction, broad spectrum antibiotics, repeat PEG placement in 7-10 days
    - Surgical exploration if patient decompensates or concern for peritonitis
  - If patient is prone to pull out, can use abdominal binder to secure tube or low profile button PEG
- Fungal tube infection:
  - Fungal colonization of tube can be a long-term complication: replace tube (polyurethane may be more resistant to fungus)

SUMMARY GUIDELINES TO AVOID COMPLICATIONS:

Procedure-Related:
- Aspiration: avoid over-sedation, minimize air insufflation, perform procedure efficiently
- Bleeding: correct coagulopathy, consider an alteration of anatomy secondary to any prior surgery
- Perforation: early recognition, consider an alteration of anatomy secondary to any prior surgery
- Prolonged ileus: wait 3-4 hours (or longer) before beginning feeding post-PEG placement; if gastric distention, uncap and decompress

Post-Procedure Related:
- Care: use mild soap and water, not hydrogen peroxide, place drain sponge over (not under) external bumper
- Infection: prophylactic antibiotics, adequate preoperative skin sterilization, set/maintain proper tension between bumpers (Do not over tighten or leave too loose)
- Leakage/Irritation: prevent infection, avoid local hydrogen peroxide, prevent excessive side torsion on PEG tube
- Buried Bumper: avoid excessive tension between bumpers, account for nutritional weight gain
- Gastric Ulceration: acid suppression, avoid lateral traction on tube
- Fistulous Tracts: elevate the head of bed during placement, utilize the 'safe tract technique' for needle injection (no air should return until entering the stomach)
- Inadvertent Removal: consider use of abdominal binder, utilize low-profile button PEG at initial placement

SECTION I ESOPHAGUS/GASTRIC

POST PEG ORDERS (IN HOSPITAL):
- NPO; Start using tube at 8 am the day after insertion after starting sterile water at 50 cc/hr for 2 hours
  - If sterile water tolerated begin tube feedings formula
- Flush tube with tap water after tube feeding begun: 30 cc every 4 hours with continuous feedings or after each bolus or intermittent feeding
- Cleanse tube exit site with soap and water once daily starting the day after tube placement
- Apply split sterile gauze dressing over external bumper once daily for first 5 days, then as needed
- Call physician for any excessive redness, drainage, or tube malfunction
- If tube was a PEG/JET: obtain KUB to confirm tube placement
  - Gastric port (options): attach to low intermittent suction, place to gravity drainage, keep plugged but may open and drain for N/V
  - Jejunal port (options): same as Gastric port

ANTICOAGULATION ISSUES: *See also Endoscopy & Procedures- Anticoagulation (Chapter 7.01)*
- Coumadin:
  - If patient has 'low risk condition' requiring anti-coagulation, then stop 3-5 days prior to procedure
  - If patient has high risk condition' requiring anti-coagulation, then stop coumadin 3-5 days prior to procedure; Heparin bridge in selected patients when INR is subtherapeutic utilizing either: LMWH at 1 mg/kg q 12 hours or unfractionated heparin gtt
- Unfractionated Heparin:
  - Discontinue heparin 4-6 hours prior to PEG; Restart post-procedure based on clinical judgment
- LMWH:
  - Discontinue LMWH at least 8 hours prior to procedure; Restart LMWH post-procedure based on clinical judgment
- Clopidogrel (Plavix):
  - Insufficient data, however, one should weigh the risk of an ischemic event (history of CVA, recent coronary stent) versus the patient's need for PEG; Consider stopping 7-10 days prior to procedure; Restart Plavix post-procedure based on clinical judgment
  - Patients on both ASA and Plavix may be at increased risk of bleeding; consider reverting to a single agent (preferably ASA)
- ASA/NSAID:
  - In the absence of pre-existing bleeding disorder, endoscopic procedures may be performed in those taking ASA/NSAIDs
- Dypyridamole (Persantine): may be continued

CARE OF PEG AFTER INSERTION (PATIENT INSTRUCTIONS):
- Site may be tender for several days; Take pain meds as prescribed; Avoid aspirin or non-steroidal medications (Advil, Motrin, etc)
- PEG tube should be clean, dry and non-tender (after initial few days)
- A healthy PEG tube site should not be sore or red
- To keep PEG site healthy, you should:
  - Carefully look at site daily
  - Wash exit site daily with mild soap and water, pat dry; You may use dressing, however this should not be necessary
  - The PEG should be freely movable in the tract; The outside bumper should be 0.5 - 1 cm from skin
  - PEG tubes can last up to a year if cared for properly
  - If the PEG tube becomes dislodged or falls out, notify your physician immediately

CARE OF PEG AFTER REMOVAL (PATIENT INSTRUCTIONS):
- Site should close rapidly, usually within 1-2 days
- Nothing to eat/drink for 4 hours after removal
- Keep site clean and dry (not unusual for the some drainage from site initially); change dressing if it becomes soiled (acid can irritate skin)
- Wash around the areas gently with soap and water and replace with dry dressing
- Avoid showering or tub baths for 1-2 days or until the site is completely healed
- If any questions or concerns, call physician

TUBE FEEDS:
- Standard tube feeds: 1 kcal/ml; Most are isotonic, and provide complete nutrition at intakes of 1,500-2,000 kcals
  - Typically they are lactose and gluten free and contain variable amounts of long/medium chain triglycerides and intact proteins

CHAPTER 1.20 PERCUTANEOUS ENDOSCOPIC GASTROSTOMY (PEG) TUBES

- Calorically-dense tube feeds: 1.5–2.0 kcal/ml
  - Most are hypertonic and don't provide enough water, so additional water needed to avoid dehydration
- Nutrition-dense tube feeds: provide extra amounts of protein or lipid; Many contain added special nutrients
- Disease specific tube feeds: designed for diabetes, pulmonary disease, renal disease, and hepatic disease
  - In general, no data supports the use of these very expensive formulas
- Diarrhea rarely results from the formula itself; can be minimized by using isotonic formula; May result from gut atrophy and will resolve
  - Check for medications containing: sorbitol, magnesium or hypertonic preparations such as potassium; Antibiotic use
- Obtain a nutrition consult if necessary

1.21 PEPTIC ULCER DISEASE (PUD): H. PYLORI, NSAIDs

(Lancet 2002;360:933-41. N Engl J Med 2002;347:1175-86. Am J Gastroenterol 1998;93:2037-46 & 2330-38)

DEFINITION:
- Ulcer: Mucosal break of the stomach or duodenum that penetrates the muscularis mucosae
- Erosion: a lesion that is superficial to the muscularis mucosae

EPIDEMIOLOGY:
- **Duodenal ulcer (DU):** ~300,000 cases per year
- **Gastric ulcer (GU):** ~75,000 cases per year
- Lifetime prevalence ~10% (Up to 60% of the world's population is estimated to harbor *H. Pylori* but only 15% will develop an ulcer)

ETIOLOGIES:
- ***H. Pylori*** **infection: (90% of DU** and 70% of GU); See epidemiology above regarding lifetime prevalence
  - *H. Pylori*: GNB with urease activity (basis for diagnostic testing): **hydrolyzes urea » ammonia (NH_3) & CO_2** (helps resist stomach acid)
  - Transmission thought to be fecal-oral or oral-oral and most infections acquired in childhood
  - Natural habitat is gastric mucosa of the antrum (gets protection from acid in the mucosa but it is not intracellular)
    - If found in duodenum, they are associated with metaplastic gastric epithelium
  - MOA: Suppresses epithelial cell immune response & generates autoantibodies which cross-react with G & D cells causing death/atrophy; This allows G cells to release gastrin without inhibition and leads to increased gastric acid secretion and ulcer formation

- **NSAIDs** (10% of DU and **15-30% of GU**, 0.1-4% UGIB) including aspirin; Up to 40% of patients may not report using these drugs
  - High-risk group requiring prevention (PPI, Misoprostol, H2As prevent GU only):
    - Age >60, Prior GI bleed, High dose NSAIDs (2× normal), Concurrent steroids, Concurrent anticoagulants
  - MOA #1: Inhibition of GI cyclooxygenase-1 (COX1), the enzyme responsible for GI prostaglandin synthesis (mucosal protectant)
    - Prostaglandins: ↑ bicarbonate and mucus secretion, ↑ mucosal blood flow, ↓ gastric secretion of H+
  - MOA #2: Most are weak acids; exposure to gastric acid = protonated and allow cross of lipid membrane entering epithelial cells
    - Once inside, it ionizes (releases H+) and gets trapped inside; also may decrease hydrophobicity of mucus gel layer
    - Result is rapid epithelial cell death, superficial hemorrhage and erosion

- Gastrinoma and other hypersecretory states such as Zollinger-Ellison Syndrome (consider if multiple recurrent ulcers) *See also Esophagus/Gastric- ZES (Chapter 1.23)*
- Malignancy (5-10% of gastric ulcers): adenocarcinoma or lymphoma
- Other: Crohn's, Eosinophilic gastritis, C1 esterase deficiency, Stress, Viral (CMV, HSV), Steroids (alone don't ↑ risk, with NSAID use ↑↑↑ risk)
- DDX of patients dyspepsia: GERD, PUD, NUD, biliary tract disease, pancreatitis, cancer; *See also Esophagus/Gastric- Dyspepsia (Chapter 1.04)*

PATHOPHYSIOLOGY:
- Although gastric acid needed for PUD formation, most do not develop even with higher than normal acid levels! (except conditions such as ZES)
  - Originally the thought was that 'Peptic Ulcer' developed by the principal components of gastric acid and pepsin exclusively
- Parietal cells produce acid, stimulated by, 1. Vagus/ACH, 2. Histamine, 3. G cell/Gastrin, 4. Proton pump *See also Esophagus/Gastric- Potpourri (Chapter 1.24)*
- Normal GI homeostasis: balance of defensive mechanisms (mucus, bicarb) and aggressive factors (*H. Pylori*, NSAIDs, acid, pepsin, smoking)
  - Insult: Exogenous (NSAIDs, Tobacco, ETOH), Endogenous (Bile), Acid & Pepsin
    - First-line defense: mucus and bicarbonate barrier
    - Second-line defense: epithelial cell mechanisms (intrinsic cell defense, extrusion of acid)
    - Third-line defense: blood-flow mediated (supply energy and removal of back-diffused H+)

CHAPTER 1.21 PEPTIC ULCER DISEASE (PUD): *H. PYLORI*, NSAIDs

- Failure of defenses = Epithelial Cell Injury
  - First-line repair: restitution
  - Second-line repair: cell replication
- Failure of repair = Acute Wound Formation
  - Third-line repair: wound healing (formation of granulation tissue, angiogenesis, remodeling of basement membrane)
- Failure of continued repair = Ulcer!

CLINICAL MANIFESTATIONS/PHYSICAL EXAM:
- Epigastric abdominal pain, **relieved with food** (duodenal) or **worsened by food** (gastric)
  - Nausea, perception of abdominal pressure/fullness or hunger sensation
- Perforated ulcer: rigid, board-like abdomen with generalized rebound tenderness
- Obstruction: nausea, vomiting, early satiety, succession splash (via retained fluid and air within distended stomach)

LABORATORY STUDIES:
- See diagnostic studies below

DIAGNOSTIC STUDIES:
- Detecting PUD: EGD more sensitive (>95%) than UGI series
  - Biopsy GU with a minimum of 8 biopsies to rule out gastric carcinoma (always!)

- Test for *H. Pylori*: Invasive (EGD with biopsy: antrum × 2, fundus × 2 & angularis × 1):
  - **Rapid urease/CLO** (sensitive and specific >95%); + *H. Pylori* infection » NH_3/CO_2 » basic pH via NH_3 & color change
    - Positive only with infections; False negatives with recent antibiotic use, bismuth-containing compounds, PPI/H2RA
  - **Biopsy/Histology** (sensitive and specific >95%); biopsy and use of hematoxylin and eosin (H&E) stain to view organism
    - Absence of chronic gastritis is good evidence of the absence of *H. Pylori*
  - **Biopsy/Culture** (highly specific only) Difficult, not clinically useful; Reserved for antibiotic sensitivities to resistant organisms

- Test for *H. Pylori*: Non-Invasive:
  - **Serology** IgG/IgA antibodies via ELISA test (90% sensitive, 70-80% specific, *not* useful in confirming eradication)
    - Titers can ↓ 3-6 months after effective treatment, or remain elevated for up to 3 years: "serologic scar"
    - Positive test doesn't always mean an ulcer is present as one can be infected with *H. Pylori* but not have an ulcer
  - **Urea Breath** Test (UBT, sensitive and specific >95%): ideal for 1° diagnosis, monitor therapy, assess re-infection 4wks after treatment
    Ingest labeled C02 » hydrolyze urea to NH_3/CO_2 » CO_2 absorbed and exhaled » labeled CO_2 collected in blood or breath
    - Positive only with infections; False negatives with recent antibiotic use, bismuth-containing compounds, PPI/H2RA
  - **Stool antigen** (HpSA, 94% sensitive, 86-92% specific; based on PCR); Useful in 1° diagnosis or confirming eradication

  - Interference with testing (causing false negatives, especially CLO test): Antibiotics, PPI, Bismuth (can suppress *H. Pylori*)
  - Ideal testing: stop antibiotics 4 weeks prior and/or PPI 2 weeks prior
  - Follow-up testing after treatment (UBT, stool antigen or endoscopy): not generally required, but advised if patient had ulcer complication

SECTION I ESOPHAGUS/GASTRIC

TREATMENTS:
- **_H. Pylori_ Eradication:** **P**PI bid & **C**larithromycin 500 mg bid & **A**moxicillin 1 g bid; **(PCA)**; All three meds × 10-14 days (>90% success rate)
  Metronidazole 500 mg bid (↑ dose to overcome resistance) can be substituted for amoxicillin in patients with penicillin allergy (PCM)
    - Document eradication after therapy with UBT or HpSA (especially in those who would not tolerate recurrence of complications such as an ulcer); Continue PPI afterwards
    - Recurrence rate after therapy with antibiotics is low: 2-10% per year (as apposed to >90% if not treated with antibiotics)
    - If _H. Pylori_ negative, treat with PPI only; Routine antibiotic therapy in ulcer patient without evidence of _H. Pylori_ is not warranted
    - Some follow up treatment with a breath test to confirm eradication (especially with recurrent symptoms)
- **Discontinue NSAIDs**
    - Prevention:
        - Identify those at high risk: history of PUD/bleeding ulcer, Concomitant steroid or anticoagulant use, Older age, Tobacco
        - H2RA. generally does not help (Famotidine at high doses, 40BID, may help)
        - Misoprostol: synthetic prostaglandin stimulating mucus/bicarbonate; may reduce ulcer formation (caution: pregnancy)
        - PPI: studies support more efficacy than H2RA and Misoprostol
        - Change to CO X 2 - before pulled from market - (~80 ↓ in PUD, ~50% ↓ in UGIB)
    - Treatment: if must continue, adding a PPI will allow ulcer healing even while NSAID use continues
- Treat with anti-secretory therapy: 8 wks for DU, 4-8 wks for GU
    - H2RA: safe and can heal 90% of ulcers at 8 weeks; can be given as single nocturnal dose rather than BID (same total daily dose); Many side effects
        - Cimetidine has most side effects: gynecomastia, impotence, binds P450, CNS (dizzy, headache); Caution with elderly
    - Sucralfate: promotes angiogenesis, best at binding ulcers at low pH so given 30-60 min before meals
        - Aluminum based, caution with renal failure as 3% is absorbed
    - Misoprostol: synthetic prostaglandin stimulating mucus/bicarbonate; may ↓ ulcer formation; primary role is prevention as above
        - However causes significant diarrhea; Prostaglandins are uterotropic and induce bleeding - never use with pregnancy!
    - PPI: Work by an irreversible complex to H+/K+ ATPase pump, which is the final step in acid production; To produce acid, parietal cells must form new pumps which can take many hours; Therefore never administer on 'as needed' basis
        - Give 30 min before meals (i.e. pumps need to be working to inactivate); Takes 3-5 days to reach steady state acid inhibition; No need to lower dose with renal insufficiency (primary liver metabolism)
    - Antacids: heal ulcers by binding bile and inhibiting pepsin; promote angiogenesis in injured mucosa
        - However, at least seven 30 cc doses daily are needed to heal ulcers! And can cause several side effects
        - Magnesium-containing agents (diarrhea), Aluminum-containing agents (constipation), Calcium-containing (acid rebound)
- Lifestyle changes: discontinue smoking (a must) and ? ETOH, diet is irrelevant contrary to old beliefs (may cause dyspepsia, but not PUD)
- Endoscopy: acutely to control UGIB, to document resolution of GU after 8-12 weeks of therapy
- Surgery: usually reserved for rare cases refractory to medical therapy (rule out surreptitious NSAID use) or for complications as below

CHAPTER 1.21 PEPTIC ULCER DISEASE (PUD): *H. PYLORI*, NSAIDs

COMPLICATIONS:
- Complications include UGIB (15-20%), perforation & penetration (6-7%), gastric outlet obstruction
- PUD-related GIB; *See also GI Bleed- UGIB & LGIB (Chapter 6.04)*
- Patients with *H. Pylori* have 3-6 fold higher incidence of gastric CA; In 1994, the WHO classified *H. Pylori* as a group I carcinogen
  - Strong association with Mucosal Associated Lymphoid Tumors (MALT); Treatment of *H. Pylori* results in regression or cure in 90% of patients; *See also Esophagus/Gastric- Gastric Cancer (Chapter 1.10)*

PROGNOSIS:
- **Repeat EGD:** 10-12 weeks to confirm healing of GU (malignancy can be easily missed, even with biopsy)
- Reoccurrence of *H. Pylori* after proper therapy is 4-6% per year for gastric and duodenal ulcers, respectively; Some suggest as high as 20%
- Treatment of *H. Pylori* (if positive) will not likely reduce the symptoms of NUD: 20% of patients at most

1.22 SCHATZKI'S RING/ESOPHAGEAL SPASM

(Gastroenterology 1999;117:229-32 & 233-54)

SCHATZKI'S RING

Definition:
- Three types of rings:
  - A: muscular in origin, occurs about 2 cm proximal to GEJ
  - B (Schatzki's): mucosal in origin, occurs at the squamocolumnar junction
  - C: nonpathologic anomaly caused by diaphragmatic indentation of the esophagus, rarely symptomatic

Etiologies:
- Cause of A & B rings: unknown; May be associated with esophageal dysmotility; B rings may be reflux related

Clinical Manifestations/Physical Exam:
- Patients usually describe intermittent solid-food dysphagia induced by hurrying a meal or anxiety
- May present initially with foreign body impaction

Diagnostic Studies:
- EGD

Treatments:
- Esophageal dilation; Repeat treatment may be necessary over time
  Dilation (selection based on stricture configuration, comfort of endoscopist, availability of equipment)
    Rule of 3's: dilate a total of three times in one session (first dilation is the one with mild resistance)
    End point is a lumen diameter of >14 mm, followed by control of reflux (PPI) if any
  - Mercury-filled tapered bougies (Maloney): axial shearing and radial forces; best for simple symmetric strictures <10 mm
  - Guidewire placed tapered polyvinyl dilators (Savary): axial shearing and radial forces; best for <10 mm, long, tortuous, post-op strictures
  - Through-the-scope balloons (TTS): only radial force; best for <10 mm, long, tortuous, post-op strictures
  Note: French sizes are circumferences sizes, divided by 3 they give the diameter in mm; So 30 Fr is 10 mm in diameter

ESOPHAGEAL SPASMS

Definition:
- Esophageal motility disorder: a motility that differs significantly from accepted normal variations

Epidemiology: (See Chapter 1.17 for details on Manometry)
- Primary Esophageal Motility Abnormalities:

Achalasia (a true disorder)	Absent distal peristalsis; Incomplete LES relaxation (residual >8 mmHg); High resting LES (>45 mmHg)
Diffuse Eso Spasm (DES)	Simultaneous contractions (>20% wet swallows); Some peristalsis; Repetitive (>3) & prolonged (>6 sec) contractions
Hypertensive peristalsis	"Nutcracker": ↑ mid/distal peristaltic amplitude (total >180 mmHg); ↑ distal peristaltic duration (>6 sec) contractions
Isolated Hypertensive LES	High-resting LES (>45 mmHg); May be incomplete relaxation (residual pressure >8 mmHg)

- Secondary Esophageal Motility Abnormalities:

Systemic Scleroderma	Loss of distal smooth muscle peristalsis (proximal is spared); Weak LES (<10 mmHg); Normal striated UES
Chagas' disease	Identical to Achalasia
Diabetes Mellitus	A variety of motility abnormalities in esophageal body
Chronic GERD	Ineffective motility; Hypotensive lower esophageal sphincter

CHAPTER 1.22 SCHATZKI'S RING/ESOPHAGEAL SPASM

Pathophysiology:
- DES: May be related to malfunction in endogenous nitric oxide synthesis and/or degradation

Clinical Manifestations/Physical Exam:
- In general: heartburn, chest pain, dysphagia
- Achalasia: *See also Esophagus/Gastric- Achalasia (Chapter 1.01)*
- DES: relatively rare disease; Approximately 3-10% of patients with unexplained chest pains or dysphagia have DES
  - Unclear if results from imbalance of inhibitory and excitatory motor innervations; Approximately 3-5% progress to achalasia

Laboratory Studies:
- Often not helpful

Diagnostic Studies:
- DES:
  - Barium Swallow: broad spectrum of severe tertiary contractions with descriptions such as: 'rosary bead' or 'corkscrew'
    - However, may be entirely normal, hence minimal specificity or sensitivity
  - Manometry findings correlate poorly with symptoms
- Manometry (with ten 5 cc liquid swallows): For complete Manometry findings, *See Chapter 1.17*

Treatments: (Except Achalasia: See Chapter 1.01)
- Supported by clinical trials: Calcium-channel blockers, Antidepressants (trazodone, imipramine)
- Positive anecdotal results: Nitrates (nitroglycerin, isosorbide dinitrate), Anticholinergic drugs (dicyclomine), Bougie dilation, Botulinum injection
- Minimal clinical support: Pneumatic dilation, Esophagectomy
- Primary symptom chest pain: CCB (diltiazem 180-240 mg/day TID or QID dosage) or TCA (imipramine 25-50 mg/hs, amitriptyline 10 mg/hs)
  - Reserve botulinum toxin (injected into LES then in a line every 1 cm proximally to create a 'medical myotomy') or nitrate (isosorbide 10 mg or sildenafil 50 mg prn basis) for nonresponders
- Primary symptom dysphagia: May consider CCB

1.23 ZOLLINGER-ELLISON SYNDROME (GASTRINOMA)

DEFINITION:
- A syndrome characterized by ulceration of the upper jejunum, hypersecretion of gastric acid, and non-beta islet cell tumors of the pancreas
- Unlike typical peptic ulcer disease, this syndrome is often progressive, persistent, and frequently life-threatening; *See also Bowel- GI Endocrine Tumors (Chapter 2.16)*

EPIDEMIOLOGY:
- Most between 30–50 y/o; Male > Female
- U.S. incidence is ~0.1–1% of all patients with duodenal ulcer (PUD)
  - May be an underestimate since symptoms similar to NSAID and *H. Pylori* disease and symptoms controlled with antisecretory drugs

ETIOLOGIES:
- Gastrin has been identified as the humoral agent responsible for the syndrome
  - Gastrin may be the link between the increased risk of carcinoids with ZES and Chronic Type A Gastritis
- Acid hypersecretion is defined as basal acid output of gastrin >10 mmol/hr

PATHOPHYSIOLOGY:
- Caused by a gastrinoma, a benign or malignant tumor of gastrin-secreting G cells
  - Located: pancreas 60-80% (non-beta islet cell tumor) or duodenum 25-35% (G-cell hyperplasia - over functioning of gastric G cells)
  - Derived from pluripotent endocrine cells; Tumors are well-differentiated
- May be sporadic or associated with MEN-1
  - 75% occur as a sporadic syndrome, occurring as an isolated condition
  - 25% association with multiple endocrine neoplasia type 1 (MEN-1): Parathyroid, Pituitary, Pancreas (ZES); Autosomal dominant

CLINICAL MANIFESTATIONS/PHYSICAL EXAM:
- Gastrin in excess stimulates high gastric acid output (See Normal physiology below under Secretin Stimulation test)
- **Severe or refractory ulcers** are mostly less than 1 cm and highest portion are in the first part (bulb) of duodenum
- Diarrhea is also prominent feature;
  - Excess acid exceeds neutralizing ability of pancreatic bicarb; Interferes with emulsification of fats and leads to a malabsorption steatorrhea
- Gastrinoma is metastatic to the liver and bone in one-third of patients
- Suspect in multiple refractory ulcers, diarrhea, history of MEN in family; *H. Pylori* is usually negative

LABORATORY STUDIES:
- Although many tests have been described, only fasting serum gastrin concentration and Secretin stimulation test are used routinely
- <u>Serum Gastrin Concentration:</u> should be drawn in a fasting state and without any antisecretory medication (see Notes below under Secretin Stimulation test)
  - A serum gastrin value greater than 1000 pg/ml is virtually diagnostic; It is almost always >150 pg/ml

CHAPTER 1.23 ZOLLINGER-ELLISON SYNDROME (GASTRINOMA)

- Secretin Stimulation Test:
  Normal physiology: G cells, located in antrum, secrete Gastrin; Parietal cell, located in fundus, secrete gastric acid (HCL)/intrinsic factor
  - Food/Antacids » alkaline environment » stimulate G cells/Gastrin » stimulate Parietal cells/gastric acid » negative feedback of gastric acid suppresses G cells
  - Secretin stimulates the release of gastrin by G cells and eventual acid production via Parietal cells; Should get feedback shutoff
    -Secretin is administered at 2 mcg/kg IV over 30 seconds to the fasting patient
    -Serum gastrin levels are measured at baseline, 2, 5, 10, 15, 20 minutes
    -A (paradoxical) rise in serum gastrin by 200 pg/ml or more is considered positive test; More than 90% sensitive and specific
    -A peak in serum gastrin level is usually seen by 10 minutes
  - Notes:
    -PUD surgery creates persistent alkaline environment, which stimulates gastrin
    -PPIs should be stopped at least five days prior to test and patient placed on H2 R' antagonist, which should be discontinued 24 hours prior to testing (again, producing a false alkaline environment and producing excessive gastrin)
    -Gastrin is metabolized by kidney and may be falsely high in renal failure
    -Atrophic Gastritis (Type A, Pernicious anemia) also produce the alkaline environment and stimulate gastrin secretion
  - **Antral G-Cell Hyperplasia:** results of test are opposite (gastrin is decreased, not changed or very slightly increased but <200 pg/ml)
    - Condition described in cluster of patients who have family history of PUD and hyperplasia of antral G cells = ↑ basal gastrin/acid levels
  - **Retained Antrum Syndrome:** rare form of hypergastrin in those with Billroth II; Secretin stimulation test is negative
    - Small cuff of antrum remains and is excluded from gastric acid, G cells release gastrin without the negative feedback

- Serum Chromogranin A:
  - A general marker for neuroendocrine tumors that does not differentiate various subtypes of tumors; Although less sensitive and specific, it may be used as a confirmatory test in difficult cases

- Calcium Infusion Study:
  - Considerably less sensitive and specific than Secretin stimulation test; Used in the rare patient when there is a strong clinical suspicion despite negative Secretin test; The test is performed by infusing calcium gluconate (5 mg/kg body weight per hour over three hours) and determining serum gastrin levels every 30 minutes for 4 hours; A gastrin level of more than 400 pg/ml is positive

DIAGNOSTIC STUDIES:
- EGD: Since gastrin is a trophic hormone, there is hyperplasia of mucosa in fundus/corpus (presenting as large gastric folds)
  - 90% develop ulcers usually in the duodenal bulb; A gastric ulcer is very rarely, if ever, seen in ZES
- Need to localize the tumor (most » less sensitive): **Octreotide scanning** (gastrinomas express somatostatin receptors), EUS, CT, MRI

TREATMENTS:
- Prior to PPIs, morbidity and mortality was associated with fulminant PUD and total gastrectomy was the only effective treatment
- Medical:
  - PPIs are the treatment of choice; Vagotomy is generally unnecessary in patients treated with PPI
- Surgical: Cure is only 5–40%
  - Patients should be offered a exploratory laparotomy with curative intent for ZES; Recommendation is based on eliminating or decreasing the need for antisecretory medical therapy and help protect against possibility of metastasis of gastrinoma tumor

1.24 POTPOURRI

GASTRIC PHYSIOLOGY (ACID SECRETION)
- Gastric juice is a combination of parietal (acid) and non-parietal secretions
  - Parietal cell, located in fundus, secrete gastric acid (HCL) and intrinsic factor (IF)
    - Stimulant receptors: Gastrin, Histamine [via enterochromaffin-like (ECL) cells], muscarinic receptors (acetylcholine)
      - Gastrin (see below) = ↑ gastric acid
      - H2R antagonists inhibit gastric acid secretion by blocking receptors = ↓ gastric acid
      - Acetylcholine via Vagus nerve act on receptor and inhibit somatostatin = ↑ gastric acid
    - Inhibitor receptors: somatostatin (via D cells) and prostaglandins
      - Prostaglandin E analogs (Misoprostol) = ↓ gastric acid production; Blockers of prostaglandins (NSAIDs) = ↑ gastric acid
    - Proton Pump: H+ ions (acid) secreted into gastric lumen in exchange for K+; PPIs work to halt this pump
  - Non-parietal cells secrete water, electrolytes and mucus
  - The volume/acidity of gastric juice produced at any time: determined by relative proportions of parietal and non-parietal secretions
- G cells, located in antrum, secrete Gastrin
  - MOA: Food (especially amino acids)/PPIs/Antacids » alkaline environment » stimulate G cells/ Gastrin » stimulate Parietal cells/gastric acid » negative feedback of gastric acid suppresses G cells
- Chief cells, located in body of stomach, secrete pepsinogen
  - Pepsinogen is converted to Pepsin in gastric lumen via gastric acid
  - In early years pepsin digest milk
  - In later life pepsin's major substrate is meat and other proteins; Amino acids from breakdown stimulate gastrin release
- Mucosal Defense Factors (Bicarbonate, Mucus, Blood flow, Prostaglandins)
  - Due to exposure to high concentrations of HCL, gastroduodenal epithelial cells would appear to be at risk for auto-digestion
  - Barrier: Surface epithelial cells secrete mucus and bicarbonate which comprises a thin alkaline protective layer
    - Barrier is so effective that the luminal pH can be 2 and the barrier pH can be 7
  - Problems occur when: Bicarb secretion suppressed; Excessive proteolysis of mucus (inflammation); Blood flow/Prostaglandin decreased
    - Prostaglandin protection: secretes mucus, stimulation of bicarb, maintenance of blood flow during injury; ↓ via NSAIDs

HICCUPS
- Spasmodic, involuntary contractions of inspiratory muscles (not just diaphragm) with simultaneous closure of the glottis (responsible for sound)
- Usually short-lived, typically after meals and subside without treatment or with simple measures such as breath-holding, water ingestion
  - Lasting longer than 48 hours or recurring episodes of protracted hiccups is defined as *chronic* (can be disabling with fatigue, diet)
- Afferent limb of the hiccups can involve vagus, phrenic and sympathetics (T6–12): hence a wide variety of intraabdominal and intrathoracic disorders have been associated with hiccups
- CNS and metabolic disorders (diabetes, renal failure) can cause chronic hiccups
- Hiccups can cause physiologic changes (such as lowered LES) and lead to reflux esophagitis
- Workup:
  - Fluoroscopy of diaphragm should be performed:
    - Unilateral involvement (usually left) then focus on course of the phrenic nerve of affected side
    - Bilateral involvement suggests an afferent or central origin
  - Labs: CBC, CMP; Abdominal X-ray (Rule out mechanical obstruction); Endoscopy (Rule out PUD, gastric cancer, infiltrating disease); CXR
  - If negative, consider CT abdomen and MRI of brain
- Therapy: Best treatment is directed toward the cause; However many times evaluation is negative and therapy directed at hiccups themselves
  - Simple maneuvers: breath-holding, swallowing water, Valsalva maneuvers, rebreathing into a bag (These rarely work for protracted hiccups)

- Stopping an episode of hiccups: trial of firm digital stimulation of the posterior pharynx (or placement of Ng tube)
- Baclofen (derivative of gamma-aminobutyric acid used as antispasticity agent in patients with tics or dystonias)
    * 5 mg TID and increased in stepwise fashion to a maximum dose of 20 mg TID (Side effects: somnolence, fatigue)
    * Must taper the medication at cessation of use
- Nefopam (10 mg IV) may be beneficial in postoperative patients

LICHEN PLANUS
- Idiopathic inflammatory disease of the skin and mucosa; involves: conjunctivia, pharynx, esophagus, stomach, rectum, bladder, vagina
- Classic cutaneous lesions: violaceous flat-tipped papules, predilection for extremities; Oral lesions may be present with no skin involvement
    * Most commonly on tongue and buccal mucosa; white streaks on violaceous background
- Esophageal Lichen Planus: rare; ♀ age 50's; Typical symptoms: dysphagia and odynophagia; reflux symptoms are uncommon
    * EGD: entire esophagus can be involved; desquamation/sloughing of mucosa with minimal trauma
    * Possible strictures, rings, webs at multiple levels
- DDX: Bullous disease (Epidermolysis bullosa, Cicatricial pemphigoid), Pill-induced, Other orogenitocutaneous (Behçet's, Steven-Johnson)
    * Fungal/Viral infections (Candida, HSV, CMV), Graft vs. Host (in transplant patients), Reflux esophagitis
- Diagnosis: history, clinical findings, biopsies with direct immunofluorescence:
    * Lichen planus: subepidermal IgM deposits; Pemphigoid: linear basement membrane IgA, IgG & C3
    * Civatte bodies (necrotic keratinocytes with anucleated remnants)
- Therapy: No established specific therapy; Systemic steroids (40–60 mg, taper 4–6 wks); Others: cyclosporine, dapsone, Imuran, FK506
    * Dilation for strictures, balloon vs. bougie: no data; Concern for Koebner phenomenon (precipitation of lesion by irritation)

EATING DISORDERS (lifetime prevalence 1% in women)
- Successful treatment requires: 1. early suspicion; 2. evaluation for complications; 3. exclusion of GI (e.g. achalasia, Crohn's) or systemic (e.g. AIDS) disorder; 4. prompt referral to a clinician experienced in treating eating disorders
- **Anorexia** DSM-IV: 1. Refusal to maintain body weight at a minimally normal weight for age/height; 2. Intense fear of gaining weight or becoming fat; 3. Disturbance in the way in which body weight or shape is experienced or denial of the seriousness of the current low body weight; 4. In postmenarcheal women, amenorrhea (i.e. absence of at least three consecutive menstrual cycles)
- **Bulimia** DSM-IV: 1. Recurrent episodes of binge eating, characterized by both eating larger meals than most people would eat during a similar period and sense of lack of control over eating during the episode; 2. Recurrent inappropriate compensatory behavior to prevent weight gain, such as self-induced vomiting, misuse of laxatives, diuretics, enemas, or other medication; fasting; or excessive exercise; 3. Binge eating and compensatory behaviors both occur, on average, at least twice a week for 3 months; 4. Body shape and weight unduly influence self-evaluation; 5. The disturbance does not occur exclusively during episodes of anorexia nervosa (Typically Bulimia patients have less body-image distortion and are more accepting of therapy)

BEZOARS
- Most common foreign bodies of the GI tract
    * Phytobezoars are much more common than Trichobezoars
- Phytobezoars: concentrations of plant and vegetable matter
    * Seen with gastric stasis, or elderly
    * Treated with enzymes, endoscopic dissolution, surgery
- Trichobezoars: contain human, animal or artificial hair; frequently mixed with vegetable matter
    * Psychological disturbance or eating disorders play a role
    * Treated with acetylcysteine (Mucomyst) mixed with cola: 140 mg/kg, then 70 mg/kq every 6 hours × 3 days; Surgery

II

SMALL BOWEL/COLON/RECTUM

2.01 ABDOMINAL PAIN: GENERAL

DEFINITION:
- No clear definitions of acute vs. chronic abdominal pain
  - Pain less than a few days that has worsened progressively until time of presentation is 'acute'
    - Characterized by severe pain, often rapid onset, that prevents bodily movement; surgical intervention may be necessary
  - Pain that has remained unchanged for months or years can be safely classified as 'chronic'
  - Pain that does not clearly fit either category may be called 'subacute' and requires consideration of differential for both acute/chronic

ETIOLOGIES:
- Most gut (visceral) nociceptors are sensitive to stretch: distention of hollow viscus (i.e. obstruction), muscular contractions (i.e. biliary/renal colic), stretching of solid organ serosa or capsule (i.e. hepatic congestion), torsion of mesentery (i.e. cecal volvulus), tension from traction of the mesentery (i.e. retroperitoneal or pancreatic tumors)

Abdominal pain may be classified into three categories: Visceral, Somatoparietal, Referred
- **Visceral pain:** occurs when noxious stimuli affect the abdominal viscus
  - Usually dull (cramping, gnawing, burning) and poorly localized to the ventral midline due to innervation being multisegmental
  - Secondary autonomic effects such as diaphoresis, restlessness, nausea, vomiting, and pallor are common
- **Somatoparietal pain:** occurs when noxious stimuli irritate the parietal peritoneum
  - Usually more intense and more precisely localized on the side of the lesion (i.e. McBurney's point inflaming the parietal peritoneum)
  - Pain is likely to be aggravated by coughing or movement
- **Referred pain:** experienced in areas remote from the site of injury
  - The remote pain site is supplied by the same neurosegment as the involved organ
  - Examples include gallbladder pain referred to right scapula, pancreatic pain referred and radiates to the mid back
    - Thoracic: pneumonia, pulmonary embolism, pneumothorax, MI, esophageal spasm or perforation
    - Neurogenic: tabes dorsalis, radicular pain (cord compression from tumor, abscess, varicella zoster)
    - Metabolic: uremia, porphyria, acute adrenal insufficiency
    - Toxins: insect bites (scorpion bite-induced pancreatitis), lead poisoning

- Common causes of acute abdominal pain in **gravid women**
  - Appendicitis, cholecystitis, pyelonephritis, ovarian cysts complicated by torsion/rupture, ectopic pregnancy
  - If suspected appendicitis proves to be a normal appendix during laparotomy, removal triples the risk of fetal loss

- Common cause of acute abdominal pain in **elderly**
  - Biliary tract disease responsible ~25% of cases; Followed by malignancy, bowel obstruction, PUD, incarcerated hernia, appendicitis

- Common cause of acute abdominal pain in **Immunocompromised/HIV**
  - All non-HIV specific diagnoses (appendicitis, cholecystitis, etc)
  - CMV leads to mucosal ischemic ulceration and perforation; HIV-associated lymphoma & Kaposi's can lead to perforation
  - AIDS cholangiopathy, papillitis, drug-induced pancreatitis (i.e. pentamidine, bactrim, didanosine, ritonavir), GVHD

- Common cause of acute abdominal pain in **SLE**
  - Lupus vasculitis ~2% of patients; Small vessels of bowel are affected leading to ulceration, perforation, infarction; Mortality >50%

CHAPTER 2.01   ABDOMINAL PAIN: GENERAL

PATHOPHYSIOLOGY:
- Types of stimuli for abdominal pain:
  - Stretching or tension
  - Inflammation
  - Ischemia
  - Neoplasms
- Classification of pain by rate of development:
  - Explosive/Excruciating (instantaneous): MI, Perforated ulcer, Ruptured aneurysm, Biliary or renal colic (passage of stone)
  - Rapid/Severe & Constant (over minutes): Acute pancreatitis, Complete bowel obstruction, Mesenteric thrombus
  - Gradual and steady (over hours): Acute cholecystitis, Diverticulitis, Acute appendicitis
  - Intermittent & Colicky (over hours): Early subacute pancreatitis, Mechanical small bowel obstruction

CLINICAL MANIFESTATIONS/PHYSICAL EXAM:
- General: Hemodynamically stable? (i.e. is there a need for resuscitation or emergent laparotomy?)
- Questions to ask: PQRST (provokes, quality, radiation, severity, time course), Alleviating/Aggravating factors, Fever/Chills, Nausea/Vomiting, Weight change
- Inspection: visually evaluate for distension, hernias, scars, hyperperistalsis
- Auscultation: Hyperperistalsis suggest obstruction, absence of bowel sounds >3 min suggest peritonitis, bruits suggest aneurysm
- Palpation: start away from the area of tenderness; Pain out of proportion suggest ischemia or infarction
- Rectal and Pelvic exam: should be done on all patients
- Iliopsoas test: pain elicited when legs fully extended in supine position suggest inflamed psoas muscle (i.e. appendicitis, psoas abscess)
- Obturator test: flexed hip at right angles to the trunk and rotating leg externally, suggest inflammation (i.e. tuboovarian abscess)

LABORATORY STUDIES:
- CBC (WBC for inflammation, H/H for blood loss, MCV for iron deficiency anemia or chronic GI blood loss or malabsorption)
- Amylase/Lipase
- LFTs
- U/A (UTI, nephrolithiasis)
- Pregnancy test
- EKG (all patients with possible myocardial infarction or >50 years of age)

DIAGNOSTIC STUDIES:
- Plain Films: quick, readily available; Reliable for bowel obstruction, viscus perforation
- Ultrasound: quick, noninvasive; Can be prone to operator expertise, obesity, gaseous abdomen
- CT: provides a detailed view of the anatomy; Always do in HIV or immunocompromised patient

TREATMENTS:
- See corresponding chapters on each condition and ***Bowel- Abdominal Pain: Acute and Chronic (Chapter 2.02 & 2.03)***

2.02 ABDOMINAL PAIN: ACUTE

DEFINITION:
- Pain less than a few days that has worsened progressively until time of presentation is 'acute'
  - Characterized by severe pain, often rapid onset, that prevents bodily movement; surgical intervention may be necessary
- Goal: early, efficient and accurate diagnosis; History and physical is key!

ETIOLOGIES:
- See also corresponding chapters on each condition:

Condition	Onset	Location	Character	Descriptor	Radiation	Intensity
Appendicitis	Gradual	Periumbilical » RLQ	Diffuse » localized	Ache	RLQ	++
Cholecystitis	Rapid	RUQ	Localized	Constricting	Scapula	++
Pancreatitis	Rapid	Epigastric/Back	Localized	Boring	Midback	++ to +++
Diverticulitis	Gradual	LLQ	Localized	Ache	None	+ to ++
Perfed PUD	Sudden	Epigastric	Localized » diffuse	Burning	None	+++
SB Obstruction	Gradual	Periumbilical	Diffuse	Crampy	None	++
Mes Ischemia	Sudden	Periumbilical	Diffuse	Agonizing	None	+++
Ruptured AA	Sudden	Abdominal/Back	Diffuse	Tearing	Back/Flank	+++
Gastroenteritis	Gradual	Periumbilical	Diffuse	Spasmodic	None	+ to ++
PID	Gradual	LLQ/RLQ, Pelvic	Localized	Ache	Upper thigh	++
Ruptured Ectopic	Sudden	LLQ/RLQ, Pelvic	Localized	Light-headed	None	++

Reprinted with permission from Glasgow RE, Mulvihill SJ. *Abdominal pain, including the acute abdomen.* In: Feldman M, Friedman LS, Sleisenger MH, Eds. *Sleisenger & Fordtran's Gastrointestinal and Liver Disease: Pathophysiology/Diagnosis/Management* 7th ed. Saunders. 2002:74.

- Extra-abdominal causes of acute abdominal pain:

Cardiac	Metabolic	Thoracic	Hematologic	Infections/Toxic	Neurologic	Miscellaneous
MI	Uremia	Pneumonitis	Sickle Cell	Herpes zoster	Radiculitis:	Muscular:
Myocarditis	DM	PE/Infarction	Hemolytic anemia	Osteomyelitis	-spinal tumors	-contusions
Endocarditis	Porphyria	Pneumothorax	Henoch-schonlein	Typhoid fever	-peripheral nerve	-hematoma
CHF	Addison's	Empyema	Acute Leukemia	Lead poisoning	-DJD of spine	-tumor
	Hyperthyroid	Esophagitis		Insect bites	Tabes dorsalis	Narcotic withdrawal
	Hyperlipidemia	Esoph Spasm		Reptile venoms		Familial Med Fever
		Boerhaave's		Hypersensitivity reactions		Psychiatric disorder

Reprinted with permission from Glasgow RE, Mulvihill SJ. *Abdominal pain, including the acute abdomen.* In: Feldman M, Friedman LS, Sleisenger MH, Eds. *Sleisenger & Fordtran's Gastrointestinal and Liver Disease: Pathophysiology/Diagnosis/Management* 7th ed. Saunders. 2002:79.

CLINICAL MANIFESTATIONS/PHYSICAL EXAM:
- Questions to ask: PQRST (Provokes, Quality, Radiation, Severity, Time course), Alleviating/Aggravating factors
- Associated symptoms: Fever/Chills, Nausea/Vomiting/Anorexia, Diarrhea/Constipation, Dysuria, Weight change, Menstruation/Pregnancy
- Past Medical History, Family History, Social History
- See Physical Exam in *Bowel- Abdominal Pain: General (Chapter 2.01)*

LABORATORY STUDIES:
- Should reflect clinical suspicion: CBC/Diff, CMP, Urinalysis, HCG, LFT/Amylase, PT/PTT (with suspected liver disease)

DIAGNOSTIC STUDIES:
- Radiographs: should reflect clinical suspicion: only 10% of abdominal radiographs reveal findings, nevertheless it is available and inexpensive and should be sought
  - Acute Abdominal Series: two views of abdomen: one supine, one upright or lateral decubitus, CXR
  - Ultrasound: imaging liver, biliary tree, spleen, pancreas, kidneys, pelvic organs
  - CT: most versatile imaging tool in evaluation of acute abdominal pain
  - MRI angiography: less invasive
  - Endoscopy
  - Diagnostic laparoscopy

TREATMENTS:
- See corresponding chapters on each condition

2.03 ABDOMINAL PAIN: CHRONIC

DEFINITION:
- Pain that has remained unchanged for months or years can be safely classified as 'chronic'
  - Divided into diagnosable (intermittent or constant) and undiagnosable
- Chronic undiagnosed abdominal pain: pain that is present for at least 6 months without diagnosis despite appropriate evaluation
  - ♀ > ♂, A history of sexual or physical abuse is common; Pain is described in vague peculiar terms; Multiple somatic complaints
- Diagnosable pain: see below

ETIOLOGIES:
- See also corresponding chapters on each condition:

Chronic Intermittent Pain:
Mechanical.
Intermittent intestinal obstruction (hernia, intussusception, adhesions, volvulus), Gallstones, Ampullary stenosis

Inflammatory:
IBD, Endometriosis/Endometritis, Acute relapsing pancreatitis, Familial Mediterranean Fever

Neurologic and Metabolic
Porphyria, Abdominal epilepsy, Diabetic radiculopathy, Nerve root compression or entrapment, Uremia

Miscellaneous:
IBS, Nonulcer dyspepsia, Chronic mesenteric ischemia, Mittelschmerz

Chronic Constant Pain:
Malignancy (primary or metastatic): gastric, pancreatic, bowel
Abscess
Chronic Pancreatitis
Psychiatric (depression, somatoform disorder)
Inexplicable (chronic intractable abdominal pain)

CLINICAL MANIFESTATIONS/PHYSICAL EXAM:
- Questions to ask: PQRST (provokes, quality, radiation, severity, time course), Alleviating/Aggravating factors
- Associated symptoms: Fever/Chills, Nausea/Vomiting/Anorexia, Diarrhea/Constipation, Dysuria, Weight change, Menstruation/Pregnancy
- Past Medical History, Family History, Social History
- See Physical Exam in *Bowel- Abdominal Pain: General (Chapter 2.01)*

LABORATORY STUDIES:
- Should reflect clinical suspicion: CBC/Diff, CMP, Urinalysis, HCG, LFT/Amylase, PT/PTT (with suspected liver disease)

DIAGNOSTIC STUDIES:
- Radiographs: should reflect clinical suspicion: only 10% of abdominal radiographs reveal findings, nevertheless it is available and inexpensive and should be sought
  - Ultrasound: imaging liver, biliary tree, spleen, pancreas, kidneys, pelvic organs
  - CT: most versatile imaging tool in evaluation of acute abdominal pain
  - MRI angiography: less invasive
  - Endoscopy
  - Diagnostic laparoscopy

TREATMENTS:
- See also corresponding chapters on each condition
- Goal: identification and cure of responsible underlying disease; Cure however, is often not possible: palliation may be worthwhile
  - Palliation: medications, endoscopic/surgery (i.e. biliary stent with cholangiocarcinoma), psychological support
- Multidisciplinary approach: anesthesia, psychiatrists, physiotherapists, pharmacists, social workers
- Use of psychopharmacological agents for functional gastrointestinal disorders (Gut 2005;54: 1332–1341); *See also Bowel- IBS (Chapter 2.17)*

2.04 ANORECTAL DISEASES

TAKE A GOOD HISTORY: Key questions:
Bowel movement quality, Anal pain (± with bowel movements), Bleeding, Prolapse/mass

HEMORRHOIDS (Gastroenterology 2004;126:1461–62 & 1463–73)
- Symptomatic involvement of vascular cushions in the anal canal that contains veins/arteries, elastic/connective tissue, and smooth muscle
- Thought to be from chronic straining at defecation and low-fiber diet
  - Increased colonic intraluminal pressure, submucosal and connective tissue support weakens with further enlargement of veins
  - As anal lining descends, the hemorrhoids are more exposed to pressure from straining and direct stool trauma
  - Results: stasis of blood, swelling, erosions, and subsequent bleeding
  - Predisposing conditions: pregnancy, constipation ± chronic straining, weight lifting

- External: originate distal to dentate line of anus (the division between squamous epithelium distally and transitional columnar epithelium proximally), they are covered by squamous epithelium
  - Usually asymptomatic; Occasional swelling and discomfort with straining
  - Acute thrombosis: sudden onset of acute, persistent pain and a lump; Occasionally ulcerate with extruding clot
  - Treatment of thrombosed hemorrhoids:
    - Early (within a day or so): excision of the clot with the involved hemorrhoidal complex (*as opposed to incision alone*)
    - Late: bowel regime, oral analgesics, warm tub baths (most resolve within 3 weeks), alternative treatment includes topical 0.3% nifedipine applied BID (↓ tonicity of sphincter)

- Internal: arise above the dentate line of anus, covered with transitional and columnar epithelium
  - Typically non-painful because they are above the anoderm without nerves; However pain occurs with incarceration
  - Degree of internal hemorrhoids
    - 1st degree: swell and bleed
    - 2nd degree: prolapse and spontaneously reduce
    - 3rd degree: prolapse and can manually be reduced
    - 4th degree: non-reducible
  - Treatment:
    - 1st & 2nd degree: Conservative with bowel regime, sitz baths
    - 2nd & 3rd degree: Office procedures: rubber band ligation, bipolar cautery, direct current electrical therapy, sclerotherapy
    - 3rd & 4th degree: Operative hemorrhoidectomy (If emergency hemorrhoidectomy needed: requires two weeks recovery)

- General Treatment:
  - Internal hemorrhoids: topical anesthetics, hydrocortisone preparations, astringents (witch-hazel, glycerine, magnesium sulfate)
    - Homeopathic: Ferguson Formula 361 Hemorrhoidal ointment, over-the-counter (Jamark Laboratories, Inc)
  - External thrombosed hemorrhoids: excision of the clot (early) or conservative (late)

SOLITARY RECTAL ULCER SYNDROME
- Chronic benign condition; Most are females under 40 years of age
- Characterized by anal pain, rectal bleeding, tenesmus, and difficult defecation
- Cause: excessive straining to defecate, intussusception/prolapse of anterior rectal wall into anal canal, mucosal ischemia/ulceration, inappropriate puborectalis contraction during defecation, history of digital rectal manipulation
- Endoscopy findings: 1 or more rectal ulcers, usually on anterior rectal wall (may be circumferential), 5-10 cm above anal verge; Ulceration may not always be present, rather scarring, localized hyperemia or nodularity may be seen
- Pathology: fibrosis of lamina propria, thickening of muscularis mucosa, distortion of crypt architecture (biopsy the margin to exclude other causes)
- DDX: Crohn's, herpes, CMV, gonorrhea, syphilis, lymphogranuloma venereum, rectal cancer/lymphoma
- Treatment: fiber supplementation, laxatives, decreasing straining, rectopexy to prevent intussusception and prolapse
  - Cauterization or surgical excision of ulcer usually leads to recurrence

ANAL FISSURES (Gastroenterology 2003;124:233-34 & 235-45)
- *Pain* with hard stools, some blood on tissue; Pain and bleeding that occurs with and after a bowel movement is a good chance of being a fissure
- Classic triad of chronic fissure: fissure present, hypertrophied anal papilla, sentinel tag
- Mechanism: an imbalance between bowel function and sphincter resistance (pushing against closed door)
  - In other words, it is a mechanical problem
  - Most occur in posterior midline and many have associated "sentinel skin tag" (represents fibrosis and excess granulation from the ulcer)
- Treatment:
  - Bowel regime: fiber/Citrucel/Metamucil, fluids, stool softeners
  Suppositories and hydrocortisone are of no value (it is a mechanical problem)
  - Sitz baths
  - Non-narcotic pain meds
  - Topical agents and smooth muscle relaxants:
  Lidocaine jelly 2% (30 mg tube)
  Nitro ointment 0.2% BID $\times$ 4-6 weeks (60 mg tube), side effects are headaches
  - Surgery may be necessary (lateral internal sphincterotomy): do manometry before surgery, incontinence can occur (2-12%)

PRURITUS ANI
- Itching around the anus; An irresistible urge to scratch; Worse at night and after bowel movements
- Etiology:
  - Excessive cleaning (vicious cycle), Skin irritants (moister, sweat, feces), Infections (pinworms, fungal)
  - Drinks (alcohol, milk, citrus, caffeine), Foods (chocolate, fruits, tomatoes, nuts, popcorn)
  - Skin disorders (psoriasis, eczema, dermatitis), Anorectal diseases: hemorrhoids, fissure, incontinence, prolapse
- Treatment:
  - Cleansing (avoid scented soaps & toilet paper; do not scrub, use unscented baby wipes or shower)
  - Warm baths, avoid further trauma (do not scratch), avoid moisture (keep clean & dry, cotton, 4×4 gauze)
  - Limited use of medications (short-term use of hydrocortisone only), Eliminate irritating foods & drinks
  - Treat any other anorectal underlying disorders

2.05 APPENDIX DISEASE & MECKEL'S DIVERTICULUM

DEFINITION:
- Appendicitis: Inflammation of the appendix
  - Carcinoid tumor: most common tumor of appendix; requires surgical removal *See also Bowel-Carcinoid Tumors (Chapter 2.08)*
- Meckel's Diverticulum: congenital omphalomesenteric mucosa remnant that may contain ectopic gastric mucosa
  - Located on antimesenteric side of ileum, usually 2 feet from IC valve, 2% of population, 2% develop diverticulitis
  - Gastric mucosa, if present, can lead to ileal ulcer and cause small intestinal bleed

EPIDEMIOLOGY:
- Peak incidence: 15–19 years old
- Highest risk groups for perforation: children <5 yrs, elderly (as high as 75%), DM and immunosuppressed patients also at risk

ETIOLOGIES:
- DDX of RLQ pain:
  - Ectopic pregnancy, Tubo-ovarian abscess, PID, Torsion of ovary, Incarcerated hernia
  - Crohn's disease, Ulcerative colitis, Infectious colitis
  - Diverticulitis, Meckel's diverticulitis, Carcinoid tumor
  - PUD, Cholecystitis (Perforation of gangrenous gallbladder and duodenal/gastric ulcers: collection of biliary/gastric fluids RLQ)
  - Mittelschmerz: pain accompanying rupture of ovarian follicle at mid-menstrual cycle; Nonsurgical ailment, but rule out appendicitis
- Two other conditions that mimic acute appendicitis:
  - Gastroenteritis, Mesenteric lymphadenitis (*Yersinia enterocolitica*)

PATHOPHYSIOLOGY:
- Appendicitis: obstruction of the appendiceal lumen
  - In young, lymphoid follicular hyperplasia is thought to be main culprit and possibly exacerbated by viral or bacterial infections
  - In older patients, most likely cause by fibrosis, fecaliths, or neoplasia

CLINICAL MANIFESTATIONS/PHYSICAL EXAM:
- Pain usually starts in the periumbilical area and later localizes to right lower quadrant
- Low-grade fever, anorexia, nausea, vomiting (usually single-episode) may occur after the onset of pain
- McBurney's point: point of maximal tenderness elicited in right lower quadrant, indicates inflammation in area
  - Located two-thirds distally from the umbilicus long the axis drawn from the umbilicus to the anterior superior iliac spine
- Psoas and obturator sign: irritation of retroperitoneal psoas (right hip extension) or internal obturator (internal rotation) by inflamed appendix
- Rovsing's sign: palpation of left lower quadrant commonly leads to right lower quadrant pain in acute appendicitis
- Charcot's triad (fever/chills, RUQ pain, jaundice) and gas in portal vein from suppurative thrombosis of portal vein due to appendix abscess
- PID differentiated by: high fever, cervical motion tenderness, cervical discharge, pain with menses

LABORATORY STUDIES:
- CBC (WBC, but 30% have normal WBC), Urinalysis (rule out urinary tract infection), Pelvic cultures and pregnancy test (sexually active women)

DIAGNOSTIC STUDIES:
- Appendicitis: most commonly ordered tests are CT and U/S; CT permits visualization of entire abdomen (15% have alternative diagnoses)
- Meckel's scan (Tc-pertechnetate scan): usefully only in young patients, rarely helps in middle-age or elderly

TREATMENTS:
- Surgery: laparoscopic appendectomy
  - A surgeon should not touch the appendix if it looks normal and the TI is inflamed: i.e. suspicion of Crohn's; Close and reevaluate for proper small bowel resection if necessary
- CT-guided drainage of appendiceal abscess: necessary with established abscess with an inaccessible appendix, as long as no sepsis
  - Appendectomy required 6-8 weeks after recovery, rate of recurrent appendicitis approaches 20%
- Antibiotics: begin presumptively and if not ruptured, discontinue

COMPLICATIONS:
- Most common complication after appendectomy: subcutaneous wound infection

PROGNOSIS:
- Surgery mortality: Nonperforated: <0.1%, Perforated: 4%
  - False-positive appendicitis diagnosis rate of 10-15% on appendectomy is within acceptable standards of surgical care
    - In 30% of these cases, some other cause of pain is identified: lymphadenitis, Meckel's diverticulum, PID, ectopic pregnancy, ileitis

2.06 BACTERIAL OVERGROWTH

DEFINITION:
- Increased number of bacteria in areas of the GI tract that usually do not provide the environment for colonization/proliferation of bacteria

EPIDEMIOLOGY:
- Depends on cause; See Factors influencing bacterial overgrowth below under Pathophysiology

ETIOLOGIES:
- Also consider in the DDX: Fructose and Lactose intolerance

PATHOPHYSIOLOGY:
- Usual bacterial presence in GI Tract: Stomach $<10^4$/ml; Jejunum $<10^5$/ml; Ileum $<10^6$/ml; Colon $<10^{10}$/ml
  - Proximal to cecal valve: nearly all aerobes; Distal to the cecal valve: nearly all anaerobes
- In health: small bowel bacteria resemble oropharyngeal flora with gram-positive, aerobic organisms
- In Bacterial Overgrowth: bacteria are mostly gram-neg (including *E. coli*), and anaerobic (including *Clostridia, Bacteroides*)
- Factors influencing Bacterial Overgrowth: structural lesions, motility, excessive bacterial load, deficiency in host defenses
  - Structural (obstruction to outflow): Surgical anastomosis, Webs, Adhesions, Strictures, Surgical diversions/blind loops, Diverticula
  - Motility (intestinal delay or stasis): Diabetes, Scleroderma, Pseudo-obstruction syndromes, Ileus, Acute enteric infection
  - Excessive bacterial load: Absence or incompetence of IC valve, Enteric fistulas (i.e. Crohn's)
  - Deficient host defenses: Acid suppression (medications/surgery), Hypochlorhydric disorders (Pernicious anemia), Immune (IgA deficiency), Malnutrition

CLINICAL MANIFESTATIONS/PHYSICAL EXAM:
- Diarrhea, anorexia, nausea, weight loss, anemia
- Obstructed patients may have bloating/pain; Small bowel diverticula may have insidious metabolic derangements
- Anemia (mostly megaloblastic/macrocytic) as result of B12 deficiency:
  - Anaerobes compete for intrinsic factor, Luminal bacteria consume B12 and produce folic acid; **Hence: ↓ B12, ↑ folate**
- **The clinical consequence of Bacterial Overgrowth, regardless of cause, is steatorrhea leading to weight loss and malabsorption**

LABORATORY STUDIES:
- Low Hb, MCV
- Low B12, High folate
  - Bacteria produce and then use up B12 (also compete with enterocytes for B12) and produce folate
- Decreased absorption of fat-soluble vitamins: ADEK
  - Same reason as fat malabsorption secondary to bacterial deconjugation of bile salts

Malabsorption of fat, carbohydrates and proteins
- Fat malabsorption (high fecal fat or steatorrhea):
  - Fat malabsorption from bacterial deconjugation of bile salts, leading to decreased concentration of bile salts needed to form micelles
- Carbohydrate malabsorption
  - From bacterial fermentation and decrease in brush-boarder enzymes from mucosal damage enhancing carbohydrate intolerance
- Protein malabsorption
  - From bacterial metabolism of protein-producing ammonia and fatty acids making less protein available and diminished brush-border peptidase levels and decreased uptake of amino acids
  - Rarely, if ever, is there a frank protein-losing enteropathy

DIAGNOSTIC STUDIES:
- Demonstrating elevated numbers of small bowel bacteria colonies and replacement of oropharyngeal organisms with predominantly colonic organisms
- Since intubation and aspiration for microbial analysis is cumbersome, Bacterial Overgrowth is considered in patients with predisposing factors and history!
  History: prior surgery, medical conditions such as osteomalacia, night blindness, easy bruising, tetany, etc. Direct aspiration from small bowel is the gold-standard for diagnosis, but again not commonly used
- Radiolabeled Breath Test: Xylose: catabolized by gram-neg aerobes and absorbed in proximal small bowel; Decreased (used)
  Glycocholic acid: released from bacterial deconjugation of radiolabelled bile acids; Increased (produced)
- Fasting Hydrogen Breath Test: Glucose (or lactulose):
  - An increase of breath hydrogen of 20 parts/million reflect small bowel or colon fermentation of lactose by ↑ concentrations of bacteria
  - Instructions: 4 wk prior: no antibiotics or Pepto; 24 hr prior: no smoking; Day of: NPO 8 hours prior, no gum chewing or mouthwash
  - Test can also be done with Fructose to check for Fructose intolerance

TREATMENTS:
- Correct underlying condition: surgery, prokinetics (prokinetics may work in scleroderma)
- Nutrition: lactose-free, low-residue, increased calories, micronutrient supplementation (B12, Fat soluble vitamins, Trace elements)
  - Lactose-free diet initially (the brush border contains lactate which is not functional with any mucosal abnormalities)
- Antibiotics: no consensus on which to use; Broad spectrum: cephalosporins; Narrow spectrum: metronidazole, fluoroquinolones
  - Recurrence is frequent, treatment for 10 days, options for treatment include:
    - Rifaximin (200 mg 2 tabs TID)
    - Augmentin (500 mg BID)
    - Metronidazole (250–500 mg TID)
    - Ciprofloxacin (500 mg BID)
    - Doxycycline (100 mg BID)
    - Bactrim DS (2 tabs BID)
    - Neomycin (500 mg BID)
- Probiotics: Saccharomyces boulardi; ? efficacy
- Promotility agents also may be useful in some individuals with underlying motility disorders

COMPLICATIONS:
- See Clinical Manifestations and Laboratory Studies above

PROGNOSIS:
- A course of therapy needs to be repeated when symptoms recur
- Rarely, longer cyclical courses of therapy may be necessary

2.07 CLOSTRIDIUM DIFFICILE

(Gastroenterology 2006;130:1311-16. Am J Gastroenterol 1997;92:739-50)

DEFINITION:
- Infectious diarrhea with *Clostridium Difficile*

EPIDEMIOLOGY:
- 20-30% of persons who take antibiotics develop diarrhea
- *C. difficile* frequency is unknown, estimated at 12/100,000 outpatients and 21/100 inpatients
  - The most severe complication, Pseudomembranous Colitis occurs in about 5-8% of all cases of *C. difficile* infections

ETIOLOGIES:
- Suspect in anyone with diarrhea:
  - Who has received antibiotics within the previous 2 months
    - Clindamycin, cephalosporins (esp. 3rd generation), Ampicillin
    - Can occur with any antibiotic, even a single-dose (including topical antibiotics)
  - Whose diarrhea began 72 hours or more after hospitalization
- Not always associated with antibiotics: Key factors appear to be alteration in colon flora that allows the organism to grow and produce toxins
  - Other factors: sporadic development or in association with chemotherapy, sepsis, etc.
  - Other factors: GI procedures/surgeries, renal failure, nursing home residents
- Control epidemics by quality hand washing with soap (not gels/foams) and infectious control programs; No need to treat asymptomatic carriers

PATHOPHYSIOLOGY:
- Overgrowth of the anaerobic gram-positive bacteria *C. difficile*, which causes disease by production of two cytotoxins: A & B
  - 3-5% have an abnormal version of toxin A not detected, so if strongly suspect, treat until endoscopy can be done to confirm
- Most commonly as a result of antibiotic therapy, which disrupts the normal colonic flora and allows *C. difficile* to grow
- Some develop *C. difficile* diarrhea and some are simply colonized (asymptomatic carriers are mostly infants):
  - Some develop higher levels of IgG antibody to toxin A (but not toxin B), thus immune response may explain the differences

CLINICAL MANIFESTATIONS/PHYSICAL EXAM:
- Diarrhea or loose stools starting typically 2 days - 8 weeks after antibiotics (most commonly 3-9 days); abdominal pain, low grade fevers
- May present with Toxic Megacolon (2 or more): HR >100/min, Temp >101.5°F (38.6°C), WBC >10,000, Hypoalbuminemia <3.0 gm/dl
- Remember, most **antibiotic associated diarrhea** is due to the antibiotic itself, See Watery Diarrhea, *Bowel- Diarrhea/Malassimilation (Chapter 2.12)*

LABORATORY STUDIES:

Test	Remarks
Endoscopy with biopsy	Diagnostic if pseudomembranes seen (creamy white/yellow patches); Best & most rapid method
Tissue culture for toxin B	'Gold standard' lab test (Cytotoxin B tissue culture assay - takes days to result)
ELISA for toxin A & B	Rapidly performed and inexpensive; Sensitivity 70-95%; Specificity is better (improved with 2-3 stool tests)
	3-5% have abnormal toxin A that may not be detected, so if strongly suspect, treat until endoscopy can be done
Latex Agglutination	Also rapidly performed and inexpensive; Detects glutamate dehydrogenase; Not as specific as ELISA
Stool Culture	Problem is that some people are asymptomatic carriers; ↑ Sensitivity, ↓ Specificity

DIAGNOSTIC STUDIES:
- Endoscopy (caution with severe disease as can be hazardous) reserved for when:
  - Rapid diagnosis is needed/lab tests delayed (findings on endoscopy yield yellow "pseudomembranes" consisting of mucus & fibrin filled with dead leukocytes)
  - Patient has ileus and stool not available
  - Other colonic diseases are in the differential

TREATMENTS:
- Antibiotics, if thought to be the cause, should be discontinued if possible
- Should expect results in 2-4 days, and resolution of diarrhea 2 weeks; Avoid narcotics and antidiarrheal as may prolong toxin exposure
- Oral Metronidazole is preferred (except children and pregnancy):
  - Oral: 250-500 mg QID or 500-750 mg TID for 10-14 days
  - IV: 500-750 mg TID or QID
- Vancomycin reserved for:
  - Patients who have failed or allergic to Metronidazole or organisms resistant to Metronidazole
  - Patient is pregnant or a child <10 y/o
  - Any evidence that *S.aureus* might be the cause
  - Oral:125 mg QID for 7-10 days or 500 mg QID (Oral Vanco is poorly absorbed thus resulting in high stool concentrations)
  - IV: useless (use oral or enema)
- Treatment of relapses, always confirm the diagnosis (Gastroenterology 2006;130:1311-16)
  - 1st: Treat again with original meds (i.e. oral Metronidazole), this is typically old spores becoming active, not resistance
  - 2nd: Vancomycin taper (all doses are 125 mg po): QID for 1week, TID × 1 week, QD × 1 week, QOD × 2 weeks, q 3 days × 2 weeks
  - 3rd: Tappered Vancomycin as above, plus one of the following
    - Florastor *(Saccharomyces boulardii)* 500 mg po BID × 1 month started during last 2 weeks of Vancomycin taper
    - Cholestyramine (4 g QD during last 2 weeks); toxin binder (binds medications too so must separated dose intervals)
  - Oral yogurt: Lactobacillus preparations–rarely or not effective
  - ? IVIG for immunocompromised or failed relapse therapy
- Vaccine: IgG to Toxin A is promising and may be used in future

COMPLICATIONS:
- Toxic megacolon: get surgery involved with toxic colon, increasing abdominal pain, development of subserosal air in colon on plain films

PROGNOSIS:
- Relapse in 10-25% of cases; Timing of relapse range from 2 to 30 days, but typically within a few days of completing therapy
- Mortality is low (2-3%), however higher among elderly or debilitated (10-20%) or fulminant colitis or toxic megacolon (30-80%)

2.08 CARCINOID TUMORS (MID-GUT)

DEFINITION:
- Carcinoids arise from enterochromaffin cells of the gastrointestinal tract *See also Bowel- GI Endocrine Tumors (Chapter 2.16)*
  - The term enterochromaffin refers to the ability to stain with potassium chromate (chromaffin), a feature of cells that contain serotonin
- Classification includes tumors of the:
  - Foregut (including the lungs, bronchi, stomach, duodenum, pancreas) *See also Esophagus/Gastric-Gastropathy (Chapter 1.13)*
  - Midgut (including the small intestine, appendix, and proximal colon)
  - Hindgut (including the distal colon, rectum, and genitourinary tract): rarely produce serotonin

EPIDEMIOLOGY:
- Carcinoid tumors are rare, but are the most common gastrointestinal neuroendocrine tumors
- Incidence: Caucasian ♂/♀: 2.5/2.5 per 100,000; African American ♂/♀: 4.5/4.0 per 100,000
- Age peak (bimodal): 15-25 and 65-75; Female predominance <50 y/o, Male predominance >50 y/o

PATHOPHYSIOLOGY:
- WHO classification (2000):
  - Well-differentiated neuroendocrine tumor; Benign behavior or uncertain malignant potential; AKA: Carcinoid
  - Well-differentiated neuroendocrine carcinoma; Low grade malignancy; AKA: Malignant carcinoid
  - Poorly-differentiated neuroendocrine carcinoma; High grade malignancy; AKA: Malignant carcinoid
- Majority of carcinoids (55%) occur in the GI tract:
  - Small intestine (45%), Rectum (20%), Appendix (16%), Colon (11%), Stomach (7%)
    Note: carcinoid is the most common tumor of appendix, but carcinoid most commonly affects small intestine
  - Small intestine: most originate in TI within 80 cm of IC value, often small (<1 cm), flat & fibrotic with submucosal location

CLINICAL MANIFESTATIONS/PHYSICAL EXAM:
- Most are asymptomatic
- Most common initial symptom: abdominal pain (30-40%)
  - Partial small bowel obstruction: extrinsic compression from mesenteric metastases/fibrosis, and/or intraluminal mass (rare)
  - Mesenteric ischemia: vasoconstrictors produced by tumor, and/or elastic vascular sclerosis of mesenteric vessels
- Carcinoid syndrome (diarrhea, right-sided valvular/fibrotic heart disease, flushing, bronchoconstriction); Only occurs in 5-20% of patients
  Flushing DDX: Carcinoid (5HIAA), Medullary cancer of thyroid (Calcitonin), Pheochromocytoma (urine VMA), Diabetes mellitus (glucose), Menopause (FSH)
- Metastases usually indicated by carcinoid syndrome symptoms: liver metastases, large retroperitoneal metastases, ovarian metastases

LABORATORY STUDIES:
- Urinary 5-HIAA (end point of serotonin metabolism): 100% specificity, 35% sensitivity; Can be influenced by food and medication use
- Blood serotonin level: may be helpful, but specificity is undetermined
- Chromogranin A (CgA): appears to be sensitive marker of neuroendocrine tumors, but specificity not been well-established
  - Levels may correlate with tumor burden; Level >5000 mcg/L associated with poor prognosis
  - Elevation not limited to carcinoid; False positive: renal failure, hepatic failure, atrophic gastritis, IBD, trauma

CHAPTER 2.08 CARCINOID TUMORS (MID-GUT)

DIAGNOSTIC STUDIES: Most patients have symptoms for 2 years before diagnosed!
- EGD: may look like an ordinary ulcer, polyp, or tumor mass; Frequently are round and yellowish
- **Octreotide scan:** 80-90% sensitivity; Positive findings predict response to octreotide therapy
- MIBG scan: MIBG is an analogue of a biogenic amine precursor, taken up by chromaffin cells; 70-84% sensitivity
  - Combination with Octreotide scan: 95% sensitivity
- PET scan: F-dopa and C-labeled 5-HTP; 65% sensitivity for F-dopa
- Bone scan: 90-100% sensitive for bone metastases (Octreotide scan only 50% sensitive for bone metastases)
- Plain films: can visualize large primary tumors or large metastases

TREATMENTS:
- EGD: lesions smaller than 1cm can generally be removed endoscopically when located in the stomach
- Systemic chemotherapy: results disappointing
- Surgical resection of primary tumor if possible: Prevents local mechanical complications, further metastases, limits carcinoid syndrome
- Treatment of Carcinoid Syndrome:
  - Flushing: avoid precipitating foods/alcohol
  - Diarrhea: Imodium, codeine, vitamin supplements, cholestyramine if ileal resection done
  - Nicotinic acid supplementation
  - Octreotide or Interferon alpha (combo no better than either alone) inhibits hormone secretion: controls diarrhea, wheezing, flushing
- Treatment of Hepatic metastases:
  - Hepatic artery embolization (chemoembolization, slightly better than embolization alone)
  - Radiofrequency ablation (used for nodules up to 4 cm)
  - ? Liver transplantation

COMPLICATIONS:
- Mid gut carcinoid can metastasis, most likely to liver; Liver metastasis can produce carcinoid-like symptoms (no detoxifying available)
  - Bronchial carcinoid can also cause carcinoid like symptoms due to direct extension of serotonin into blood (bypassing liver)
- Metastases-risk based on size of primary: 0.5-1 cm: 15%, 1-1.5 cm: 61%, >1.5 cm: 84%

PROGNOSIS:
- Overall 5 year survival with local tumors: 95% or with regional lymph nodes: 67%; Inoperable liver metastasis, 5 year survival: 20-50%
  - "Out of the woods" theory does not apply: 75% have recurrence within 25 years
- Poor prognostic indicators:
  - Liver metastases, Carcinoid heart disease, Significant weight loss, Extra abdominal metastases
  - High 5-HIAA or CgA levels, Age >75 years

2.09 CELIAC & TROPICAL SPRUE

(Gastroenterology 2006;131:1977-80 & 2001;120:1526-40)

CELIAC SPRUE

Definition:
- Intestinal reaction to alpha-gliadin in gluten » loss of villi & absorptive area
- Gluten sensitive enteropathy, multisystem disease

Epidemiology:
- 1% of population or 1 in 200 persons; Under diagnosed in U.S.
- All Races, All Ages, All Genders
- Inherited (70% of twins, 10% of relatives); **First degree relative is a risk factor**

Etiologies:
- Antibodies directed against connective tissue or surface component of smooth muscle fibers
- Associated disorders (many autoimmune):
  - Endocrine (DM, Thyroid, Addison's, Osteopenia, Amenorrhea, Infertility)
  - Mixed connective tissue disease (Sjogren's, RA)
  - Pulmonary (Asthma, Sarcoid)
  - Neurological (Seizures, Dementia, Peripheral neuropathy)
  - Skin (Dermatitis, Atopy, Psoriasis)
  - Malignancy (Lymphoma, Esophageal, Oropharyngeal)
  - Others: **Down syndrome,** Psychiatric disorders, Liver disease, IgA deficiency, IBD

Pathophysiology:
- Genetics: HLA-DQ2 (95% of patients) and HLA-DQ8; Absence of the DQ gene rules out celiac disease with 99% confidence
  - However, DQ2 and 8 are present in 20-30% of the general Western population, suggesting other factors play a role
- Environment: can affect any age of patients and since 70% (not 100%) of twins get the disease both suggest an environmental component
- Histological stages: Type 0 (pre-infiltrative), Type 1 (infiltrative), Type 2 (hyperplastic), Type 3 (destructive), Type 4 (hypoplastic)
  - Type 3 usually begins symptoms; Type 4 is irreversible and is found in those not responding to gluten-free diet and lymphoma

Clinical Manifestations/Physical Exam:
- Classic: **Malabsorption** leading to ± diarrhea, foul smelling stools, cramps, and weight loss
- Silent: Atypical
- Multisystemic: Neurologic, Oral (dental enamel, aphthous ulcers), Labs (Iron deficiency anemia, ↑ amylase/ESR, ↓ Albumin, Hyposplenism)
- Rash: **Dermatitis Hepatoformis**
- May be confused with IBS due to non-specific symptoms

Laboratory Studies:
- General: Iron deficiency anemia, ↓ calcium, abnormal LFTs, ↑ amylase/ESR, ↓ Albumin; High fecal fat

- Anti Gliadin IgG: 75% sensitivity (i.e. basically not a good test compared to the others)
  - May also be found in 10-20% of patients with other disease that affect the small intestinal mucosa
  - Helpful for monitoring outcome: always becomes negative with the regrowth of jejunal villi in patients after gluten-free diet

- Anti Endomysial IgA: 100% specificity, 85% sensitivity (untreated patients)
  - Can persist in low titiers in 10-25% of patients who are treated despite normal histology, or become negative with adherence to gluten-free diet

- Anti-transglutaminase IgA (tTG IgA): 100% specificity, 90% sensitivity - best sensitivity and specificity
  - Endomysial and transglutaminase can be false negative in those with IgA deficiency (approximately 2.5% of the population; Hence IgA level should always be ordered with serology) and those with mild enteropathy (positivity correlates with degree of enteropathy) and children less than 2 years old
  - IgG based labs available, but ? specificity and sensitivity

- Any serological tests for celiac disease should be confirmed with a small bowel biopsy
  - Whether or not patients with serologic abnormalities and normal biopsy results should be treated remains controversial

CHAPTER 2.09 CELIAC & TROPICAL SPRUE

Diagnostic Studies:
- Clinical suspicion leads to Biopsy or Serology; If Serology + that leads additionally to biopsy
- EGD classically demonstrates duodenal scalloping, reduced folds, mucosal groves and mosaic appearance prompting for small bowel biopsy which is key
  - Jejunal mucosa may be more accurate than duodenal biopsy
  - If presence of the disease is to be proved, it is crucial that patients not be receiving a gluten-free diet
  - Biopsy shows increased **intraepithelial lymphocytes** (similar to Microscopic Colitis)

Treatments:
- Gluten-free diet: removal of wheat, rye and barley; Nutrition consult for education
  - Oats do not contain gluten but are often contaminated with gluten during processing
  - Rice, corn, and millet do not contain gluten
- Lactose-free diet initially (the brush border contains lactate which is not functional with sprue)
- Those with continued diarrhea should be examined for other causes of diarrhea
  DDX of non-responders:
  - Incorrect diagnosis (IBS?), Continuing gluten intake (restaurants?), Bacterial overgrowth, IBD/Microscopic colitis
  - Pancreatic insufficiency, Lymphoma, Autoimmune enteropathy, Refractory sprue
- Rarely refractory cases, see below under Prognosis

Complications:
- Malignancy: Squamous cell cancer of esophagus, Small bowel adenocarcinoma, Intestinal and extraintestinal lymphoma (T-cell)
- Rarely a functional asplenia can occur, consider Pneumovax
- Risk of untreated Celiac disease: Infertility, Miscarriage, Epilepsy, Intestinal Lymphoma

Prognosis:
- Conditions to consider if previously responsive patients begin to deteriorate:
  - Noncompliance: with gluten-free diet (most common)
  - Lymphoma (T-cell): most common malignancy complicating celiac disease; Requires high index of suspicion
    - **Think about in patients not responding to diet therapy or recurrent weight loss despite diet therapy**
    - EGD, CT & exploratory laparotomy may be necessary
  - Refractory Sprue: Patients do not respond to gluten-free diet, either at onset of diagnosis or becoming refractory with diet adherence
    - No other cause found after thorough investigation
    - Some respond to steroids, azathioprine and cyclosporine; Absence of Paneth cells is a poor prognostic sign
    - Severe complications include ulcerative jejunitis, collagenous sprue (below), and lymphoma
  - Collagenous Sprue: subset of Refractory Sprue; Usually refractory to all forms of therapy other than parenteral alimentation
    - Characterized by development of thick band of collagen-like material beneath the basement membrane of epithelial cells

TROPICAL SPRUE

Definition:
- A distinctive malabsorptive and megaloblastic anemia illness that can manifest as an acute or chronic illness in those who have been to a tropical climate

Epidemiology:
- Endemic in Puerto Rico, Cuba, Dominican Republic, Haiti, Central America, Venezuela, Columbia

Etiologies:
- DDX: *Giardia, Strongyloides, Isospora belli, Capillaria philippinensis, Metagonimus yokogawai*

Pathophysiology:
- Histologically, the mucosa has shortening and broadening of villi with lengthening of crypts and increased chronic inflammatory cells
  - Fat staining shows accumulation of lipid droplets adjacent to the surface epithelium

Clinical Manifestations/Physical Exam:
- Can manifest as acute or chronic illness
- Chronic course, usually requiring 2–4 years of residence in a tropical area, occurring in three stages:
  1. Fatigue, malaise, abdominal cramps with or without diarrhea, and steatorrhea
  2. Various gastrointestinal complaints: dyspepsia, diarrhea, and manifestations of malabsorptive deficiencies
  3. Characterized by macrocytic anemia and pancytopenia
- Acute tropical sprue is not dependent on length of stay, the clinical stages are compressed and the onset is rapid

Diagnostic Studies:
- EGD: scalloping of duodenum has been reported
  - Biopsy shows short blunted villi, crypt elongation, chronic inflammatory infiltrate

Treatments:
- Folic acid 5 mg/day for 1 year, and
- Antibiotics usually result in a response within weeks; Tetracycline 250 mg 4/day for up to 6 months
- Vitamin B12 may be given if symptoms have been present for more than 4 months

NOTES

2.10 COLORECTAL CANCER

(Gastroenterology 2006;130:1872-85. N Engl J Med 2006;355:2533-41. Gastrointest Endosc 2006;63:546-57. Gastroenterology 2003;124:544-60 & 2000;118:1233-34 & 1235-57. Am J Gastroenterol 2000;95:3053-63)

DEFINITION:
- Colorectal cancer (CRC) includes both colon (**Sporadic** and Familial) and rectal cancer
  - Colon cancers: adenocarcinoma ≥95%; The rest are lymphomas, malignant carcinoid, leiomyosarcomas, Kaposi's sarcoma
  - Rectal cancers: rectum is immobile, lacks serosal covering and therefore more commonly spreads contiguously by direct extension

- Familial Colon Cancer Syndromes (Inherited Colon Cancer Syndromes): Gastro 2001;121:195-97 & 198-213
  - **Familial Adenomatous Polyposis (FAP);** Autosomal dominant; Lifetime risk of CRC 100%; Sporadic cases (patient first in family to develop FAP) 30%
    - Extracolonic features: fundic gland polyps, duodenal adenomas, desmoid tumors, osteomas (jaw), multiple teeth, eye disorders
    - **Attenuated Adenomatous Polyposis Coli (AAPC):** later onset, CRC ~ age 50, fewer adenomas (right sided)
    - **Gardner's Syndrome** (FAP with extracolonic manifestations, above)
    - ↑ risk of cancers: thyroid, pancreatic, duodenal, ampullary, gastric
  - **Hereditary Nonpolyposis Colorectal Cancer (HNPCC);** Autosomal dominant; Lifetime risk CRC (most right side) 80%
    - 'Nonpolyposis' is misleading, really should use: **Lynch Syndrome I** (CRC alone), **Lynch Syndrome II** (CRC and other malignancies)
    - 3-2-1 rule (Amsterdam II criteria): 3 relatives with CRC (one first degree), 2 generations involved, 1 patient diagnosed <50 yrs
    - ↑ risk extracolonic cancer: endometrium (60%), Stomach (20%), Urinary (15%), Small bowel (10%), ovarian, hepatobiliary
  - **Hamartomatous Polyp Syndromes (Peutz-Jeghers Syndrome, Juvenile Polyposis);** Autosomal dominant (STK11/LKB1 gene)
    - Mucocutaneous pigmentation; Have ↑ CRC risk (not as high as FAP) along with breast, pancreas, stomach, ovary cancer
    - Other differential in this category: Cowden's disease and the Bannayan-Ruvalcaba-Riley syndrome

EPIDEMIOLOGY:
- CRC leading cause of death in U.S., after CAD; Second leading cause of death from malignancy, after lung cancer; M = F
  - Lifetime risk of CRC is 1 in 18 (5.5%); Most (75%) of people have no risk factors! New cases per year 150,000; Deaths per year 57,000
  - Risk Factors:
    - Age >60, First and second degree relative with CRC or adenomas- see Screening below (lifetime risk is increased to 15% from 5.5%)
    - Environmental: ↓ Fiber, Fruits & Vegetables, ↑ Red meats, ↑ Fat, Obesity (? diabetes), ↓ physical activity, smoking, IBD after 8 yrs
  - Prevalence of adenomas varies, depending on study: ranging from 20-50%
- Rectal cancer accounts for 40% of CRC; Annual incidence 43,000; Annual mortality 7,000; 90% are older than 50 years (5% <40 years)

ETIOLOGIES:

	Sporadic CRC	HNPCC	FAP
Causes of CRC	65-85%	5%	1%
Mean age	69	44	39
Arise from adenoma	Yes, few	Yes, few	Yes, 100-1000's
Distribution	Distal to splenic flex (65%)	Proximal to splenic flex (70%)	Throughout entire colon/rectum
Genetic abnormalities	Polygenic (multiple)	MSH2, MSH6, MLH1	APC
Variants	—	Lynch syndromes	Gardner's, AAPC (1-100 polyps)
Mode of inheritance	Unknown	Autosomal dominant	Autosomal dominant

Modified from Toribara N: *Colorectal cancer.* In McNally P (ed): *GI & Liver Secrets,* 2nd ed. Philadelphia, Hanley & Belfus, 2001, pp 335.

CHAPTER 2.10 COLORECTAL CANCER

PATHOPHYSIOLOGY:
- Cancer is caused by accumulation of heritable mutations in cellular DNA, resulting in uncontrolled cell growth
- Typically it takes 5-10 years for a adenoma to develop into cancer
  - Protrude into bowel lumen with stalk (pedunculated) or directly from the bowel wall (sessile)
  - Severe dysplasia (carcinoma in situ, intramucosal carcinoma)
  - Malignant polyp (focus of carcinoma has invaded beyond the muscularis mucosa into submucosa)
- Metastases (25% of patients): CRC metastasizes to liver, peritoneal cavity, lungs; Rectal cancer metastasizes to lungs
- Pathologic classification of colorectal polyps; Definitions:
  - Neoplasia: abnormal disorganized growth of tissue or organ usually forming a distinct mass (a tumor); Can be benign or malignant
  - Dysplasia: an abnormality of the appearance of cells indicative of an early step towards transforming to neoplasia (pre-neoplastic)
  - Adenoma: a collection of growths (-oma) of glandular origin; These are benign but have the potential to transform to malignancy

Neoplastic	Non-Neoplastic	Prevalence of Polyps Based on Age:	
Benign ("premalignant"):	Hyperplastic	50 yrs	30%
Tubular Adenoma	Inflammatory	60 yrs	40-50%
Tubulovillous Adenoma	Lymphoid	70 yrs	50-65%
Severe Dysplasia (old terms:	Hamartoma		
Intramucosal cancer,	Juvenile		
Carcinoma in situ)			
Malignant:			
Polyp or Tumor: Invasive			
Adenocarcinoma			

CLINICAL MANIFESTATIONS/PHYSICAL EXAM:
- Two conditions that should raise suspicion for CRC: unexplained iron deficiency anemia or sepsis with *Streptococcus bovis*
- Early lesions are often asymptomatic
  - Early symptoms: occult bleeding, iron deficient anemia, change in bowel habits
  - Late symptoms: obstruction, fistula (pneumaturia), weight loss, fever/chills/sweats

LABORATORY STUDIES:
- CEA, if high at diagnosis (60% of time), it provides a convenient method for assessing effectiveness of surgery and early detection
  - Note: CEA is excreted in bile, so elevated levels difficult to interpret with biliary obstruction or hepatic dysfunction

DIAGNOSTIC STUDIES:
- Fecal occult blood testing (FOBT) with sigmoidoscopy; Barium enemas (only in skilled hands); CT colonography
- Colonoscopy (especially before any CRC surgery to exclude synchronous lesions that may influence the operation)
- Preoperative CT (look for metastatic disease)
- In rectal cancer, transrectal ultrasound helps to determine depth of invasion and hence utility of adjunct radiation therapy

SECTION II SMALL BOWEL/COLON/RECTUM

SCREENING FOR COLORECTAL CANCER:
Note: missed polyps during endoscopy (depending on size): 6-25%; Colonoscope withdraw time should be 6-10 min; Endoscopy report should comment on quality of bowel prep as well

- **Average Risk** (No history of polyps and no history of relatives with polyps/cancer): Start screening at age 50 (Age 45 if African American)
  -Flexible sigmoidoscopy q 5 yrs *and*
  FOBT q 1 yr (Usually done at home with 3 consecutive stool smears; One + smear (office or home) makes test positive » Colonoscopy)
  -Barium Enema   q 5 yr (double contrast)
  -Colonoscopy   q 10 yr
  -Fecal DNA   Maybe in the future

- **Increased Risk** (A personal history of polyps or if a family member has polyps or cancer as below; *See also IBD- Ulcerative Colitis (Chapter 3.04)* for IBD surveillance)
  (Family history of first-degree relative [FDR]: parent/siblings/child at least doubles risk of CRC)
  (Second-degree relative [SDR]: grandparent, aunt/uncle, cousin)

-1 FDR or 2 SDR	>60 at diagnosis	Colonoscopy beginning at age 40, q 10 yr
-1 FDR or 2 SDR	≤60 at diagnosis	Colonoscopy beginning at age 40 or 10 years earlier than youngest relatives diagnosis, q 3-5 yr
-2 or more FDR	Any age	Colonoscopy beginning at age 40 or 10 years earlier than youngest relatives diagnosis, q 3-5 yr

- **High Risk** (Family history of FAP or HNPCC)
  FAP (Endoscopy with both end-viewing and ampullary side-viewing instruments for upper endoscopy with antral and duodenal biopsies)
  -Screen starting at age 9-12, Cscope or Flex Sig q 1 yr; Screen: TSH, LFT for other malignancies too
  -APC gene testing: test for mutations starting at age 9-12; Helps guide genetic counseling

  HNPCC
  -Screen starting at age 21 (or 10 yrs younger than 1st relative): Colonoscopy q 6 mon-2 yr (no greater than every 2 years)
  -Also should be screened for: Endometrial biopsy (at diagnosis); Transvaginal U/S & CA125 (begin age 25-35, q 1 yr);
  -Urine cytology (begin age 30, q 1-2 yrs); Genetic counseling (at diagnosis)

SURVEILLANCE: POST-POLYPECTOMY

Risk Factor	Surveillance Interval
1-2 adenomas, or <1 cm, or tubular adenomas	5-10 years
Large sessile adenoma (>2 cm)	3-6 months (ensure removal)
Inadequate colon prep	Repeat 2-6 months
≥3 total, or ≥1 cm or advanced adenoma (villous component or high grade dysplasia)	3 years (<3 years if >10 total polyps)

- Note: if out of norm, should be more aggressive; i.e. multiple polyps return in 1 year, or large sessile polyps 2-6 months (ensure removal), etc
- If, for example 10% of colon is not seen due to inadequate prep, the guidelines are vague about when to repeat; Use clinical judgment
- Guidelines *do* suggest that one should reschedule the colonoscopy if prep is inadequate; however the quantification of retained stool is not mentioned

CHAPTER 2.10 COLORECTAL CANCER

SURVEILLANCE: POST OPERATIVE FOR COLORECTAL CANCER RESECTION
(Gastroenterology 2006;130:1865-71)
- If well prepped colonoscopy was performed preoperatively, repeat colonoscopy at 1 year; the yield of colonoscopy will demonstrate:
  - 2-3% for anastomotic recurrence, 3-4% for metachronous cancer, 25-33% for adenomas
  - If 1 year follow-up is normal, a repeat colonoscopy should be done in 3 years followed by 5 years if all are normal; earlier depending on findings
- If preoperative colonoscopy was not done, surveillance should be done at 3-6 months postoperatively to exclude synchronous disease
- CEA positive tumors: reasonable to check levels q 2 months for first 6 months, then q 4 months for 2 years, and then q 6 months for 5 years
- Rectal cancer follow-up: every 3-6 month intervals for 2-3 years (utilizing rigid proctoscopy, flexible proctoscopy, or endoscopic ultrasound)

TREATMENTS:
- In general:
  - Colon: surgery and chemotherapy rather than radiation (radiation not normally used due to tendency for hematogenous metastases)
    —Malignant polyps that indicate a colectomy:
    - Sessile growth or short stalk (<3 mm), residual villous adenoma, stalk invasion, lymphatic or vascular permeation, poor differentiation, invasive carcinoma at or near the polyp resection margin
    —Conservative approach for:
    - Polyp completely excised (properly processed in lab and resected margin not involved, not poorly differentiated), no evidence of vascular/lymphatic involvement
  - Rectal: surgery & adjuvant radiation ± chemotherapy (due to its relative immobility and tendency for direct extension metastases)
    - Abdominal-perineal resection (APR): 10% of patients, poor sphincter function
    - Low anterior resection (LAR): 85% of patients, sphincter preserving resection
  - Anal: chemotherapy and radiation (surgery is generally not used or for salvage only)
- Surgery: Stage I & II Colon; Stage I Rectal Cancer
- Adjuvant Chemo-radiation therapy: Stage II Colon; Stage III Rectal
- Adjuvant Chemo therapy: Stage III Colon

PROGNOSIS:

Stage	T	N	M	5 yr Survival (%)	Dukes Classification (Old)	5 yr Survival (%)
I	T1 or T2	N0	M0	90-95	A: Limited to mucosa	95-100
II	T3 or T4	N0	M0	75-80	B1: Into muscularis propria	80-85
III	Any T	N1-3	M0	35-70	B2: Through serosa	75
IV	Any T	Any N	M1	<10	C1: 1-4 LN positive	65
(T1: Confined to (sub) mucosa)					C2: >4 LN positive	42
(T2: Invades muscularis propria)					D: distant mets	5

(T3: Invades serosa)
(T4: Invades adjacent organs)
(N: Lymph nodes: N1 = 1-3; N2 ≥ 4; N3 = Any node along vascular trunk)
(M: Metastases)

2.11 CONSTIPATION

(Gastroenterology 2006;130:1480-91. N Engl J Med 2003;349:1360-68. Gastroenterology 2000;119: 1761-78)

DEFINITION:
- Historically less than 2-3 bowel movements/week; Excessive difficulty straining at defecation
- Rome III for functional constipation: see below under Diagnostic Studies
- Dyschezia: difficulty in defecating

EPIDEMIOLOGY:
- 5-30% of population report symptoms; Prevalence increases with age

ETIOLOGIES:

Causes	Example
Idiopathic/Functional	Chronic idiopathic: Impaired colonic transit, IBS
Structural	Colonic or anorectal: cancer, stricture
Metabolic/Endocrine	Hypokalemia, Hypercalcemia, Hypocalcemia, Uremia, Hypothyroid, DM
Collagen vascular disorders	Scleroderma, Amyloidosis
Inherited muscular disorders	Familial visceral myopathy
Colonic disorders	Colonic inertia
Enteric neuro disorders	Hirschsprung's, Chronic intestinal pseudo-obstruction
Nonenteric neuro disorders	Parkinson's, Spinal cord injury, MS, Scleroderma (fibrotic/non-contractile)
Anorectal disorders	Anal stricture, Rectocele
Psychological	Anorexia nervosa
Medications	Opiates & antihypertensives such as calcium channel blockers (most common causes), antacids (calcium, aluminum), anti-cholinergics, antispasmodics, anticonvulsants, antidepressants, diuretics, iron

- Classification based upon transit time:
  - Normal transit constipation: perception of disordered evacuation; Fiber supplementation may help
  - Slow transit constipation: malfunction of neural network; i.e. infection, endocrine, drug, scleroderma; Fiber may worsen
  - Obstructive defecation: mechanical; i.e. Hirschsprung's, Pelvic floor dysfunction; Fiber may worsen

- Anorectal dysfunction:
  - Anismus/spastic pelvic floor syndrome: spasticity of levator ani, abnormal angulated recto-anal axis; Functional problem
  - Impaired rectal sensation: decrease in urge to defecate
  - Megarectum: long-term fecal impaction, often seen in children, physically/mentally impaired elderly; Occasionally with neuro disorder
  - Rectocele: stool directed away from anal canal into rectocele during straining, leading to retention of feces in pouch

PATHOPHYSIOLOGY:
- The colon absorbs approximately 100 mL of fluid and 1 mEq of sodium and chloride from 1,500 mL of chyme daily
  - If necessary, the absorptive capacity can increased to 5-6 L and 800-1000 mEq of sodium and chloride per day
- Healthy subjects: average mouth-to-cecum time is 6 hrs, average transit through right, left and sigmoid colon is 12 hrs each (36 hrs total)
- Normally:
  - First sensing in rectum via stretch receptors in the muscularis propria initiate a spinal reflex arc: relaxation of internal anal sphincter

CHAPTER 2.11 CONSTIPATION

- Then relaxation of striated muscles of pelvic floor (puborectalis, pubococcygeus), rectoanal angle opens from 90 to 130°
- Final relaxation of external anal sphincter and passage of stool, often with concomitant diaphragm & abdominal muscle contraction
- Serotonin & Motility: 5-HT receptors located on both cholinergic neurons enhancing contraction and inhibitory neurons reducing contractions
- Colonic inertia: isolated dysfunction of propulsive forces of the colon, whereas other test of upper GI motility are normal

CLINICAL MANIFESTATIONS/PHYSICAL EXAM:
- Red flags: bloody stools, weight loss, risks for CRC, signs of systemic illness
- Digital rectal exam should be performed

LABORATORY STUDIES:
- Check stool for occult blood, CBC, electrolytes (calcium), TSH

DIAGNOSTIC STUDIES:
- Proposed workup:
  - Sigmoidoscopy/Colonoscopy as indicated: consider food, symptom, activity diary
  - Empiric Therapy: diet, fiber, medications
    - Responds: continue ± modify treatment
    - No response: Evaluate patient: colon transit study, anorectal manometry, defecography; Treatment based on results
- Colonic transit study: Metcalf study: Tablet (24 markers) on day 1, 2, 3; X-ray day 4 and 7 (No laxatives or enemas before test)
  - Normally 80% pass by day 5, nearly all by day 7; In other words, more than 20% of retained markers indicates prolonged transit; General findings:
    - Normal transit (majority of markers passed)
    - Colonic inertia (markers remain and are evenly distributed throughout colon)
    - Defecatory disorder (markers related in left lower colon/rectum)
- Anorectal manometry ± Balloon expulsion
- Defecatory: Best at detecting rectocele
  - Some centers have replaced with Pelvic MRI test
- If an entire workup is negative, then patient is considered to have **functional constipation; Rome III criteria:**
  1. At least 2 of the following:
     - Straining during ≥25% of defecations
     - Lumpy/hard stools ≥25% of defecations
     - Sense of incomplete evacuation or anorectal obstruction ≥25% of defecations
     - Manual maneuvers to facilitate defecation ≥25% of defecations
     - Fewer than 3 BMs per week
  2. Loose stools rarely present without use of laxatives
  3. There are insufficient criteria to diagnose IBS

TREATMENTS:
- General Classes of Medications:
  - Bulk-forming/Dietary fiber: goal of 25-35 gm/day (cereals, fruits, vegetables, bran); Rule out fecal impaction/obstruction first
    - Increases stool weight and accelerates colonic transit, hence most efficient in normal transit constipation
    - All have high water binding capacity so patients should drink plenty of water
    - Psyllium (Metamucil), Wheat Dextrin (Benefiber): plant husks/natural occurring; Most fiber (3 gm) per serving
      - Can be fermented by colonic bacteria and cause gas/bloating, but can have benefits such as lowering cholesterol level
    - Methylcellulose (Citrucel): synthetic; Fiber (2 gm) per serving
      - Not fermented by colonic bacteria and causes less gas/bloating, but no natural benefits

SECTION II SMALL BOWEL/COLON/RECTUM

- Laxatives/Cathartics: Increase water content of stool via: osmotic retention (trapping solute/inhibiting absorption) or stimulating intestinal secretion
  - Lactulose/Sorbitol (Osmotic laxative): may increase gas
  - Mag/Phos Sulfates (Osmotic laxative): not used with elderly/cardiac/CRF patients (can cause high mg, phos)
  - Polyethelene glycol (Osmotic laxative): Golytely, Miralax
  - Castor or Mineral Oil (Secretion laxative): Aspiration lung injury can occur (there are better options); Use only as enema
  - Docusate sodium (Secretion laxative): Colace; stimulates mild fluid secretion, little effect on stool volume/motility
  - Myth: chronic use of stimulant laxatives is harmful to the colon and will lead to cathartic colon or increased colon cancer risk (no evidence)
- Prokinetics: enhance intrinsic motor function of gut
  - Metoclopramide: much less effective in stimulating colonic contractions as compared to upper GI tract
  - Cisapride: restricted due to side effect of torsade de pointes
- Enemas: reliable results in fecal impaction, and megarectum (prevent recurrent impaction with scheduled bowel training)
  - Tap water, soap suds, mineral oil
- 5-HT4: agonist stimulate GI transit
  - Tegaserod (Zelnorm): For constipation in both men/women (FDA restricted 2007)
  - 6 mg BID or TID; Start with trial of up to 12 weeks and reassess
- Chloride channel activation: increasing intestinal fluid secretion and motility
  - Lubiprostone (Amitiza): Indicated for functional or idiopathic constipation

- Chronic Constipation:
  - Dietary modification with fiber; exercise accelerates colonic transit time
  - Use of Bulk-forming/Dietary fiber and/or Laxatives/Cathartics (see above)

- Acute Constipation: Rule of thumb: 'begin with "afterload" before "preload" or "inotropy"'
  - Afterload: Bisacodyl (Dulcolax) tabs 10-15 mg po or 10 mg PR or Glycerin PR OTC
  Bisacodyl (Fleets) enema (1 unit); Alternatives: soap suds (1500 ml), tap water (500 ml), mineral oil (150-250 ml)
  - Preload: Milk of Magnesia (30 ml po qhs)
  - Inotropy: Magnesium Citrate, 18 g/10 oz po (Caution: not in elderly/cardiac/CRF patients!)
  Senna, 25 mg po QD or BID
  - Alternatives:
    - Lactulose (30 cc po q 6-8 hr); Sorbitol 25 ml of 75% solution po TID; Polyethelene glycol; Manual disimpaction

- Biofeedback is another behavioral approach that can be used in patients with severe chronic constipation (with dyssynergic defecation)
  - Can correct inappropriate contraction of pelvic floor muscles and external anal sphincter during defecation

COMPLICATIONS:

- Subtotal colectomy with ileorectal anastomosis can ameliorate incapacitating constipation in carefully selected patients; Criteria for surgery:
  - The patient has chronic, severe, and disabling symptoms from constipation that are unresponsive to medical therapy
  - The patient has slow colonic transit of the inertia pattern
  - The patient does not have intestinal pseudoobstruction, as demonstrated by radiologic or manometric studies
  - The patient has normal anorectal function (Pelvic floor dysfunction is ruled out)
  - The patient does not have abdominal pain as a prominent symptom
    - Complications of surgery can include small bowel obstruction and prolonged ileus
    - Most report significant improvement in quality of life after a brief post-op period of diarrhea

- Melanosis Coli: staining of the colonic wall due to chronic laxative use
  - Most likely culprit is Senna (anthraquinones) i.e. Ex-lax
  - Develops in months but may take a year or more to go away after stopping laxatives
  - Polyps, for whatever reason, do not develop melanosis coli (i.e. a natural chromoendoscopy!)

NOTES

2.12 DIARRHEA/MALASSIMILATION

(Gastroenterology 1999;116:1461-63 & 1464-84)

DEFINITION:
- **Stool output more than 200 g/day** or increased frequency & decreased consistency of stool (can be altered by diet, so these are imperfect criteria but the best we have)
- Note, is the patients complaint really diarrhea? Always ask about fecal incontinence "do you have accidents?"; Many complain of diarrhea due to embarrassment
- MOA: incomplete absorption of fluid; Normal stool 25% solid, 75% water; Normal fecal water output 80 ml/day representing 1% of GI fluid load
  - Fluid load 9-10 L/day: 2 L food/drink, 1.5 L saliva, 2.5 L gastric juice, 1.5 L bile, 2.5 L pancreatic juice; Jejunum/ileum absorb most
  - Colon absorbs more than 90% of fluid reaching it, leaving only 1% of original fluid entering the jejunum to be excreted in stool

Classify and categorize diarrhea via: **Acute or Chronic,** followed by:	Inflammatory Watery (Osmotic/Secretory) Malassimilation (Fatty Diarrhea) Motility/Functional

INFLAMMATORY (fever, hematochezia, abdominal pain)
- Infectious • Radiation enteritis • IBD (Ulcerative colitis, Crohn's) • Ischemic colitis

Infectious - *See also Bowel- Diarrheal Infections (Chapter 2.13)* for specifics on each bug
- **Acute**
  - Cytotonic/Preformed toxins/Enterotoxin ("food poisoning"; typical onset <24 hrs):
    - *S. aureus; C. perfringens; B. cereus*
  - Viral gastroenteritis often has nausea/vomiting, (no high fever, severe abdominal pain, or bloody diarrhea; Brief/self-limiting
    - *Rotovirus; Norwalk; Adenovirus; Astrovirus*
  - Non-Invasive Bacteria
    Cytotonic: toxin activation of intracellular enzymes: watery diarrhea; **(No fecal WBC or Blood)**
    - Enterotoxigenic *E. coli* (ETEC); Enteropathogenic *E. coli* (EPEC); *Vibrio cholera*
    Cytotoxic: toxins cause structural injury: mucosal inflammation and bleeding; **(+ fecal WBC** (inflammatory) **and blood)**
    - Enterohemorrhagic *E. coli 0157:H7* (EHEC); *C. difficile*
  - Invasive Bacteria **(+ fecal WBC and blood)**
    - *Campylobacter* (most common); *Salmonella; Shigella;* Enteroinvasive *E. coli* (EIEC); *Vibrio parahemolyticus; Yersinia*
  - Parasites (erratic shedding, need 3 collections for O&P for best chance of detection)
    - *Giardia; Entamoeba histolytica*
  - Opportunistic:
    - *Cryptosporidia, Isospora, Microsporidia, Cyclospora,* MAC, CMV
- **Chronic**
  - *Giardia, E. hystolytica, C. difficile,* Opportunistic organisms listed above

WATERY DIARRHEA:
Osmotic: (↓ diarrhea with fasting, **osmotic gap >50,** normal fecal fat)
  Ingestion of a poorly absorbed substance
- **Medications:** antacids (containing mag and/or phos), lactulose, sorbitol (i.e. 'sugar-free' products or elixir medicines), antibiotics
  - Antibiotic associated diarrhea: 1. *C. difficile* or 2. Osmotic diarrhea secondary to impaired colon fermentation of carbohydrates (CHO):
    Normally CHO not absorbed in small bowel, undergo colon fermentation to organic acids, which are absorbed and provide mucosal cell energy to absorb water and ions; Antibiotics reduce colon bacteria = ↓ fermentation of organic acids and mucosal energy = net ↓ water reabsorption; Also unabsorbed CHO can cause osmotic diarrhea

CHAPTER 2.12 DIARRHEA/MALASSIMILATION

- **Lactose intolerance:** primary and secondary mucosal abnormalities, viral/bacterial enteritis, bowel resection; Clinical: bloating, flatulence, discomfort, diarrhea
  - Diagnosis: lactose hydrogen breath test or empiric lactose free diet
  - Treatment: lactose-free diet, use of lactaid milk and lactase enzyme tablets

Secretory: (no change in diarrhea with fasting, **normal osmotic gap,** large volume)
Failure to absorb electrolytes or stimulation of electrolyte secretion

- **Hormonal:** *See also Bowel- GI Endocrine Tumors (Chapter 2.16)*
  - Diabetes (Fasting blood sugar), Thyroid (TSH), Addison's (ACTH stim), Hyperparathyroid (PTH), Multiple myeloma (SPEP), AIDS (HIV)
  - Neuroendocrine tumors are rare: Carcinoid (Urine 5-HIAA, Serotonin), Insulinoma (Insulin), Zollinger-Ellison (Gastrin), VIPoma/Verner-Morrison (VIP), Medullary Ca of thyroid (Calcitonin), Amyloid (fat pad biopsy), Pheochromocytoma (Urine Metanephrine), Glucagonoma (Glucagon), Mastocytosis (Histamine/C1esterase)
- **Laxative abuse/Stimulants** (phenolphthalein)
- **Colitis:** Diverticulitis; *Microscopic:* Lymphocytic colitis, Collagenous Colitis; *Macroscopic:* Crohn's, Ulcerative Colitis *See also Inflammatory Bowel Disease- Section II*
- Other: Villous adenoma/Colon carcinoma or Idiopathic bile salt malabsorption

MALASSIMILATION (FATTY DIARRHEA):
(↓ diarrhea with fasting, **osmotic gap >50,** ↑ fecal fat; deficiency in fat-soluble vitamins)

Maldigestion: (problem in the lumen/pancreas, breaking up food)
- **Bile Salt Deficiency**
  - Bacterial overgrowth (i.e. blind loops) » deconjugation of bile salts
  - Ileal disease (i.e. Crohn's/fistulas, surgery) » interruption of enterohepatic circulation
  - Postcholecystectomy » no local storage » bile concentration in colon (laxative effect); treat with binders (Cholestyramine)
- **Pancreatic Insufficiency:**
  - Diagnosis with secretin pancreatic function test, however most resort to trial of pancreatic enzymes

Malabsorption: (problem at the mucosal level, nutrient absorption)
- **Mucosal abnormalities**
  - Celiac Sprue: *See also Bowel- Celiac Sprue (Chapter 2.09)*
  - Tropical Sprue: Occurs in residents of the tropics;
  - Whipple's Disease: due to infection with *Tropheryma whippelii* (g+ bacilli); Typically middle-age white males: diarrhea, arthralgias, weight loss, abdominal pain; Therapy: prolonged course of antibiotics; *See also Bowel- Whipple's Disease (Chapter 2.25)*
  - Intestinal Lymphoma (lymph obstruction)
- Other: Short bowel syndrome; Bacterial overgrowth; Mesenteric ischemia

MOTILITY/FUNCTIONAL:
- **IBS** (10–22% of adults): abdominal pain and changes in bowel habits; pain relief with bowel movement; incomplete evacuation; *See also Bowel- IBS (Chapter 2.17)*
- Rheumatological: Scleroderma (pseudo-obstruction); Endocrinopathies: DM, Hyperthyroidism, Addison's (hyperdefecation)

ACUTE DIARRHEA (<3–4 WEEKS OF DIARRHEA) WORK UP:
- Severe dehydration, fever, duration >5 days, mucus/pus/blood in bowel movement, abdominal pain, recent travel, recent antibiotic use?
  - No to all: Observation and rehydrate as needed
  - Yes to any: check Fecal WBC's; FOBT; *C. difficile* toxin
    - Negative Fecal WBCs, Negative FOBT
      - Stool O&P × 3
        - Pos O&P: Parasitic infection
        - Neg O&P: Med-induced (i.e. Antibiotic associated), Viral, Enterotoxic Bacteria
    - Positive Fecal WBC or Positive FOBT
      - Stool Culture ± Flex sig
        - Pos Culture: Cytotoxic or Invasive Bacterial
        - Neg Culture with positive Flex Sig findings/biopsy: IBD, radiation, ischemia
    - Positive *C. difficile* toxin: Pseudomembranous colitis

CHRONIC DIARRHEA (>3–4 WEEKS OF DIARRHEA) WORK UP:
- History: Onset (abrupt/gradual), Pattern (continuous/intermittent), Duration
  Epidemiology (travel/food/water)
  Stool (watery/bloody/fatty)
  Abdominal pain (IBD/IBS/ischemia), Weight loss (malabsorption/neoplasm)
  Aggravating factors (**lactose**/NPO response/stress), Previous evaluations
  Iatrogenic (**medications**/radiation/surgery), Factitious (laxatives)
  Systemic disease (thyroid/diabetes/mixed connective tissue disease/Ig deficiency)
- Exam: General (fluid balance/nutrition), Skin (flushing/rashes), Thyroid, Abdomen (HSM/Mass/Ascites), Anorectal (sphincter/FOBT)
- Blood: CBC (anemia/leukocytosis), Chemistry (electrolyte status/protein/albumin)
- Stool: Weight, Electrolytes (gap), FOBT, WBC (inflammation/Infection), Laxative screen (phenolphthalein), Fat: *See also Bowel- Potpourri (Chapter 2.26)*

Stool Osmotic Gap = Stool Osm (290) − [2 × (stool Na + K)]
(For stool Osm use standard 290, measured can be influenced by water, urine, or sitting in lab)

Categorize: *Inflammatory, Watery (Osmotic/Secretory), Fatty*

Inflammatory: (+WBC & FOBT); Stool culture indicated for bloody diarrhea since bacterial pathogens likely
- Exclude Structural » Small bowel series, Colonoscopy with biopsy, CT scan of abdomen, Small bowel biopsy ± aspirate: quantitative culture
- Exclude Infection » Bacterial pathogens: *Aeromonas, Plesiomonas, Tuberculosis;* Others: Parasites, Viruses

Osmotic: (↓ diarrhea with fasting, ↑ osmotic gap >50, normal Fecal fat)
- Stool analysis » Low pH (<5.6): carbohydrate malabsorption producing fatty acids
  Dietary review, Lactose breath test
  Normal pH (7): ingestion of poorly absorbed cations/anions, no pH effect
  High Mg output: inadvertent ingestion vs. laxative abuse

Secretory: (no change with fasting, normal osmotic gap, large volume, normal fecal fat, negative WBC/FOBT)
- Exclude Infection » Bacterial pathogens: *Aeromonas, Plesiomonas,* O&P, *Giardia* antigen, *Coccidia, Microsporidia, Cholera*
- Exclude Structural » Small bowel series, Colonoscopy with biopsy, CT scan of abdomen, Small bowel biopsy ± aspirate: quantitative culture
- Selective testing » Plasma peptides (gastrin, calcitonin, VIP, somatostatin), Urine (5-HIAA, Histamine, Metanephrine), Other (TSH, ACTH stimulation, SPEP/Immunoglobulins)
- Cholestyramine (Questran) trial for bile acid diarrhea
- Note: 25% patients fail to reveal cause, most resolve 1–2 years without recurrence, hence preferable to treat symptomatically, not retest

Fatty: (↓ diarrhea with fasting, ↑ osmotic gap >50, + Fecal fat)
- Exclude Structural » Small bowel series, CT scan of abdomen, Small bowel biopsy ± aspirate: quantitative culture
- Exclude Pancreatic » Secretin pancreatic function test, Stool chymotrypsin activity; Most resort to therapeutic trial of pancreatic enzymes
- Exclude Bile Deficiency » Bacterial overgrowth (hydrogen breath test)

CHAPTER 2.12 DIARRHEA/MALASSIMILATION

TREATMENT:
- Rest, fluids, electrolyte replacement, stop offending agents (i.e. lactose products, Sorbitol in elixirs, Metformin in diabetics, etc)
- Initial absorbents
  - Attapulgite (Kaopectate): 60-120 mg po q 3-4 hr
  - Bismuth subsalicylate (Pepto-Bismol): 30 mg po q 6 hr (caution: Salicylate toxicity)
- Opioids (antiperistaltic): may precipitate toxic megacolon in invasive bacterial colitis
  - Loperamide HCL (Imodium): 2-4 mg po q 6 hr
  - Diphenoxylate HCL (Lomotil): 2.5-5 mg po q 6 hr
  - Codeine: 15-60 mg po q 6 hr
  - Morphine: 2-20 mg po q 6 hr
  - Tincture of Opium: 2-20 drops po q 6 hr
- Adrenergic agonist:
  - Clonidine 0.1-0.3 mg po q 8 hr (restores the 'sympathetic brake')
- Somatostatin analog:
  - Octreotide 50-250 mcg SQ q 8 hr
- Bile acid-binding resin:
  - Cholestyramine 4 gm po q 6-24 hr
- **Most do not need antibiotics,** however **Moderate-Severe** diarrhea or fever, blood, pus or immunocompromised: empiric fluoroquinolone × 3 days

2.13 DIARRHEAL INFECTIONS

(Am J Gastroenterol 1997;1962-75)

Infectious Diarrhea: Worldwide 1 billion cases/year and death rates are second only to cardiovascular disease! Note: normally the stool does not have any PMNs on microscopic examination, likewise there may be many false negatives during inspection for PMNs

CLUES TO ETIOLOGY: Ask about water: city vs. well water
Dairy: *Staph aureus, Campylobacter, Salmonella, Yersina*
Seafood/Shellfish: *Norwalk, Vibrio sp., Campylobacter*
Undercooked hamburger: EHEC *(E. coli 0157:H7)*
Guillain-Barre' syndrome: *Campylobacter jejuni*
HUS/TTP: EHEC *(E. coli* 0157:H7), *Shigella*

Fried rice: *Bacillus cereus*
Poultry: *Campylobacter, Salmonella*
Lunchmeat: *Listeria*
Reactive arthritis: *Shigella, Salmonella, Yersina, Campylobacter*
Toxic Megacolon: *Shigella*

CLINICAL FEATURES OF INFECTIOUS DIARRHEA:

Small bowel:
Pathogens: *Salmonella, Vibrio Cholerae, ETEC, EPEC, Yersina, Rotavirus, Norwalk virus, Adenovirus, Giardia, Cryptosporidium*
Location of pain: Mid abdomen or diffuse
Volume of stool: Large
Type of stool: Watery
Fecal leukocytes: Rare
Other: Dehydration, malabsorption

Large bowel:
Pathogens: *Campylobacter, Salmonella, Shigella, Yersina, EIEC, EHEC, C. difficile, E.histolytica, CMV*
Location of pain: Lower abdomen or rectum
Volume of stool: Small
Type of stool: Mucoid/Blood
Fecal leukocytes: Common
Other: Tenesmus if proctitis

ACUTE INFECTIOUS DIARRHEA
- Cytotonic/Preformed toxins/Enterotoxin ("food poisoning"; typical onset <24 hrs):
  - **S. aureus, C. perfringens, B. cereus**
- Viral gastroenteritis is responsible for 75% of infectious diarrhea
  Often presents with nausea/vomiting without high fever, severe abdominal pain, or bloody diarrhea
  Brief/self-limiting
  Note: Alcohol hand gel does not prevent the spread of viruses (or *C. difficile* spores) - Must use old fashion soap and water
  - ***Rotovirus:*** most common worldwide, spread via fecal-oral; symptoms in 72 hrs and last 5 days; death from dehydration
  - ***Norwalk:*** outbreaks via contaminated food, water, person-to-person; symptoms in 48 hrs and last 3 days
- Non-Invasive Bacteria
  Cytotonic: toxin activation of intracellular enzymes: watery diarrhea; (No fecal WBC or Blood)
  - **Enterotoxigenic *E. coli* (ETEC):** travelers diarrhea; empiric antibiotics given for severe cases
  - **Enteropathogenic *E. coli* (EPEC):** pediatrics/infants; antibiotics effective although resistance to TMP-SMX is emerging
  - ***Vibrio cholera:*** can cause profuse diarrhea (up to 1liter/hr) and vomiting, leading to hypotension, renal failure, death
    - Stool is described as 'rice water': water with mucus flecks; Need IV hydration with electrolyte repletion; Treated with tetracycline, doxycycline, TMP-SMX, or erythromycin

CHAPTER 2.13 DIARRHEAL INFECTIONS

Cytotoxic: toxins cause structural injury: mucosal inflammation and bleeding; (+ fecal WBC (inflammatory) and blood)
- **Enterohemorrhagic *E. coli* 0157:H7 (EHEC):** watery turned bloody and typically NO fever; easily killed with heat/cooking
  - Can cause ischemic colitis via initiation of coagulation cascade; Some diagnosed ischemic colitis likely represent EHEC; Need contact isolation and personal contacts should be tested for EHEC; Can lead to HUS with antibiotics
- ***C. difficile,*** consider with any recent hospitalization or antibiotic use! *See also Bowel- Clostridium Difficile (Chapter 2.07)*

■ Invasive Bacteria (+ fecal WBC and blood)
- **Campylobacter:** most common U.S. infectious diarrhea cause; watery to bloody lasting 7 days; Complication: HUS, Guillain-Barre
  - Most don't need antibiotics; indicated with symptoms >7 days or pregnancy: erythromycin (early) or fluoroquinolones (late)

- **Salmonella:** range from gastroenteritis (watery to bloody) to typhoid fever; RLQ pain (ileal location of infection)
  - Also carried in pets/reptiles or people; Risk with multiple systemic conditions (HIV, Leukemia, Sickle cell)
  - Risk is five F's: Flies, Food, Fingers, Feces, Fomites
  - Do not treat with antibiotics unless severe, neonates, elderly, immunosuppressed or prostheses

- **Shigella:** person-to-person spread or contaminated water/food; Respiratory and seizures (children) complaints common
  - Complications include difficult to distinguish from IBD and arthritis in HLA B27 patients
  - Antibiotics decrease duration/mortality: fluoroquinolones (Cipro), TMP-SMX, or ampicillin for 5 days

- **Enteroinvasive *E. coli* (EIEC):** fever, abdominal pain, watery turned bloody with leukocytes (i.e. dysentery) in 10%
  - Resistance to TMP-SMX is common, but not to fluoroquinolones

- ***Vibrio parahemolyticus:*** watery turned bloody; lasts 2–5 days and antibiotics usually not necessary

- **Yersinia:** Infection occurs in terminal ileum; Many animals harbor the organism; Complications: rash, arthritis, hemochromatosis
  - Antibiotics of no benefit, unless severe, bacteremia, or distant infections
  - Yersina ileocolitis can simulate Crohn's and RLQ tenderness and lymphadenitis can simulate appendicitis

- **Others:** *Aeromonas, Plesiomonas* (both are water borne, such as with shellfish)
  - Self limited diarrhea can cause colitis and mimic UC (or trigger it?); Treat if severe

■ Parasites (erratic shedding, need 3 collections for O&P for best chance of detection)
- **Giardia:** acquired by water (lakes/streams) or person-to-person (daycare); organism attaches to small bowel and damage mucosa
  - Symptoms of watery diarrhea, cramps, nausea, bloating; Treatment with metronidazole 250 mg TID for 5–7 days

- ***Entamoeba histolytica:*** most common cause of dysentery in world; Acquired via ingestion contaminated food/water
  - Symptoms in 7–21 days: bloody diarrhea, pain, fever, tenesmus; Check PCR for DNA with stool samples
  - Ulcers vary from mild to severe with undermined edges leading to 'flask-shaped' ulcer
  - Can penetrate bowel wall and enter portal circulation and cause liver abscess
  - Most (90%) are asymptomatic carriers and still need treatment
  - Treatment is metronidazole 750 mg TID for 7–10 days

- **Cryptosporidia:** waterborne organism causing watery diarrhea
  - Treatment is nitazoxanide for 14 days

■ Opportunistic:
- ***Cryptosporidia, Isospora, Microsporidia, Cyclospora, MAC, CMV***

CHRONIC INFECTIONS DIARRHEA
- *Giardia, E. hystolytica, C. difficile,* **Opportunistic** organisms above

TIPS ON TREATING INFECTIOUS DIARRHEA:
- Antibiotics are most helpful if given within 3 days of illness to shorten duration:
  - When to prescribe: Moderate/Severe illness, High fever (>39°), Dysentery (bloody mucoid), Immunosuppressed
  - Fluoroquinolones are generally drug of choice

FOOD POISONING:

Symptoms	Incubation	Possible Agents
Acute nausea, vomiting	6 hr	Preformed toxins of *Staphylococcus aureus, Bacillus cereus*
Watery diarrhea	6-72 hrs	*C. perfringens, B. cereus, ETEC, V. cholerae, Giardia*
Inflammatory ileocolitis (dysentery)	16-72hrs	*Salmonella, Shigella, Campylobacter, EIEC, EHEC, V. parahaemolyticus, Yersina*

TRAVELER'S DIARRHEA:
- 80-90% bacterial, 10-20% parasites/viruses/toxins
  - Small intestine (ETEC) 40-60%; Colon invasive bacteria *(Campylobacter, Salmonella, Shigella, Aeromonas)* 15-30%; Unknown 20%
- Symptoms: watery diarrhea, bloating, fatigue
- Bloody diarrhea and fever are uncommon (these suggest invasive organism and need for prompt evaluation)
- Prophylaxis:
  - Bismuth (2 Tabs QID)
  - Probiotics: *S. boulardii, Lactobacillus*
  - Antibiotics: ? if worth cost and resistant bugs
- Treatment:
  - Rehydration, antidiarrheals or bismuth
  - Rifaximin (Xifaxan) 200 mg po TID × 3 days
  - Fluoroquinolone (Cipro 500 mg daily), resistance with TMP-SMX
  - Persistence: Antigiardial treatment ± further evaluation with endoscopy
- Persistent travelers diarrhea: Giardia, Ameba, Salmonella, Yersina, Unmasked celiac sprue, Bacterial overgrowth, Post-infectious IBS

ORAL SOLUTIONS:
- In the diarrhea state, there is a net efflux of sodium; Oral solutions containing glucose allow small bowel to reabsorb glucose *with* sodium
  - Solutions containing too much or too little glucose can work in detrimental ways
  - Many sports drinks, ginger ale, apple juice and chicken broth have too little or too much sodium and too high an osmolality
  - Rice water (boiling rice and drinking water after cooling) has nearly the right concentrations of sodium/glucose for rehydration

NOTES

2.14 DIVERTICULOSIS & DIVERTICULITIS

(Am J Gastroenterol 1999;94:3110-21)

DIVERTICULOSIS

Definition:
- Acquired herniations of mucosa and submucosa through the colonic wall

Epidemiology:
- Affects 5-15% of persons over the age of 45 and 65-80% of persons over the age of 80

Pathophysiology:
- May be a consequence of a low-fiber diet » decreased stool volume » colonic mucosa contracting against small, hard stools » greater intraluminal pressure » each diverticula is a result of herniation of mucosa through a point of weakness at the muscular colonic wall
- More common on **Left side** than on right side of colon (descending and sigmoid)
- Western diets high in refined carbohydrates and low in dietary fiber may be a contributor
- Western style toilets result in increased intraluminal pressures, compared to knee-chest position (3rd world countries)

Clinical Manifestations/Physical Exam:
- Usually asymptomatic
  - Can be complicated by diverticulitis (20%) or bleeding (2nd most common colonic bleed source after vascular lesions)
- If symptoms such as abdominal pain and altered bowel habits, consider IBS (avoid the term "painful diverticulosis")

Diagnostic Studies:
- Sigmoidoscopy/Colonoscopy
- Barium enema: demonstrate diverticula, but not inflammation

Treatments:
- High fiber diet and antispasmotics are unproven, but commonly prescribed and probably the best treatment to date
- Little evidence supports the advice of refraining from certain foods such as seeds and nuts (actually eliminates many high fiber foods)

Complications:
- Majority remain asymptomatic; complications of diverticular bleeding: 3-5%; *See also GI Bleed-Diverticular Bleeding (Chapter 6.02)*

DIVERTICULITIS

Definition:
- Inflammation of diverticula
- Classification stage: I. Small confined pericolonic abscesses
  - II. Larger confined pericolonic abscess
  - III. Generalized suppurative peritonitis (perforated diverticulitis) but obstructing fecolith doesn't allow feces contamination
  - IV. Fecal peritonitis

Epidemiology:
- Approximately 20% of patients with diverticula have an episode of symptomatic diverticulitis

Etiologies:
- DDX elderly: ischemia, carcinoma, volvulus, obstruction, penetrating ulcer, nephrolithiasis/urosepsis, *C. difficile*
- DDX middle-age/younger: appendicitis, salpingitis, IBD, penetrating ulcer, urosepsis

Pathophysiology:
- Retention of undigested food and bacteria in diverticulum » fecalith formation » obstruction » compromise of diverticulum's blood supply, infection, perforation
- Microperforation (localized infection) or Macroperforation (abscess and/or peritonitis)
- Histologically diverticulitis is not accompanied by mucosal inflammation

CHAPTER 2.14 DIVERTICULOSIS & DIVERTICULITIS

Clinical Manifestations/Physical Exam:
- Note, in elderly and patients on steroids, abdominal exam and usual signs are unreliable
- Abrupt **LLQ abdominal pain, fever,** nausea, vomiting, altered bowels: diarrhea > constipation
- Mild: **LLQ tenderness, ± palpable mass** (from phlegmonous reaction), ± positive FOBT
- Diverticuli in other colic sites can mimic other diseases such as Transverse colon: PUD; Right colon: appendicitis
- Clues:
  - Dysuria, urinary frequency and urgency reflect bladder irritation
  - Pneumaturia, fecaluria, or recurrent UTIs suggest colovesical fistula
- Ruptured peridiverticular abscess or uninflamed diverticulum causes peritonitis and septic shock
  - Most commonly in elderly and immunosuppressed; High mortality

Laboratory Studies:
- **Leukocytosis** (along with fever, help distinguish from the spasm of IBS)

Diagnostic Studies:
- Plain abdominal radiographs to rule out free air, ileus, or obstruction/mass effect
- Abdominal CT may show thickening of bowel wall (falsely negative in 20%): **Preferred imaging modality**
  - Consider in cases with: palpable mass/suspect pericolic abscess, clinical toxicity, failure of medical therapy, corticosteroid use
- Sigmoidoscopy/Colonoscopy *relative* contraindication in acute setting because of increased risk for overt perforation; Sometime must be done
  - Exclude perforation and examine when in doubt (rectal bleeding): exclude ischemic bowel, Crohn's, carcinoma
  - Colonoscopy recommended 2–6 weeks after resolution to rule out neoplasm
- Contrast enema: mild-moderate cases when diagnosis is in doubt, water-soluble contrast; Otherwise delay for 6–8 weeks

Treatments:
- Mild (outpatient):
  - Oral antibiotics (GNB/Anaerobes): TMP-SMX & Metronidazole with liquid diet × 7–10 days; Cipro or Cephalexin may be substituted for TMP-SMX
- Severe (inpatient):
  - NPO, IVF, Ng if ileus, CT abdomen
  - IV antibiotics (GNR: *E. coli, Klebsiella, Pseudomonas* & Anerobic: *B.fragilis, Clostridium*): Cefotetan/Metronidazole or Ampicillin/Gentamycin/Metronidazole or Cipro/Metronidazole
  - Pain control: meperidine is preferred to morphine sulfate (which causes colonic spasm)
- Abscess drainage percutaneously or surgically
- Surgery if medical therapy fails: perforation/peritonitis/abscess/sepsis, fistula, obstruction, recurrent disease (≥2 episodes)

Complications:
- Fistula (bowel, bladder, skin, vagina): most common colovesicular fistula, often have pneumaturia, reflux of contrast on enema = surgery
- Stricture: usually longer, 3–6 cm and smooth contours (Malignant <3 cm with abrupt shoulders on each end, IBD/Ischemia 6–10 cm)
- Other: abscess, obstruction, peritonitis from perforation

2.15 FECAL INCONTINENCE

(Am J Gastroenterol 2004;99:1585-04)

DEFINITION:
- Continuous or recurrent uncontrolled passage of fecal material (>10 mL) for at least one month in an individual older than 3 or 4 years old
- Considering definitions used among various studies, it is reasonable to divide fecal incontinence into major and minor:
  - Minor incontinence is the inadvertent escape of flatus or partial soiling of undergarments with liquid stool
  - Major incontinence is the involuntary excretion of feces

EPIDEMIOLOGY:
- Prevalence estimated between 11-15% of community-dwelling adults and up to 40% among nursing home residents
- Often mistaken as 'diarrhea'; A detailed history of diarrhea should include questions about fecal incontinence

ETIOLOGIES:
- Anal sphincter injury (i.e. obstetrical trauma or post surgical)
- Neurological (Multiple sclerosis, Parkinson's, Alzheimer's, Stroke, Diabetic neuropathy, Cauda equine)
- Pudendal nerve injury/neuropathy (may be due to obstetric trauma, or severe constipation resulting in the nerve being stretched)
- Other: perianal sepsis, systemic scleroisis (fibrosis of internal anal sphincter), radiation proctitis (stiff rectum overwhelms normal continence)

PATHOPHYSIOLOGY:
- Physiology of defecation: Begins with colonic high-amplitude propagated contraction » Rectal distention: » Desire to defecate:
  - » Involuntary: Internal sphincter relaxation
  - » Voluntary: Suitable posture, Raise intra-abdominal pressure, Relaxation of puborectalis and external sphincter:
    - » Fecal expulsion
- Passive incontinence: involuntary leak, aware only after the leak: lower resting pressures of anal sphincters
- Urge incontinence: can't get to restroom in time, brief warning: decreased squeeze pressures and durations
- Rectal Seepage: involuntary seepage, otherwise normal
- Nocturnal incontinence: occurs in patients with diabetes or scleroderma: suggest internal sphincter weakness

CLINICAL MANIFESTATIONS/PHYSICAL EXAM:
- History of Obstetrics with forceps = higher prevalence
- Associated urinary incontinence = damage to pelvic floor
- Rectal exam: feel for resting and squeeze tone, test for anal wink, inspect for prolapsing hemorrhoids or other obvious pathology

LABORATORY STUDIES:
- Not helpful

DIAGNOSTIC STUDIES:
- Proposed workup: History, Exam, Clinical grading:
  - Suspected prolapse » Clinically confirmed: Surgery (If not clinically confirmed, consider defography/pelvic MRI to confirm)
  - Local anorectal problems » Appropriate treatment
  - Diarrhea with incontinence » Flex Sig/Colonoscopy/Barium enema/Metabolic profile
    - If negative treat with Loperamide or others » If no improvement, follow Obstetric/Surgical/Neurological Injury route

- Obstetric/Surgical/Neurological Injury » Anorectal Manometry (Gastro 1999;116:732–60) and Anal U/S
  ± Balloon expulsion test
  ± PNTML (Pudendal Nerve Terminal Latency)
  * Normal » ? Fictitious
  * Weak Sphincter/Defect & normal PNTML » Surgery and Biofeedback
  * Weak Sphincter/Defect & abnormal PNTML » Biofeedback or Colostomy
  * Impaired Sensation » Biofeedback
  * Dyssynergic Defecation ± Impaired Evacuation » Biofeedback to improve dyssynergia

TREATMENTS:
- As above under Diagnostic Studies
- Treat underlying cause: i.e. diarrhea, colitis
- Diet: increase fiber (bulking agent) in some and reduce in others (decreases work of colon), lactose, decrease caffeine intake
- Medications: Loperamide, Lomotil, Cholestyramine, Estrogen, Codeine
- Biofeedback: strengthen anal sphincters
- Surgery

COMPLICATIONS:
- Can be one of the most devastating of all physical disabilities because it can affect self-confidence and lead to social isolation

PROGNOSIS:
- Surgical Sphincteroplasty: ? long term outcome

2.16 GI ENDOCRINE TUMORS

GENERAL:
- Most are classified as functional or non-functional depending if the clinical syndrome is due to a hormone release
  - Non-functioning tumors are generally reported as incidental finding during surgery or autopsy
- GI endocrine tumors are uncommon; **Most to least common:** carcinoid, gastrinomas, insulinomas, VIPoma, glucagonoma, somatostatinoma
- Their origin is thought to be from endodermal stem cells of the neuroendocrine system; most are slow growing
- Detection of tumors is difficult: <1 cm have a detection rate of <10% and >3 cm have a detection rate of ~50%
  - Any imaging modality (CT, U/S, MRI) detect <40% of all tumors
- Somatostatin receptors are present in: 90% of Gastrinomas, VIPomas, Glucagonomas, Somatostatinomas; >75% Carcinoids
  - This is the basis for radiolabeled somatostatin analoge (i.e. octreotide) scintigraphy or octreotide scanning (except with Insulinomas)
  - This is also the basis of therapy to alleviate symptoms and slow tumor growth
- These tumors may occur in sporadic (nonfamilial) form or as part of MEN Syndrome Type 1 (pituitary, parathyroid, pancreas)

CARCINOID TUMORS: *See Bowel- Carcinoid Tumors (Chapter 2.08)*

ZOLLINGER-ELLISON SYNDROME (GASTRINOMA): *See Esophagus/Gastric- ZES (Chapter 1.23)*

INSULINOMA
Definition:
- Insulin secreting tumors that cause symptoms of hypoglycemia (almost always originate in the beta-cells of the pancreas)

Epidemiology:
- Patients are typically (60%) female and age range from 20–75 years

Pathophysiology:
- Beta-cell tumors that arise in or adjacent to the pancreas; Mostly are solitary (2% multiple) and arise evenly in head, body, tail
- Should raise the question of MEN-1

Clinical Manifestations/Physical Exam:
- Signs and symptoms of hypoglycemia, including neurological manifestations ("neuroglycopenic symptoms"): confusion, diplopia, dizziness
- Catecholamine-mediated (from hypoglycemia): anxiety, weakness, fatigue, headache, palpitations, sweating especially during fasting
- Weight gain in 40% because patients learn to eat to control the symptoms
- If you don't think about symptoms and the possibility of an Insulinoma, you won't diagnose it (25% are not diagnosed for 3 years)

Laboratory Studies:
- Fasting glucose and insulin levels (See Diagnostic Sudies below)
- Possibly:
  - Sulfonylurea levels
  - Antibodies to insulin
  - C-peptide: exogenous insulin has no C-peptide, so Insulinoma patients have high or normal C-peptide levels
  - Plasma proinsulin levels: in most patients with Insulinomas, proinsulin comprises more than 20% of the circulating insulin

Diagnostic Studies:
- Combination of: low fasting glucose level and inappropriately high plasma insulin level (Only 65% of patients present with these findings)
  - If negative and diagnosis still considered: 72-hour fast with blood glucose and insulin levels, including when symptoms develop
    - Test is positive in 75% of patients in 24 hours and virtually 100% in 72 hours
- Caution: other causes of hypoglycemia need to be excluded: exogenous insulin use, sulfonylurea use, autoantibodies to insulin
- CT scan: most tumors are small, so detection is 50%
- EUS: detects 80–90%
- MRI: detects liver metastases in 80%, which is important for determining candidacy for surgical resection
- Other:
  - Angiography with venous sampling for insulin has a sensitivity of 80%
  - Octreotide scanning: 50% detection due to the lower level of somatostatin receptors on Insulinomas

Treatments:
- Reverse hypoglycemic symptoms: Octreotide inhibits insulin secretion in the short term
  - Diazoxide inhibits insulin release and enhances glycogenolysis (effective 60%); Treatment of choice for those with metastases
- Surgical resection: definitive treatment and best option in those without metastases; Cure in 70–95%
  - If no tumor found upon exploration, then stepwise distal pancreatectomy is performed until frozen section indicates tumor removal
  - If pathology indicates still no tumor, then 80% pancreatectomy is performed to preserve endocrine/exocrine function
- Chemotherapy is an option for some with metastases, along with symptoms control as above

Prognosis:
- Malignancy occurs in 5–10% and frequently have metastasized to liver at time of diagnosis

VIPOMA

Definition:
- The production of VIP caused by a neuroendocrine tumor typically located in the pancreas
- VIPoma Syndrome ("Verner-Morrison or WDHA Syndrome") characterized by: severe Watery Diarrhea, Hypokalemia, & Achlorhydria (WDHA)
  - Other tumors (carcinoid, pheochromocytoma) may produce VIP, but rarely cause the syndrome

Pathophysiology:
- Most (90%) of VIPomas are pancreatic tumors: solitary, non-B islet cell, occur in the tail (75%)
- VIP induces intestinal water and chloride secretion and inhibits gastric acid secretion

Clinical Manifestations/Physical Exam:
- Severe secretory (persists despite fasting) diarrhea and dehydration
  - Stool volume exceeds 1 L/day in all and 3 L/day in most (75% of patients); Resembles cholera
- Erythematous flushing of head and trunk in 20%
- Hyperglycemia in 30%: VIP and Hypokalemia induced glycogenolysis in the liver

Laboratory Studies:
- Low K (frequently <2.5 mEq/L)
- Increased plasma level of VIP

Diagnostic Studies:
- CT or MRI to localize tumor and assess for metastases
- EUS and Octreotide scanning may have role

Treatments:
- Correct dehydration and electrolyte abnormalities: IVF of 5 L/day and aggressive replacement of potassium may be needed
- Octreotide controls diarrhea in 90% and is the treatment of choice
  - Steroids may be necessary or tried to control diarrhea
- Surgery relieves symptoms and is a cure in 30%
- Metastatic disease: chemotherapy and hepatic artery embolization

Prognosis:
- Malignancy occurs in 75% and 50% have metastasized to liver at time of diagnosis

SECTION II SMALL BOWEL/COLON/RECTUM

GLUCAGONOMA

Definition:
- A rare pancreatic alpha-cell tumor that over produce glucagons resulting in a syndrome of dermatitis, glucose intolerance, weight loss, anemia

Epidemiology:
- Most patients are middle to late age (45–70 years)

Pathophysiology:
- A pancreatic alpha-cell tumor that is solitary and large (most are 5–6 cm at time of diagnosis); Most (65%) occur in head of pancreas
- Glucagon stimulates glycogenolysis, gluconeogenesis, lipolysis, ketogenesis, and insulin secretion
  - Inhibits pancreatic and gastric secretions and intestinal motility

Clinical Manifestations/Physical Exam:
- Dermatitis: "necrolytic migratory erythema"; usually develops 7 years before diagnosis starting in intertriginous areas (groin, buttocks, thighs)
  - Erythematous lesions spread laterally becoming raised with superficial central blistering or bullous formation; Crusting after rupture
  - A sequence that waxes and wanes of erythema, bullous formation, epidermal separation, crusting, hyperpigmentation
- Glucose intolerance or DM: weight loss from the catabolic effect of glucagons
- Other: glossitis, angular stomatitis, dystrophic nails, hair thinning, risk of thromboembolic disease (25%) and severe diarrhea (15%)

Laboratory Studies:
- Plasma glucagons level >1000 pg/mL
- High glucagon level (but <500 pg/mL)
  - DDX: CRF, ESLD, septicemia, DKA, severe burns, prolonged starvation, acromegally, pancreatitis

Diagnostic Studies:
- CT of abdomen to localize tumor

Treatments:
- Nutrition support and control of hyperglycemia
- Octreotide controls symptoms: dermatitis, weight loss, diarrhea, abdominal pain (not diabetes)
- Surgery for non-metastatic disease (but cure is only 20%); Risk of thromboemoblic disease is high
- Metastatic disease: no clear evidence that supports the use of chemotherapy

Prognosis:
- Metastases in 75% at time of diagnosis (liver, bone, mesentery)

SOMATOSTATINOMA

Definition:
- A tumor producing somatostatin giving rise to a syndrome of diabetes, gallbladder disease, and steatorrhea

Epidemiology:
- Very rare entity occurring in middle age patients (40–60 years) and many are found incidentally during surgery for gallbladder disease

Pathophysiology:
- Occur in the endocrine pancreas (delta-cells): 60%; Duodenum or jejunum: 40%; Most are large solitary tumors
- Somatostatin inhibits insulin release, gallbladder motility, and secretion of pancreatic enzymes and bicarbonate
  - Other tumors that secrete somatostatin: small cell lung cancer, medullary thyroid carcinoma, pheochromocytomas, paragangliomas
- These tumors are NOT associated with MEN-I; Possibly associated with MEN-2B (found in some with pheochromocytoma, neurofibromatosis)

Clinical Manifestations/Physical Exam:
- More common symptoms with pancreatic tumors (they have higher levels of somatostatin)
  - Diabetes: 50%, Gallbladder: 65% (cholelithiasis, acalculous cholecystitis, obstructive jaundice/tumor invasion), Steatorrhea 35%

Diagnostic Studies:
- CT of abdomen to localize tumor

Treatments:
- Correct any nutritional deficiencies and diabetic control (typically mild so responds to oral hypoglycemic agents or low dose insulin)
- Surgery is curative, but 85% present with metastatic disease
- Metastatic disease: no clear evidence that supports the use of chemotherapy

Prognosis:
- Metastases in 85% at time of diagnosis

2.17 IRRITABLE BOWEL SYNDROME (IBS)

(Gastroenterology 2006;130:1480-91 & 2002;123:2105-07 & 2108-31)

DEFINITION:
- A group of functional bowel disorders which abdominal discomfort or pain is associated with defecation or change in bowel habits, and with features of disordered defecation; As of now, no specific discriminatory findings or diagnostic tests for IBS
    - Subtypes: Constipation predominant, Diarrhea predominant, Alternating between constipation and diarrhea
    - Hallmark symptoms (not otherwise explained by other structural or biochemical abnormalities):
        - Lower abdominal pain/discomfort
        - Altered bowel function (urgency, altered stool consistency or frequency, incomplete evaluation)
        - Bloating
    - Disease severity (less than 5% considered Severe)

Clinical	Mild	Moderate	Severe
Constant symptoms	0	+	+++
Healthcare use	+	++	+++
Illness behavior	0	+	+++
Psychiatric diagnosis	0	+	+++

- Chronic continuous diarrhea in the absence of pain is not IBS, although it may be functional in nature

EPIDEMIOLOGY:
- Up to 20% of U.S. population reports symptoms of IBS; Most common GI diagnosis; Affects predominantly women (~70%)
- Fewer than 25% seek medical evaluation and treatment for their symptoms
- IBS patients are more likely to see other physicians frequently or undergo surgery than non-IBS patients
- Economic impact: 2 billion in direct healthcare costs per year and 20 billion in indirect costs (loss of work & school)

ETIOLOGIES:
- The effect of stress on gut function is universal, and patients with IBS appear to have greater reactivity to stress compared to healthy patients
    - In other words, IBS patients appear to have lower visceral pain threshold
- Differential diagnosis:
    - Malabsorption (celiac, postgastrectomy, pancreatic insufficiency); Dietary factors (lactose intolerance, caffeine/alcohol, fatty foods)
    - Infection/bacterial overgrowth (bacterial/*campylobacter*, parasites/*giardia*); IBD; Psychological (panic disorder, depression, somatization)
    - Gynecological disorders (endometriosis); Other (GI endocrine tumors, HIV-associated infections)
- Bloating differential diagnosis:
    Lactose intake, carbonated drinks, bulking agents (Metamucil), bacterial overgrowth, constipation

PATHOPHYSIOLOGY:
- Evolution of thought process (1950's to 2000's)
    - Abnormal gut motility » Visceral hypersensitivity » Brain-gut interaction » 5HT mediated sensitivity
- Enteric Nervous System, like CNS, has integrated circuits for program library, feedback, reflexes, information processing
    - Disregulation of CNS-ENS interaction: visceral hypersensitivy and abnormal colonic motility (hallmarks of functional GI disorders)
- Serotonin (5HT - neurotransmitter in both gut/brain at every level) has role in mediating visceral hypersensitivity and the peristaltic reflex
    - 95% of 5HT is found in gut, with 90% localized within enterochromaffin cells of the mucosa
    - IBS patients have higher post-prandial levels and they remain higher for longer periods of time
- Post-infectious: IBS may be a shift in host-gut microbial relationships: ? if IBS leads to gastroenteritis, or gastroenteritis leads to IBS
    - IBS patients may develop symptoms after an acute episode of bacterial gastroenteritis
    - IBS, on the other hand, may predispose patients to bacterial gastroenteritis
- Some believe there may be an association between IBS and Celiac disease and serologic studies should be recommended for IBS patients

CHAPTER 2.17 IRRITABLE BOWEL SYNDROME (IBS)

CLINICAL MANIFESTATIONS/PHYSICAL EXAM:
- Rome III Criteria: Subtyping IBS by predominant stool pattern
  Constipation predominant (IBS-C): hard or lumpy stools ≥25% of bowel movements and loose (mushy) or watery stools <25% of bowel movements
  Diarrhea predominant (IBS-D): loose (mushy) or watery stools ≥25% of bowel movements and hard or lumpy stools <25% of bowel movements
  Mixed predominant (IBS-M): hard or lumpy stools ≥25% of bowel movements and loose (mushy) or watery stools ≥25% of bowel movements
  Unsubtyped IBS: insufficient abnormality of stool consistency to meet criteria for IBS-C, IBS-D, or IBS-M

- Postinfectious IBS: acute onset of symptoms after a bout of gastroenteritis (30% IBS patients report this phenomenon)
  - 50% recover within 6 years

LABORATORY STUDIES:
- Rule out anatomic disorders; screening:
  - CBC, Chemistry panel including LFTs, ESR, TSH, FOBT, Stool O&P, Celiac panel (especially with diarrhea predominant)
  - Additional studies based on presenting symptoms (See Diagnostic Studies below)

DIAGNOSTIC STUDIES:
- **Rome III:** Recurrent abdominal pain or discomfort at least 3 days per month in the last 3 months associated with 2 or more of the following:
  - Improvement with defecation
  - Onset associated with change in frequency of stool
  - Onset associated with a change in form (appearance) of stool
    (Discomfort means an uncomfortable sensation not described as pain)

- **Red Flags** (symptoms not typical of IBS and should prompt an evaluation for organic disease):
  - Anemia, Fever, Persistent diarrhea, Severe constipation, Rectal bleeding, Weight loss
  - Nocturnal symptoms (pain/bowel function), Family history of GI cancer/IBD/Celiac, New onset of symptoms >50 yrs old

- Algorithm: Identify symptoms of IBS and eliminate alarm symptoms/signs (Rome III & Alarm symptoms criteria) »
  Do physical and limited series of initial lab tests to exclude structural, metabolic, infectious disease (as above under Laboratory Studies)
  Make a confident diagnosis: IBS-C; IBS-D; IBS-M; Pain/Gas/Bloating

  - IBS-C: Trial of fiber/increased roughage (bulking agents), Osmotic laxative »
    * If no response:
      * Infrequent BM: Colonic transit study
      * Obstructive symptoms: Anorectal motility/sensory/balloon expulsion test, Defecography/Pelvic MRI

  - IBS-D: Loperamide(Imodium)/Lomotil » (Always ask about incontinence, this may simply be fecal incontinence) »
    * If no response:
      * Lactose/Bacterial overgrowth testing, Stool for giardia/fat/osmolality, Celiac antibodies, Biopsy of small bowel, large bowel (microscopic colitis)

  - Pain/Gas/Bloating: Anticholinergic, Antidepressant, Psychological treatment »
    * If no response:
      * Plain X-ray of abdomen during exacerbation, Small bowel follow through, CT/MR, Pelvic ultrasound

  - Initiate treatment plan for your diagnosis: IBS-C; IBS-D; IBS-M; Pain/Gas/Bleeding »
    * Follow up 3–6 weeks

SECTION II SMALL BOWEL/COLON/RECTUM

TREATMENTS:
- Outcomes in IBS patients can be improved when physicians:
  - Establish long-term relationship with a positive diagnosis: patients need validation of symptoms *after* a physical exam or evaluation
    - Actively listen to concerns; respond to patient concerns and expectations
  - Set realistic goals: Patients need to know what they can expect; *IBS can be managed, not cured*
  - Provide Explanation:
    - Intestines overreact to variety of stimuli (food/hormones/medications/stress) which produce spasm/enhanced sensitivity
    - Identify behavior stressors that exacerbate symptoms
- Treatment (general):
  Constipation » laxatives/bulking agents; Diarrhea » anti-diarrheals; Pain » anti-spasmatics; Failure » psychiatric/psychotropics
- Laxatives & Bulking agents: symptomatic treatment of constipation
  - Osmotic laxatives ($MgSO_4$ 2–4 tbsp/day, Lactulose 10–20 g/BID, Polyethylene glycol 17 g in 8 oz water daily)
  - Stimulant laxatives (Bisacodyl/Dulcolax)
  - Fiber: supplement 20–30 gm per day; accelerates colonic transit, decreases intracolonic pressure, does not reduce contractility (some laxatives and bulking agents can exacerbate abdominal pain and bloating) *See also Bowel- Constipation (Chapter 2.11)*
- Antidiarrheals: symptomatic treatment of diarrhea
  (Slows intestinal transit and enhances intestinal water and ion absorption resulting in increased stool consistency & decreased stool frequency)
  - Loperamide (Imodium) does not cross blood-brain barrier; 2–4 mg prn (maximum 12/day)
  - Several other options: *See also Bowel- Diarrhea/Malassimilation (Chapter 2.12)*
- Antispasmotics: symptomatic treatment of abdominal pain; Caution in elderly patients due to anti-cholinergic effects
  (Smooth-muscle relaxants via anticholinergic effects and/or direct action on smooth muscle)
  - Dicyclomine HCL (Bentyl)
  - Hyoscyamine sulfate (Short acting: NuLev, Levsin, Anaspaz; Long acting: Levbid)
  - Chlordiazepoxide/Clidinium (Librax): often works well for men or younger patients
- Serotonin modulators
  - 5HT3 antagonist (Alosetron/Lotronex): For diarrhea predominant: decreased small bowel and colon transit, decreased small bowel secretions
    - 0.5–1 mg BID; restricted approved for women only
    - Side effects: ischemic colitis (withdrawn from market 2000 for ischemic colitis, returned with restricted use 2002)
  - 5HT3 agonist (Tegaserod/Zelnorm): For constipation predominant: ↑ peristalsis, ↑ small bowel secretions
    - 6 mg BID; for women only; commonly used in TID dosing unless diarrhea then QD or BID
    - Side effects: diarrhea and headache (FDA restricted 2007)
- Psychotropic agents: (Gut 2005;54:1332–41)
  Can have neuromodulatory and analgesic properties, especially in gut; potential benefit even in absence of psychiatric co-morbidity
  Most common mistake is not increasing dose 10–25 mg q 7 days prn; treatment continued for 6–12 months before tapering
  Benefit occurs no sooner than 3–4 weeks and side effects, if they occur, usually tend to diminish in 1–2 weeks
  - TCAs: offer benefit for abdominal pain and diarrhea ± depression (if older, get baseline EKG to make sure QTC is not >450 msec)
    Amitriptyline start at 25 mg qhs (max 300 mg/day for depression) or Nortriptyline start at 10 mg qhs (max 150 mg/day for depression)
    Imipramine start at 25 mg qhs (max 300 mg/day for depression) or Desipramine start at 10 mg qhs (max 300 mg/day for depression)
  - SSRIs: offer benefit for constipation predominant (can cause diarrhea) ± depression/panic/anxiety/OCD; begin with small dose and increase PRN; SSRIs don't offer pain relief like TCAs

CHAPTER 2.17 IRRITABLE BOWEL SYNDROME (IBS)

- Psychological treatments:
  - Cognitive behavior therapy: attempts to change way patients perceive/react to symptoms, use of diaries, increases control over symptoms
  - Interpersonal psychotherapy: Identifies and addresses difficulties in relationships
  - Hypnosis: Suggestions are used to reduce gut sensations
  - Relaxation training: uses imagery and relaxation techniques to reduce autonomic arousal and stimulate muscular relaxation

2.18 ISCHEMIC COLITIS

(Gastroenterology 2000;118:951–53 & 954–68)

DEFINITION:
- The most common form of intestinal ischemic injury

EPIDEMIOLOGY:
- Most are older than 60; The incidence is underestimated because many suffer only mild or transient damage and don't seek medical attention

ETIOLOGIES:
- Usually a **non-occlusive** low-flow state or thrombosis of IMA; Often times there is a low cardiac output ± high doses of vasoconstrictors
  - Risk factors: post-op valve surgery, hemodialysis with hypotensive episodes
  - **Often no recognizable cause**
- Can result from alterations in systemic circulation or anatomic or functional changes in the local mesenteric vasculature
  - Risk factors: older age, vasculitidies, sickle cell, cocaine use, infection, long distance runners; Rarely embolus, hypercoagulable states
- **DDX:** perforated viscus, small bowel obstruction, cecal volvulus, incarcerated hernia, dissecting aortic aneurysm, pancreatitis/cholecystitis
  - Often confused with IBD or gastrointestinal infections (*CMV, E. coli, C. difficile*)

PATHOPHYSIOLOGY:
- Mesenteric circulation (or splanchnic circulation):
  - Inflow with three major arteries: celiac axis (stomach, duodenum, spleen, liver), superior mesenteric artery or SMA (duodenum, entire small bowel, right colon), inferior mesenteric artery or IMA (left colon and rectum); Rectum also supplied by iliac arteries (dual supply)
    - Three major systemic-splanchnic collaterals anastomose major mesenteric arteries and their branches:
      Pancreaticoduodenal (Celiac-SMA), Arch of Riolan (SMA-IMA), Marginal Drummond (SMA-IMA)
  - Outflow with two major veins: superior mesenteric vein (SMV) and inferior mesenteric vein (IMV)
    - The SMV and splenic vein form the portal vein, which enters the liver hilum; The IMV and short gastric veins join the splenic vein
- "Watershed" areas (splenic flexure to sigmoid) are most susceptible; Rectum rarely involved due to dual blood supply (clue)
- Disease spectrum:
  - Reversible colopathy (35%), chronic ulcerating colitis (20%), transient colitis (15%), gangrene (15%), stricture (10%), fulminant colitis (<5%)

CLINICAL MANIFESTATIONS/PHYSICAL EXAM:
- Usually crampy LLQ pain associated with urge to defecate, subsequently passing guaiac positive or overtly bloody/maroon diarrhea
- Nausea, vomiting, tachycardia, and fever with abdominal distention or peritoneal signs should raise clinical suspicion for infarction

LABORATORY STUDIES:
- May be normal
- ↑ WBC ± left shift, AST, Amylase, LDH and CK
- Metabolic acidosis and ↑ lactate (late)

DIAGNOSTIC STUDIES:
- Imaging studies:
  - **Plain radiographs:** Important for secondary causes of ischemia and other causes of acute abdominal pain (obstruction/perforation)
    - Normal prior to infarction, followed by
      - **"Thumbprinting"** (submucosal hemorrhage/edema in bowel wall), bowel wall thickening & ileus in later stage disease
    - Pneumatosis intestinalis: air in bowel wall indicates usually pre- or actual bowel infarction (late finding)
    - SBO: dilated loops of bowel with/without air-fluid levels
    - Pancreatitis: sentinel loop of jejunum or colon cut off sign
    - Pneumobilia: air in biliary tree: emphysematous cholangitis or intra-abdominal sepsis caused by gas-forming bacteria
    - Perforation: free air under diaphragm
    - Some X-rays may show 'airless abdomen' due to spasming and air being squeezed out
- **Primary test:** Flex sig or Colonoscopy within 48 hrs if no peritonitis (to confirm KUB findings of thumbprinting)
  - Segmental colonic involvement: erythema, friability, ulceration, and/or necrosis
- Consider and exclude: GI infections, IBD, diverticulitis, pancreatitis
- Angiography often not needed (predisposing non-occlusive factors are not demonstrable once ischemic injury occurred)
  - Rarely angiography is needed for severe ischemic colitis or right-sided involvement which may or may not include the small bowel

TREATMENTS:
- Bowel rest, IVF & optimize cardiac function
  - Avoid vasoconstrictors, digitalis therapy, and vasopressors when possible if needed
- Broad spectrum Antibiotics (controversial), blood transfusions if needed
- Serial abdominal exams
- Surgery for infarction, fulminant colitis, or obstruction due to ischemic stricture

COMPLICATIONS:
- Strictures can occur as healing occurs (may require surgical correction)

PROGNOSIS:
- Resolution within 48 hrs with conservative measures occurs in over 50% of cases (healing without stricture in 1-2 weeks)
  - Severely injured colon may require 1-6 months to heal completely

2.19 ISCHEMIC SMALL BOWEL

(Gastroenterology 2000;118:951-53 & 954-68)

DEFINITION:
- Ischemic injury of the intestine resulting from deprivation of oxygen and nutrients necessary for cellular integrity

EPIDEMIOLOGY:
- Responsible for about 0.1% of admissions to tertiary care centers (or 1 per 1,000)

ETIOLOGIES:
- **SMA embolism (50%):** From left atrium or left ventricle
  - Risk factors: older age, atrial fibrillation, valvular disease, myxoma, CHF/low-flow states, MI, arrhythmias, angiography
- **SMA thrombosis** (15%): usually at the site of atherosclerosis which many times is at the origin of artery
  - Risk factors: older age, low-flow states (hypotension, arrhythmia, MI, CHF), atherosclerosis, hypercoagulable state, vasculitis
- **Mesenteric venous thrombosis** (5-10%): of which 95% occur in the SMV
  - Risk factors:
    - Hypercoagulable states (personal/family history, protein C & S deficiency, antiphospholipid, sickle cell)
    - Abdominal inflammation/infection (peritonitis, appendicitis, pancreatitis, diverticulitis, abscess, Crohn's, vasculitis, trauma)
    - Portal HTN/Cirrhosis, malignant obstruction
- **Non-occlusive mesenteric ischemia** (20%): Low cardiac output ± high doses of vasoconstrictors
  - Risk factors:
    - Low-flow states (CHF, MI, pulmonary edema, arrhythmia, shock, sepsis, pancreatitis, burns, hemorrhage)
    - Vasospasm (cocaine, digoxin)
    - Pre-existing disease (DM, Lipids, Vasculopathy, IBD)
- **Focal segmental ischemia of the small bowel** (5%): vascular occlusion to small segments of the small bowel
  - Risk factors: vasculitis, atheromatous emboli, strangulated hernias, radiation therapy
- **DDX:** perforated viscus, small bowel obstruction, cecal volvulus, incarcerated hernia, dissecting aortic aneurysm, pancreatitis/cholecystitis

PATHOPHYSIOLOGY:
- Mesenteric circulation (or splanchnic circulation):
  - Inflow with three major arteries: celiac axis (stomach, duodenum, spleen, liver), superior mesenteric artery or SMA (duodenum, entire small bowel, right colon), inferior mesenteric artery or IMA (left colon and rectum); Rectum also supplied by iliac arteries (dual supply)
    - Three major systemic-splanchnic collaterals anastomose major mesenteric arteries and their branches:
      Pancreaticoduodenal (Celiac-SMA), Arch of Riolan (SMA-IMA), Marginal Drummond (SMA-IMA)
  - Outflow with two major veins: superior mesenteric vein (SMV) and inferior mesenteric vein (IMV)
    - The SMV and splenic vein form the portal vein, which enters the liver hilum; The IMV and short gastric veins join the splenic vein

CLINICAL MANIFESTATIONS/PHYSICAL EXAM:
- Sudden onset of abdominal **pain out of proportion** to abdominal palpation/tenderness on exam
- Nonspecific complaints: fever, nausea, vomiting, abdominal distention, diarrhea
- "Intestinal angina" (usually seen with SMA thrombosis):
  - Postprandial abdominal pain & early satiety occurring weeks to months prior to the onset of acute pain; patients fear eating (sitophobia)
- Abdominal distention without pain (usually with non-occlusive disease)
- GI bleed (the right colon is supplied by the SMA where embolism and thrombosis predominate)
- As ischemia progresses ileus develops, bowel sounds diminish, and abdominal distention ensues
- Physical exam may be unremarkable/normal; Can mistake them for psychological cases; Ask yourself: are they at risk for ischemia?
- Peritoneal signs suggest possible bowel infarction

CHAPTER 2.19 ISCHEMIC SMALL BOWEL

LABORATORY STUDIES:
- May be normal
- ↑ WBC ± left shift, AST, Amylase, LDH and CK
- Metabolic acidosis and ↑ lactate (late finding)
- Bacteremia (i.e. *Bacteroides* with mesenteric venous thrombosis)
- + FOBT (65–75% of cases)

DIAGNOSTIC STUDIES:
- Imaging studies:
  - **Plain radiographs:** Important for secondary causes of ischemia and other causes of acute abdominal pain (obstruction/perforation)
    - Normal prior to infarction, followed by
      - **"Thumbprinting"** (submucosal hemorrhage/edema in bowel wall), bowel wall thickening & ileus in later stage disease
    - Pneumatosis intestinalis: air in bowel wall indicates usually pre- or actual bowel infarction (late finding)
    - SBO: dilated loops of bowel with/without air-fluid levels
    - Pancreatitis: sentinel loop of jejunum or colon cut off sign
    - Pneumobilia: air in biliary tree: emphysematous cholangitis or intra-abdominal sepsis caused by gas-forming bacteria
    - Perforation: free air under diaphragm
    - Some X-rays may show 'airless abdomen' due to spasming and air being squeezed out
  - **Mesenteric Doppler U/S:** useful for identifying venous and proximal arterial occlusion – Best for chronic ischemia
  - **Abd CT (or MRI):** early signs nonspecific: bowel wall thickening & pneumatosis; best test to detect mesenteric venous thrombosis
  - **DO not perform** barium studies for anticipated CT and/or surgery or conventional endoscopy for purposes of small bowel ischemia
  - **Angiography:** gold standard; proceed if clinical suspicion is high even if X-ray/CT negative

TREATMENTS:
- Volume resuscitation, **optimization of hemodynamics,** discontinue vasopressors if possible
- **Antibiotics** for infarctions, sepsis
- Anticoagulation: for arterial and venous thrombosis, embolic disease (not for non-occlusive mesenteric ischemia)
- Intraarterial infusion of thrombolytic agent for acute arterial embolism
- Intraarterial bolus Tolazoline (short-acting vasodilator) followed by infusion of Papaverine (long-acting vasodilator) for non-occlusive mesenteric ischemia
- Surgery: embolectomy for acute arterial embolism; Revascularization for acute SMA thrombosis; Resection of infracted bowel

PROGNOSIS:
- Mortality 20–70% (mortality <10% if recognized before peritoneal signs)
- The best predictor of survival is diagnosing ischemia prior to actual infarction

2.20 MEGACOLON (OGILVIE'S SYNDROME)

(Gastrointest Endosc 2002;56:789-92)

DEFINITION:
- Ogilvie's Syndrome (Acute Colonic Pseudo-obstruction): acute non-toxic megacolon without evidence of more distal colonic obstruction
  - Usually dilation of cecum and/or right side of colon
- Acute Toxic Megacolon: serious, life-threatening complication (usually late) of IBD or pseudomembranous colitis or Typhlitis or Ischemia
  - Typhlitis: necrotizing of cecum in setting of neutropenia (usually seen in chemotherapy or immunosuppression)
    - Infection usually follows with ensuing necrosis, colonic dilation, perforation; Death 50%, typically due to perforation
- Toxic vs. Nontoxic Megacolon *See also IBD- Ulcerative Colitis (Chapter 3.04)*
  Clinical situation is best predictor of various cause of toxic and nontoxic acute megacolon
  - Toxic Megacolon: usually involves entire colon in patients with UC
    - Two or more: HR >100/min, Temp >101.5°F (38.6°C), WBC >10,000, Hypoalbuminemia <3.0 gm/dl
  - Thumbprinting on KUB suggest ischemia
- Congenital: Hirschsprung's: aganglionosis of rectum, beginning at dentate line and extending cephlad
  - So the dilated appearing colon is normal & trying to accommodate, the distal portion that looks 'normal' is the problem (denervated)
- Acquired megacolon: Idiopathic, DM, Amyloidsosis, Scleroderma, Parkinson's, Muscular dystrophy, Chaga's disease

EPIDEMIOLOGY:
- Ogilvies: More common in men over the age of 60
- Toxic Megacolon: Precise incidence is unknown as the incidence of IBD has decreased; *C. difficile* occurs in 1% of all hospitalized patients

ETIOLOGIES:
- Ogilvie's: recent surgery/anesthesia, medications, DM, neurologic disorders, COPD, CHF, uremia, underlying infections, electrolyte abnormalities
  - Medications causes: NSAIDs, Opiates, Antidepressants, Antipsychotics, Antiseizure, CCB, Antiparkinsons, Antacids, Cationic supplements

PATHOPHYSIOLOGY:
- Ogilvie's syndrome is theorized to be a dilation from a physiologic response to an autonomic imbalance; May be true by proof of neostigmine therapy

CLINICAL MANIFESTATIONS/PHYSICAL EXAM:
- Ogilvie's: typically post-op with distended abdomen; abdominal pain minimal, increasing as syndrome progresses; occasional diarrhea
  - Patients usually on or recently weaned from ventilator; Low grade fevers, leukocytosis
  - Nausea and vomiting; patients (50%) still pass flatus; bowel sounds high pitched and quite active during early phase
  - Perforation <10%, but death in 15-30%; Death rarely from perforation, rather from multiorgan system failure
    - Cecal diameter: does not predict perforation; Some perforate <12, others don't >24 cm?
    - Rate and duration of cecal dilation are more important factors!
- Toxic megacolon due to IBD: usually UC flare with increased abdominal pain, bloating, distention, fever
  - Hypotension, hypovolemia, tachycardia, leukocytosis, electrolyte abnormalities, hypoalbuminemia, mental status changes

CHAPTER 2.20 MEGACOLON (OGILVIE'S SYNDROME)

LABORATORY STUDIES:
- ↑WBC ↓ Hb, Electrolyte disturbances, Hypoalbuminemia

DIAGNOSTIC STUDIES:
- Radiographs:
  - Ogilvie's: entire colon distension
  - Inflammatory (IBD, Infectious/C. *difficile*): may reveal colonic wall thickening, ulceration, thumbprinting, loss of haustral folds
  - Obstructive (tumor, diverticular, sigmoid vovulus): air-fluid levels; Likely need barium enema/ endsocopy to exclude obstruction
  - Metabolic/Medication: get history and correlate with X-ray
- HIrschsrung's: rectal biopsy demonstrating no myenteric neurons and high acetylcholinesterase

TREATMENTS:
- First step in acute megacolon, evaluate the cause and rule out obstruction, colitis and ischemia via radiographs and endoscopy
  - Ogilvie's: usually non-blood diarrhea (clue)
  - Inflammatory (IBD, Infectious/C. *difficile*): acute toxic picture, history of diarrhea, hematochezia, weight loss, diet and antibiotic history
  - Obstructive (tumor, diverticular, sigmoid vovulus): anemia, change in bowel habit, lower abdominal pain, low-grade fever
  - Metabolic/Medication: replete/hydration
- Ogilvie's: NPO, IVF, Ng & Rectal tubes, Correct lytes, Discontinue medicinal causes, Mobilization (bed to chair), Enemas (? ↑ perforation risk)
  - If above unsuccessful, and no obstruction/vovulus; Consider neostigmine 2.5 mg IV over 3-5 min
    - Cholinesterase inhibitor = cholinertic stimulation of colon (watch for bradycardia)
  - Serial KUBs; May need colonic decompression: colonoscopy, percutaneous decompression tube, surgical cecostomy
- Toxic Megacolon due to IBD: resuscitation: IVF, replace electrolytes, transfusions; Bowel rest with Ng tube; IV antibiotics and steroids; Avoid narcotics
  - Close monitoring of physical exam, labs, serial KUBs to assess need for early surgery
  - Surgery: early if perforation, peritonitis, or rapid deterioration despite medical therapy
  - Complications in up to 50% of surviving patients: sepsis, wound infections, abscess, fistula, delayed wound healing
  - Mortality: 11-40% depending on perforation; 90% if hypoalbuminemia
  - Observations suggest that more conservative surgery is appropriate in acute setting!
  - If recovery, usually relapse within several weeks or months; Elective surgery may be scheduled 1-4 weeks after stabilization

2.21 NUTRITION: MALNUTRITION & OBESITY

(Gastroenterology 2002;123:879-81 & 882-32)

DEFINITIONS:
- Nutritional status: reflects how well nutrient intake contributes to body composition and function in the face of existing metabolic needs
  - Four major components: water, protein, mineral, and fat; The first three compose the lean body mass (LBM)
- Malnutrition: refers to states of overnutrition (obesity) or undernutrition relative to body requirements, resulting in dysfunction
  - Marasmus: protein-calorie undernutrition associated with physical wasting, but preservation of visceral and serum proteins
  - Hypoalbuminemic: malnutrition occurring with stressed metabolism and common in hospitalized patients
- Body Mass Index (BMI) = wt (kg)/ht^2 (m)
  - Normal: 18.5-24.9; Overweight: 25-29.9; Obesity: 30-39.9; Morbid Obesity: 40-49.9; Super obesity: >50
  - Obesity related comorbidities/diseases:
    - Cardiomyopathy, Coronary artery disease, Dyslipidemia, Hypertension, Diabetes, Infertility, Fatty Liver
    - GERD, Gallstones, Chronic fatigue, Urinary stress incontinence, Deep vein thrombosis/Pulmonary embolus/Venous stasis
    - Degenerative joint disease, Immobility, Depression, Malignancies, Dyspnea, Obstructive sleep apnea
- Closer assessment if: poor intake for longer than 1-2 weeks; Weight loss of more than 10%; Weight less than 80% of desirable weight
  - Ideal body weight:
    - ♂ = 106 lb for first 5', plus 6 lb for each additional inch
    - ♀ = 100 lb for first 5', plus 5 lb for each additional inch
- See also: *Bowel- Short Bowel Syndrome (Chapter 2.23)* and Eating disorders in *Esophagus/Gastric-Potpourri (Chapter 1.24)*

PATHOPHYSIOLOGY:
- Intestinal epithelial cells are renewed and turned over every 48-72 hours
- Absorption:
  - Iron and folate in Duodenum
  - Vitamin B12 and bile salts in Ileum
    - B12 from food is bound to R-protein in stomach; Pancreas enzyme cleave R-Protein in duodenum; B12 then binds to intrinsic factor
  - All others (carbohydrates, fats, proteins, calcium, magnesium, trace elements, vitamins, etc) throughout entire small bowel
- Carbohydrates (Starch, Sucrose/Sugar, Lactose):
  - Starch requires amylase to convert to maltase; Maltase, Sucrase and Lactose are absorbed in the brush border of small bowel
- Protein:
  - Require endo/exopeptidases from intestine and pancreas; Proteins are absorbed in the brush border of small bowel
- Fat:
  - Requires pancreas (lipolysis), Liver (bile salts), Jejunal mucosa (absorption) and lymphatics for transport (Fats are not transported via portal system)
  - A deficiency in any of the above, will cause fat malabsorption
- Note, the bowel ages very well (better than the rest of you!) and there is little decrease in capacity to absorb nutrients

CHAPTER 2.21 NUTRITION: MALNUTRITION & OBESITY

Micronutrient	Deficiency	Toxicity
Vitamin A	Follicular hyperkeratosis, night blindness	Dermatitis, cirrhosis, hair loss, joint/bone pain, edema, hypercalcemia
Vitamin D	Rickets, osteomalacia, hypophosphatemia, weakness	Fatigue, headache, hypercalcemia, bone decalcification
Vitamin E	Hemolytic anemia, myopathy, ataxia, ophthalmoplegia	Rare; possible interference with Vit. K (coags), headache, myopathy
Vitamin K	Bruisability, prolonged prothrombin time	Rapid IV infusion: flushing, cardiovascular collapse
Vitamin C	Scurvy: poor wound healing, gingivitis, dental defects	Diarrhea, possible hyperoxaluria, Interference: glucose, FOBT
B1 (thiamine)	Dry beriberi (**polyneuropathy**): anorexia, low temp Wet beriberi (high output CHF): **lactic acidosis** Wernicke-Korsakoff: ataxia, **nystagmus,** memory loss	Large dose IV: anorexia, ataxia, ileus, headache, irritability
B2 (riboflavin)	Seborrheic dermatitis, cheilosis, geographic tongue	None
B3 (niacin)	Anorexia, lethargy, burning sensations, glossitis, headache Pellagra: diarrhea, pigmented dermatitis, dementia	Hyperglycemia, Hyperuricemia, GI upset, liver dysfunction
B6 (pyridoxine)	Peripheral neuritis, seborrhea, glossitis/stomatitis, anemia	Metabolic dependency, sensory neuropathy
B12 (cobalamin)	Glossitis, paresthesias/CNS change, megaloblastic anemia	None
Folic acid	Glossitis, diarrhea, megaloblastic anemia	Antagonizes antiepileptic drugs, decreases zinc absorption
Biotin	Scaly dermatitis, hair loss, papillae, myalgia	None
Pantothenic acid	Malaise, GI upset, cramps, paresthesias	Diarrhea
Calcium	Paresthesias, tetany, seizures, osteopenia, arrhythmia	Hypercalciuria, GI upset, lethargy
Phosphorus	Hemolysis, muscle weakness, ophthalmoplegia, osteopenia	Diarrhea
Magnesium	**Paresthesias, tetany, seizures, arrhythmia**	Diarrhea, muscle weakness, arrhythmia
Iron	Fatigue, dyspnea, glossitis, anemia, koilonychia	Iron overload (hepatic, cardiac)
Iodine	Goiter, Hypothyroidism	Goiter, Hypo/Hyperthyroidism
Zinc	Lethargy, **rash,** loss of taste/smell, poor wound healing	Impaired copper/iron metabolism, reduced HDL, immunosuppression
Copper	Anemia, **neuro/weakness,** connective tissue weakness	GI upset/hemorrhagic gastritis, hepatic damage
Chromium	Glucose intolerance, neuropathy, hyperlipidemia	None
Selenium	Keshan **cardiomyopathy, muscle weakness (myositis)**	GI upset
Manganese	**Night blindness, headache,** weight loss, dermatitis	**Cholestasis, extrapyramidal symptoms, MRI: basal ganglia lesion**
Molybdenum	Possible headache, vomiting, CNS changes	Impaired copper metabolism, possible gout
Fluoride	Increased dental caries	Teeth mottling, possible bone integrity/fluorosis

SECTION II SMALL BOWEL/COLON/RECTUM

DIAGNOSTIC STUDIES:
- Closer assessment if: poor intake for longer 1-2 weeks; Weight loss of more than 10%; Weight less than 80% of desirable weight
  - See ideal body weights above under Definitions
- Labs: electrolytes, vitamins and trace elements

TREATMENTS:
- Types of commonly prescribed diets:
  - Clear liquid: supplies fluid and calories in a form that requires minimal digestion, stimulation or elimination via GI tract
    - Provides about 600 calories & 150 gm carbohydrate, but inadequate protein, vitamins, and minerals
    - Hyperosmolar in nature and diluting may minimize any GI symptoms; If needed >3 days, consult dietician
  - Full liquid diet: Often used in progressing from clear liquids to solid foods
    - Provides >2000 calories & 70 gm of protein; May be adequate in all nutrients (except fiber) especially if high-protein
- Medical therapy for Obesity:
  - Dietary restrictions of calories (while maintaining adequate protein and fluid electrolytes)
    - Gradual weight reduction by behavior modifications, including diet and activity changes: total lifestyle modification
- Surgical therapy for Obesity:
  - Gastric bypass surgery (mortality 0.3-1.6%; perioperative complications 10%) Indications:
    - Failure of major weight-loss program plus morbid obesity (BMI >40)
    - Failure of major weight-loss program plus BMI >35 and obesity related comorbidities (listed above under Definitions)
  - Nutritional deficiencies with gastric bypass surgery: fat malabsorption, deficiencies in B12, Folate, Fat-soluble vitamins, Iron (anemia)
  - Recommended supplements: Multivitamin to include Iron 325 BID, Folate, Calcium 1500 mg/day

NOTES

2.22 NUTRITION: TOTAL PARENTERAL NUTRITION (TPN) & REFEEDING SYNDROME

(Gastroenterology 2001;121:966-69 & 970-1001)

GENERAL NUTRITION QUESTIONS/ANSWERS:
- Ask yourself:
  - How long has the patient been without nutrition?
  - How malnourished is the patient?
  - Can you use the GI tract? If not, when can you use it?
- Best predictive value of malnutrition is weight loss in preceding 3 months:
  - Severe protein-calorie malnutrition: loss of >20% of baseline weight; Begin supplemental nutrition immediately if NPO
  - Moderate protein-calorie malnutrition: loss of 10-20% of baseline weight; Begin supplemental nutrition within 2-3 days after NPO
  - Mild protein-calorie malnutrition: loss of <10% of baseline weight; Begin supplemental nutrition within 3-5 days after NPO
  - No protein-calorie malnutrition: no loss of baseline weight; Begin supplemental nutrition within 7-10 days after NPO; As long as fluids and electrolytes are maintained
- Enteral (tube feed) vs. Parenteral (TPN): If the gut works, use it!
  - If the problem is dysphagia, gastroparesis, unwillingness to eat then the enteral route is indicated
    - For gastrostomy tubes and feeding formulas, *See also Esophagus/Gastric- PEG Tubes (Chapter 1.20)*
  - If the problem is digestion or absorption, then parenteral route is indicated

STEPS FOR WRITING TPN/PPN:
1. Determine protein (PRO) Requirements (1st bag with full protein); (Max with PPN: 30 g/L)
2. Determine energy (CHO) requirements (1st bag with half kcals for TPN, PPN can start full kcals); (Max with PPN: 700/L)
3. First bag of TPN should be 2-in-1 solution (PRO and CHO only, no FAT); So CHO/FAT: 100/0%
   First bag of PPN can be 3-in-1 solution; So CHO/FAT: 40/60%
4. Determine % CHO and FAT kcals for subsequent bags; Standard CHO/FAT is TPN: 70/30%; PPN: 40/60%
5. Determine volume
6. Check compatibility of 3-in-1 (PRO, CHO and FAT) solutions to prevent instability
7. Determine Electrolytes; Make adjustments daily; See back of TPN order form at some institutions
8. Determine calcium:phosphorous product (not to exceed 200)
9. Add adult vitamins, multiple trace elements and 120 mcg selenium daily if not included
10. Additions:
    - Heparin: (prevent thrombus) 1 unit per ml total volume for TPN, 2 units per ml total volume for PPN
    - Famotidine (prevent stress ulcers): 40 mg/day standard, 20 mg/day renal dose
    - Insulin: (for BS control): A safe starting point is 0.1 units of insulin per 1 g of dextrose (i.e. CHO)
      - Calculation example: Say your TPN contains the following: 1200 total calories, CHO/FAT: 70/30%, PRO 100 g
        - First subtract PRO kcals (which is 4 kcals/g): 100 g $\times$ 4 kcal/g = 400; So 1200 − 400 = 800 kcals
        - Then remove FAT kcals: 800 kcals $\times$ 0.70 for 70% dextrose = 560 kcals
        - Finally CHO provides 3.4 kcals/g: 560 kcals/3.4 kcals/g = 165 g of dextrose; So 165 g $\times$ 0.1 units/g = 16.5 units insulin in TPN
11. Determine rate:
    - Divide volume by 24 hrs for continuous infusion
    - Cycling TPN for home (typically done with 1 hour taper down) from 24 hrs to 20 hrs to 16 hrs to 12 hrs (goal) over several days: 20 hr (2200-1800); 16 hr (2200-1400); 12 hr (2200-1000)
      - Main rate = total volume / (Cycle hrs − $1/2$ hour); 1st hour taper rate = Main rate /2
      - So, for example a 2600 ml solution cycled over 12 hours:
        - From 2200-0900 infuse TPN at 226 ml/hr $\times$ 11 hrs, then from 0900-1000 infuse 113 ml/hr $\times$ 1 hrs
        - At 1000, discontinue TPN and flush catheter; Accu-checks at 2300, 0400, 1100
12. Complete any TPN ancillary form if necessary

CHAPTER 2.22 NUTRITION: TOTAL PARENTERAL NUTRITION (TPN) & REFEEDING SYNDROME

Addendum (Reminders) of above steps (1–12) for writing for PPN:
Calculate volume first, then PRO and CHO (kcals) because of the limits; Always add Fat initially to help with ease of tonicity of periperal infusion I.e. Total volume of PPN is 2000 ml; CHO/FAT: 40/60%; kcals: 1400 (max 700/L); PRO: 60 (max 30 g/L); Heparin 2 units/ml

BODY MASS INDEX:
BMI = wt (kg)/ht^2 (m)

IDEAL BODY WEIGHT:
IBW (males) = 106 lb for first 5′, plus 6 lb for each additional inch
IBW (female) = 100 lb for first 5′, plus 5 lb for each additional inch

ENERGY OR KCALS (CHO) REQUIREMENTS:
CHO provides 3.4 kcal/g
Minimum: 100–150 g/day
I.e. CHO = 400 kcals 400/3.4 = 117 g/day

PROTEIN (PRO) REQUIREMENTS:
PRO provides 4 kcal/g
Volume of protein: standard 10% is 100 g/L, concentrated 15% is 150 g/L

BMI	CHO kcals/kg/day			PRO Grams/day
<25 (Normal)	25–35 kcals/kg	CURRENT (dry)	weight/day	1.5 g/kg CURRENT (dry) weight/day
<25–29.9 (Over wt)	20–25 kcals/kg	CURRENT (dry)	weight/day	1.7 g/kg IDEAL weight/day
30–34.9 (Obese)	15–20 kcals/kg	CURRENT (dry)	weight/day	2.0 g/kg IDEAL weight/day
≥35 (Morbid Obese)	10–15 kcals/kg	CURRENT (dry)	weight/day	2.0 g/kg IDEAL weight/day

VOLUME CALCULATIONS:
(Rule of thumb: think about how much a patient would need if giving simple IVFs to keep euvolemic)

Minimal vol (mL) = (g PRO × 10 [6.7 for 15% concentration]) + (CHO calories/2.38) + (FAT calories/3.0) + (~ 200 mL for electrolytes, vitamins, minerals)

—Think about how much volume patient needs/can't have: Is CRF/CHF a risk of fluid overloaded: use 15% concentration; Is patient a young person that needs fluid?
—Don't forget to take into account that 1500–2000 ml for urine/day and 500–1000 for insensible losses/day

EXAMPLE: goal is 100 g PRO and 1200 kcals energy (CHO), using 15% (concentrated, ie. 150 g in 1 L)
PRO: 100 g × 6.7 = 670 ml needed for PRO portion; 100 g PRO at 4 kcal/g = 400 kcals coming from PRO portion

CHO: 1200 kcals − 400 (PRO portion) = 800 kcals coming from CHO portion; 800/2.38 vol per kcal = 336

MISC: add 200 ml for vit/minerals/lytes

. . . so: 670 + 336 + 200 = 1200 ml of total volume for a hemodialysis patient using a concentrated solution; If young patient, may need to add additional 1000–2000 ml for urine/insensible losses

COMPATIBILITY RANGE FOR 3-IN-1 SOLUTIONS:
Protein (PRO) = 20–60 g/L
Dextrose (CHO) = 40–250 g/L (136–850 kcals/L)
Fat (FAT) = 20–60 g/L (200–600 kcals/L)

CALCULATION OF CA:PHOS PRODUCT:
mEq Ca/L x mEq Phos/L = X (X should not exceed 200)
The precipitate can be lethal via emboli
3 ways to correct: ↓ Ca or Phos, or ↑ volume

SECTION II SMALL BOWEL/COLON/RECTUM

ELECTROLYTES & MINERALS:
FDA mandates 13 water-soluble and fat-soluble vitamins including vitamin K and Vitamin C be added
Trace elements are available in combinations of 4, 5, 6, or 7 elements; Those without selenium should not be used longterm

Mineral added individually: Normal requirement (good starting point)
- Calcium: 9-22 mEq (start with 10 mEq)
- Magnesium: 8-24 mEq (start with 10 mEq)
- Phosphate: 15-30 mM (start with NaP04: 30 mM; as KP04: 0 mM; Rule of thumb, best to use Na, rather than K); 4.4 mEq = 3 mM
- Potassium: 60-120 mEq (start with KCl: 30 mM; as KAcetate: 30 mM; Rule of thumb, best to split if labs normal; If need ↑ CO_2, then use ↑ Acetate)
- Sodium: 100-150 mEq (start with NaCl: 60 mEq; as NaAcetate: 60 mEq; Rule of thumb, make equivalent to D5 $^1/_2$NS);
  - Remember: NS = 156 Na/L, $^1/_2$ NS = 77 Na/L
    - Example: 2000 ml total volume: For $^1/_2$ NS want 77 Na/L; So, total ~150 mEq of Na in 2 L: 30 mM as NaPO4, 60 mEq as NaCl, 60 mEq as NaAcetate
- Iron: can't give with 3-in-1 (i.e. those with FAT) because will precipitate out

BLOOD SUGAR MANAGEMENT:
Accu-checks: 6 am, 12 noon, 6 pm, 12 midnight
TPN: 1st bag at $^1/_2$ calories and gradually advance to goal over next 2-3 days if blood sugar remains <150
PPN: Accu-checks not necessary unless history of DM or exhibiting glucose intolerance
Cyclic TPN: Accu-check 1 hr after start of infusion, mid-cycle check at least 6 hrs prior to completion and 1 hr after cycle complete (Do not give insulin with post 1 hr Accu-check)
SSI: <60 (amp D50); 150-199 (4 units); 200-249 (8 units); 250-299 (12 units); 300-349 (16 units); >350 (stop TPN; Start D5 $^1/_2$ NS at same rate as TPN)

D5 & Lytes: (Change TPN/PPN to D5/Lytes for suspected catheter infections)
D5: 50 g of dextrose/L; 3.4 kcals/g dextrose
Example: Volume is 2200 = 2.2 L × 50 = 110 g dextrose; 110 g × 3.4 = 374 total kcals
Filling out TPN form: No PRO/FAT, 374 kcals, Volume 2200 (same); All other electrolytes stay the same

COMPLICATIONS:
- Catheter related infections are the most common complication
  - Inpatient catheters should be removed without attempts at treatment
  - Outpatients with long-term catheters can have attempted therapy
- PICC lines have ↑ thrombotic complications as compared to the 1-4% of central venous catheters (i.e. subclavian); Hickman is best
- Metabolic bone disease has been reported with those receiving home TPN
- Hepatobiliary disease: takes the form of increased LFTs, cholestasis, sludge and gallstones, and hepatocellular disease

STOPPING TPN:
Decrease infusion rate by half (i.e. from 150 cc/hr to 75 cc/hr) for one hour and then stop; Avoids rebound hypoglycemia

CHAPTER 2.22   NUTRITION: TOTAL PARENTERAL NUTRITION (TPN) & REFEEDING SYNDROME

REFEEDING SYNDROME:
- Seen after a patient develops moderate-severe malnutrition and then is abruptly provided with full caloric meal in the form of food, enteral nutrition, or peripheral nutrition
- Defined as development of Hypokalemia, Hypophosphatemia, Hypomagnesemia
  - Insulin production suddenly rises with carbohydrate load moving potassium, phosphorus and magnesium into cells
  - The kidneys reabsorb sodium and water, leading to expansion of extracellular fluid space, anasarca, CHF
- Overall abnormalities include: muscle weakness, respiratory failure/acidosis, cardiac arrhythmias/hypotension, ketoacidosis, osmotic diuresis, prerenal azotemia, and hyperosmolar nonketotic coma; Sudden death can result
- In order to prevent refeeding syndrome, patient who are at risk should initially be started on a hypocaloric feeding (usually <1000 kcal) with carbohydrate component restricted substantially
- Can be avoided by use of:
  - Parenteral thiamine (100mg/day for 3 days),
  - Slow initiation of feed with liberal amounts of potassium, magnesium, and phosphate
  - Attention to intake and output records and laboratory results

2.23 SHORT BOWEL SYNDROME

(Gut 2006;55:1-12. Gastroenterology 2003;124:1105-10 & 1111-34)

DEFINITION:
- A malabsorptive state that often follows massive resection of the small intestine
- The definition is a functional one: the extent or location of resection is independent of the degree of malabsorption
  - In general- patients develop symptoms when <200 cm of functional bowel remains
- Intestinal failure: describes the state when GI function is inadequate to maintain the nutrient and hydration status of a person without intravenous or enteral supplementation

ETIOLOGIES:
- Most common causes:
  - Adults: Crohn's, Malignancy, Radiation enteritis, Vascular insufficiency, Trauma
  - Children: Crohn's, Intestinal tumors, Radiation enteritis
  - Infants: Necrotizing enterocolitis, Intestinal atresia, Volvulus, Meconium ileus, Hirschsprung's

PATHOPHYSIOLOGY:
- Small bowel: Total length 390-690 cm (13-23 ft); 30 cm equals ~1 ft
  - Duodenum (5%) 50 cm (1.5 ft); Jejunum (35%) 160-280 cm (4-9 ft); Ileum (60%) 240-420 cm (8-14 ft)
  - Colon 150-180 cm (5-6 ft)
- Small bowel: absorbs about 10 L/day of ingested and secreted liquids
  - In general, patients develop symptoms when <200 cm of functional bowel remains
  - Majority of nutrient digestion/absorption is complete within first 100 cm of jejunum
  - Most will be able to maintain nutrient balance using oral feeds if 100 cm of jejunum is intact
- Jejunal epithelium: relatively porous, allowing free and rapid flux of water and electrolytes - primary digestive and absorptive site
  - Characteristic long villi create a large absorptive area
  - Most carbohydrate, protein, water-soluble vitamins are absorbed in upper 200 cm of jejunum; Fat absorption occurs over a larger area
- Ileum epithelium: site of significant reabsorption of fluid and electrolytes
  - Much less porous, hence potential for back diffusion of fluids and electrolytes is lower; shorter villi and reduced surface area
  - Adaptation: able to undergo massive adaptation via lengthening and function of villi - dependant on enteral nutrition!
    - Glucagon-like peptide II is major hormone involved in stimulating adaptation - stimulated primarily by fat
  - Ulcer disease initially due to hypergastrinemia: intestinal negative feedback for inhibiting gastrin secretion and reducing acid is interrupted
    - PUD and esophagitis are common
  - B12 intrinsic factor absorbed in ileum, therefore can result in B12 deficiency especially if >60 cm resected
  - Bile salts absorbed in ileum, therefore can result in bile acid malabsorption/decreased bile salts with malabsorption of fat-soluble vitamins
    - More than 100 cm of resected ileum results in disruption of the enterohepatic circulation (bile salt deficiency and fat malabsorption)
    - The delivery of unabsorbed bile acids to the colon can lead to secretory diarrhea (Cholerheic enteropathy); Also leads to hyperabsorption of oxalate, leading to hyperoxaluria and kidney stone formation
  - The jejunum secretes a large amount of fluid in response to any hypertonic feeds - this is reabsorbed primarily by the ileum
    - If a substantial portion of ileum (>100 cm) is resected, fluid and electrolyte loss will occur
    - This results in intolerance to large bolus feeds or feeds containing high concentrations of simple carbohydrates
- Ileocecal valve: major barrier to reflux of colonic material from the colon to small intestine; regulator of ileal contents exiting to colon
  - Resection is associated with bacterial overgrowth-a major feature of short bowel syndrome

CHAPTER 2.23 SHORT BOWEL SYNDROME

- Colon is important too:
  - The presence of a colon is clearly a benefit in a patient with short bowel syndrome because of its ability to absorb water, electrolytes, short chain fatty acids
  - Colonic brake: signals small bowel to slow down; If no colon, no colonic break
  - Those without a colon and <100 cm of jejunum are likely to require life-long TPN

CLINICAL MANIFESTATIONS/PHYSICAL EXAM:
- Symptoms associated with bowel resection are highly dependant upon the physiology of the remaining small bowel
  - See Pathophysiology above
- Diarrhea: a major cause is the osmotic load generated by malabsorbed carbohydrates; especially true with simple carbohydrates
  - In colon, further breakdown via bacteria create additional osmotic loads and fluid losses
  - Many carbohydrates may be recovered by absorption of short-chain fatty acids in the colon
  - Proteins and fats do not create a large osmotic load
    - Since proteins and fats are a dense source of calories, they are an ideal source of calories and help with adaptation

LABORATORY STUDIES:
- Plasma citrulline level (a non-protein amino acid produced by intestinal mucosa)
- Electrolytes and minerals
  - B12, calcium, magnesium, zinc, selenium, fat soluble vitamins (ADEK) should be monitored every 3 months

DIAGNOSTIC STUDIES:
- A surgical history and knowledge of remaining anatomy is the best diagnostic study
- CT scans or Barium studies may help delineate

TREATMENTS:
- Focus at replacing nutrients due to loss of overall bowel absorptive surface
  - May need specialized center for intestinal rehabilitation
- Likelihood of resuming an oral diet:
  - Most with a jejunal length >200 cm and intact colon can eventually be managed on oral intake alone
    - Note: length of small bowel may be underestimated during surgery due to spasm of bowel
    - Intestinal adaptation is individual – it is not unreasonable to try to convert a patient to oral diet
    - One study suggest a plasma citrulline level <20 micromol/L is predictive of those who have intestinal failure
  - The segment of remaining intestine is important for anticipating adaptation and determining any metabolic consequences
    - See above under Pathophysiology for characteristics of jejunum, ileum and colon
  - Presence of a colon
    - Those with no colon and small bowel resection is poorly tolerated and likely require long-term TPN
- Initial therapy: Usually with TPN after surgery to balance fluid/electrolyte loss;
  - Fluid loss can be dramatic, usually replace ml-for-ml of fluid loss (including ostomy); Include H2 blocker in formula
  - Predictors of permanent TPN:
    - <50 cm of small bowel with colon or <100-150 cm without colon
    - Residual small bowel disease (Crohn's, ischemia, etc)
- Enteral therapy: directed at stimulating intestinal adaptation (villus hyperplasia resulting in longer villi and absorptive area)
  - Parenteral route can provide calories, nutrients, etc-but won't promote adaptation
    - Starts enteral feeds as soon as fluid/electrolyte losses have diminished or been controlled
    - Antimotility drugs may be used
    - Oral feeds: initially continuous and then frequent small meals (every 2-3 hours)
    - TPN should be continued during the transition to enteral feeds
  - MOA: enteral feeds stimulates mucosal epithelium, also GI secretions from stomach/pancreas/intestine release trophic secretions

SECTION II SMALL BOWEL/COLON/RECTUM

- Feeds
  - High carbohydrate formula feeds are a disadvantage due to the high osmotic load (especially simple carbohydrates)
  - Protein hydrolysate diets often contain a higher more physiologic percentage of fat and are better tolerated
  - Dietary fats decrease the osmotic load to the small bowel and help stimulate adaptation (40% of calories should be fat)
  - Extra vitamins and minerals based upon the absorptive characteristics of the segment of small bowel resected
  - Fiber supplementation may decrease the watery nature of the stools by absorbing stool water
  - Lactose restriction is not important: most is absorbed in the proximal bowel and may provide a source of fat/calcium
  - Avoid hypertonic beverages (i.e. sodas and fruit juices)
  - Oxalate restriction is important in those malabsorbing fat with a colon to prevent kidney stone formation

  High Oxalate foods that should be avoided:
  Drinks: draft beer, juices with berries or tomatoes, cocoa/ovaltine, instant coffee
  Fruits/Vegetables: beans, beets, carrots, celery, swiss chard, chives, french fries, okra, berries, sweet potato, tangerines
  Bread/Pasta: grits, soybean crackers, wheat germ
  Miscellaneous: nuts, pretzels, chocolate, vegetable soup

- PPIs have been shown to decrease GI fluid loss via inhibition of acid secretion and prevent ulcer disease
  - High gastric acid also deactivate pancreatic enzymes
- Cholestyramine may be needed to bind malabsorbed bile acids, especially after ileal resections and help decrease secretory diarrhea
- Low B12 levels require life-long supplementation via monthly intramuscular injections
- Evaluate for bacterial overgrowth, especially without an ileocecal valve
- Octreotide reduces fluid loss; increases small bowel transit but fortunately tachyphylaxis develops; may predispose to gallstones as well
- Small bowel transplant, reserved for late in course and when TPN is considered a higher mortality risk (i.e. TPN complicated by liver disease)
  - Complications: sepsis, rejection, CMV infection, lymphoproliferative disease
- Bianchi procedure: narrowing a dilated intestinal segment; The dilated bowel may be contributing to poor motility and enhancing bacterial overgrowth
  - Performed if dilated bowel segment is significantly impairing ability to digest and absorb nutrients because of symptoms of bacterial overgrowth

COMPLICATIONS:
- Liver disease associated with TPN: steatohepatitis and cholestasis
  - Rarely leads to cirrhosis and portal hypertension
- Gallstones: gallbladder stasis due to lack of enteral feedings is a contributor
- Bacterial overgrowth: dilations of small intestine, poor motility, lack of ileocecal valve
- D-Lactic acidosis: result of carbohydrate overload in colon, disturbs normal pattern of colonic fermentation, leads to formation of D-Lactate in blood
  - Neurological symptoms: headache, dizziness, seizure-like, coma
  - May need low carbohydrate diets and antibiotic therapy to decrease bacterial load
- Kidney stones: Increased malabsorbed fat binds calcium and leaves oxalate unopposed, therefore hyperoxaluria and stone formation
  - Treated with low oxalate diet and cholestyramine with calcium carbonate supplementation (1–4 g/day) to bind oxalate in lumen
- Esophagitis, gastritis, duodenitis: loss of intestine results in loss of normal hormonal feedback loops that suppress gastrin; Treat with PPI
- Bone disease: osteopenia/osteoporosis; Patients should be monitored with DEXA scan

PROGNOSIS:
- Long term (5 year) TPN prognosis is generally good (85%) as long as it is associated with centers structures for such patients
- For small bowel resections (with intact colon) and fatty acid/bile salt diarrhea, **See also IBD- Potpourri (Chapter 3.05)**

NOTES

2.24 SMALL BOWEL TUMORS

DEFINITION:
- Tumors of the small bowel; Fortunately primary neoplasia of the small bowel is rare

EPIDEMIOLOGY:
- Small bowel comprises >75% of the length and >90% of the mucosal surface area of the gut, yet the small bowel is the least common site of primary cancer
- Prevalence:
  - 3-6% of all GI tumors, 75% of these are malignant
  - Therefore small bowel cancer accounts for 1-2% of GI malignancies and 0.1-0.3% of all malignancies
- Incidence: 10 in 1 million; Low, reasons:
  - Small bowel is alkaline, therefore not allowing activation of certain carcinogens; Lots of lymphatic tissue with protective IgA production
  - Faster transient time with less exposure to carcinogens, small bowel has higher cell turnover with fewer stem cells (carcinogen target cells)
  - Benzpyrene hydroxylase present in high concentrations: converts benzpyrene, a known carcinogen in food, to less toxic metabolite
- Risk factors: older age, male, African American, ? Diet
- Inheritable conditions with increased risk of small bowel tumors:
  - Adenomatous polyposis coli (FAP, Gardner's): associated with colorectal and duodenal adenomas
  - Peutz-Jeghers Syndrome: associated with hamartomas of GI tract; Also increased incident of small bowel adenocarcinoma
  - Hereditary nonpolyposis colon cancer (HNPCC) or Lynch II syndrome; Increased incident of small bowel adenocarcinoma
  - Von Recklinghausen's Disease (Neurofibromatosis type 1): associated with occasional schwannomas
  - Crohn's Disease
- Immunosuppressed condition with increased risk:
  - HIV: will likely be the leading cause of primary GI lymphomas (usually high-grade B-cell non-Hodgkins); Kaposi's sarcoma too
  - Immunosuppression: cyclosporine is associated with increased incidence of small bowel lymphoma in transplant patients
- Impaired mucosal barrier with increased risk:
  - Crohn's disease (adenocarcinoma), Celiac disease (T-cell lymphoma), *H. Pylori* (gastric lymphoma, MALT)

ETIOLOGIES: Terminology; See also Treatment below for further definitions

Tissue of Origin	Benign	Malignant	How Common	Site of Primary Tumor
Mucosa	Adenoma	Adenocarcinoma	20-70% (most common)	Duodenum, jejunum
Enterochromaffin	—	Carcinoid	1-4%	Ileum
Lymphoid	—	Lymphoma (T-cell with Celiac)	3-50%	Ileum, jejunum
Mesenchymal	Benign GIST (Gastrointestinal Stromal Tumor)	Malignant GIST	1% (rare)	Stomach (most common)
Smooth muscle	Leiomyomas	Leiomyosarcomas	Note: GIST previously misclassified in Smooth muscle group	
Vascular	Hemangioma Lymphangioma —	Angiosarcoma Lymphangiosarcoma Kaposi sarcoma		
Connective tissue	Fibroma	Fibrosarcoma		
Nerve	Neurofibroma Schwann cell tumor	Neurofibrosarcoma Malignant schwannoma		
Fat	Lipoma	Liposarcoma		

- Tumors that Metastasize *to* small bowel: melanoma > ovarian > bladder > breast > lung

CHAPTER 2.24 SMALL BOWEL TUMORS

CLINICAL MANIFESTATIONS/PHYSICAL EXAM:
See also Treatments below for further manifestations
- Presenting symptoms are vague and nonspecific, leading to delay in diagnosis (mean duration of symptoms 3-12 months)
- Abdominal pain 67%, GI bleed (occult, melena) 41%, Weight loss 38%, N/V 33%
- Less frequent: Bowel obstruction, Intussusception, Palpable mass, Painless jaundice (periampullary), Perforation (especially lymphomas)

LABORATORY STUDIES:
- Carcinoid tumors: Serum serotonin and urine 5-HIAA levels, *See also Bowel- Carcinoid Tumors (Chapter 2.08)*

DIAGNOSTIC STUDIES:
- Plain Radiographs: can show obstruction, but not helpful in localizing or diagnosing the cause
- Endoscopy: primary means of assessing the upper GI tract
  - GISTs (average size at presentation 4.5 cm) are submucosal and routine biopsy are usually non-diagnostic
    - EUS/FNA is helpful for determining submucosal nature of tumor and extent of gastric wall invasion
- Barium studies: Enteroclysis (95%) has better sensitivity than Small Bowel Follow-Through (60%)
  - CT enterography will likely replace in the future
- CT scan sensitivities: 100% duodenum, 17% jejunum, 70% ileum; Can also show presence of metastatic disease
- MRI: can be useful

TREATMENTS:
- Types of Adenomas and their treatment:
  - Tubular Adenoma: low malignant potential, may be asymptomatic or bleeding
    Therapy: endoscopic polypectomy or local surgical excision
  - Villous Adenoma: moderate malignant potential, may present with bleeding or obstruction
    Therapy: endoscopic polypectomy or local surgical excision
  - Brunner's Gland Adenoma: hyperplasia of the glands of first portion of duodenum with no malignant potential; Usually asymptomatic
    Therapy: endoscopic resection if symptomatic
- Adenocarcinoma:
  - Wide resection, including lymphadenectomy; Adjuvant chemotherapy not clearly defined
- GISTs: arise from interstitial cells of Cajal (intestinal pacemakers), previously misclassification used the terms leiomyoma, leiomyosarcomas
  - May have many myogenic features, neural features, both muscle and nerve (mixed GIST), or lack differentiation (non-specific GIST)
  - Therapy: surgical resection; Usually no spread via lymph, so resection of nodes not needed
  - Resistant to most chemotherapy/radiation is a problem
    However, Imatinib (Gleevec) is the only effective chemotherapy with 70% tumor response
- Carcinoid: usually rapid spread to liver, via secretion of humoral factors and draining into portal system; *See also Bowel- Carcinoid Tumors (Chapter 2.08)*
  - Cutaneous flushing, secretory watery diarrhea, bronchospasm
  - Serotonin metabolized to 5-hydroxyindoleacetic acid (5-HIAA), increased levels in urine (>200 mg/day)
  - Diagnosis: Serum serotonin and urine 5-HIAA levels, CT scan, Indium-111 octreotide imaging
  - Therapy: Surgical resection with segmental lymphadenectomy;
      Octreotide (decrease serotonin level, symptom control, lifesaving in serotonin crisis)

PROGNOSIS:
- Adenocarcinoma: periampullary 35% 5-year survival, elsewhere in bowel <20%
- Leiomyosarcoma: 30-40% 5-year survival
- Lymphoma: 10-50% 5-year survival, average 30%

2.25 WHIPPLE'S DISEASE

(N Engl J Med 2007;356:55-66)

DEFINITION:
- An extremely rare infectious illness that causes an intestinal malabsorption process
  - Can have numerous other potential manifestations including rheumatological, cardiopulmonary, and neurological

EPIDEMIOLOGY:
- Extremely Rare; 1907-1987 only 696 cases reported
- Predilection: white males in their fourth or fifth decade with exposure to soil & animals (i.e. farms)

ETIOLOGIES:
- Etiologic agent identified in 1992: *Tropheryma whipplei;* Gram-positive bacillus, PAS positive, Acid-fast negative
  - Thought to be related to other soil-borne Actinomyces
- Patients appear to have lack of immune response
- Accumulation of massive numbers of organisms in GI tract
- Subsequent impaired nutrient absorption

CLINICAL MANIFESTATIONS/PHYSICAL EXAM:
- Four cardinal clinical manifestations: arthralgia, weight loss, diarrhea, abdominal pain
  - Arthralgias may be present for years before diagnosis (clue)
- General manifestations: Fever in >50%, Hyperpigmentation and Lymphadenopathy
- Rheumatologic manifestations: arthralgias in 67% and most have symptoms more than 5 years; large/small joints, non-deforming
- Pulmonary manifestations: chest pain, shortness of breath, cough
- Cardiac manifestations (>50%): CHF, pericarditis, valvular heart disease, infective endocarditis
- Renal manifestations: focal embolic glomerulonephritis from endocarditis or direct bacillus involvement
- Neuro manifestations (10%): dementia/cognitive dysfunction
  - Pathognomonic: Oculomasticatory Myorrhythmia (Slow rhythmic and synchronized contractions of ocular, facial, or other muscles)

LABORATORY STUDIES:
- IgM and IgG (Serology) antibodies have high specificity and moderate sensitivity: Titers above 1:400 specific for Whipple's
  - Low sensitivity might reflect impurities and/or cross-reactivity by other microorganisms
- The advent of PCR gene amplification has aided in the diagnosis of Whipple's
  - Highly sensitive and specific, PCR is expensive, has potential risk of DNA cross-contamination, and is technically demanding

DIAGNOSTIC STUDIES:
- EGD
  - Endoscopy: multiple whitish-yellow small plaques diffusely distributed in intestinal mucosa (may represent accumulation of chyle in obstructed lymphatic channels) Not pathognomonic, DDX: Intestinal lymphangiectasia, Waldenstrom's disease

- Small bowel biopsy: Extensive PAS-positive (periodic acid-Schiff) staining with villous atrophy followed by AFB staining (Ziehl-Neelsen stain) that is negative
  - Most relevant microscopic finding: foamy-apparent (containing collections of fine rod-shaped particles corresponding to intact or partially degraded bacteria) macrophages infiltrating the lamina propria and staining PAS-positive
  - DDX of PAS positive: Whipple's (AFB−), *Mycobacterium* (AFB +), *Histoplasmosis,* Macroglobulinemia, EDTA therapy

TREATMENTS:

- Goal: Eradicate infection and avoid relapse
  Many investigators believe that the duration of the treatments correlates with length of remission
  (Rationale for prolonged therapy: complete eradication to reduce likelihood of relapse); Controversial

Initial IV Therapy × 2 Weeks	Followed by Oral Therapy × 1–2 Years (Minimum)
Penicillin G (1.2 mill U/day) & Streptomycin (1 gm/day)	Trimethoprim (160 mg)-Sulfamethoxazole (800 mg) po BID
Third-generation cephalosporin (i.e. Ceftriaxone 2 gm/day)	Trimethoprim (160 mg)-Sulfamethoxazole (800 mg) po BID

COMPLICATIONS:

- Relapses, especially with Neuro manifestations; Hence the reason for the long course of antibiotic therapy

2.26 POTPOURRI

FECAL FAT
- Best *screening test:* Qualitative with Sudan stain is really only valuable as a screening test for those patients excreting >20 g/day
- Best quantitative test: 72 hr stool collection; Intake of 100 gm of fat per day is necessary for accurate results; Normal excretion is 6–8 g/day
  - Therefore if >8 gm of fecal fat present, steatorrhea secondary to malabsorption is confirmed, see topic below about differentiation
- Physiologic conditions with increased excretion: high fiber diet (>100 gm/day), ingestion of solid-form dietary fat (i.e. whole peanuts, Olestra)

DIFFERENTIATING MALABSORPTION CAUSED BY SMALL BOWEL ENTEROPATHY VS. PANCREATIC INSUFFICIENCY (D-XYLOSE TEST):
- D-Xylose test: normally D-xylose is absorbed completely in small bowel without help of pancreatic enzymes and excreted unchanged in urine
- Test: 25 gm oral dose of D-Xylose, urine collected for 5 hours
  - Normal test: urine excretion is >5 gm of D-xylose and this excludes small bowel disease (Celiac, Whipple's, bacterial overgrowth, etc)
    -These patients are often empirically treated with pancreatic enzymes, resolution of symptoms is both therapeutic and diagnostic of a pancreatic process
  - Positive test (<5 gm in urine): small bowel disease, so if low D-Xylose in urine with steatorrhea, do a small bowel biopsy or test for bacterial overgrowth to help diagnose small bowel enteropathy
    -False Positive: delayed gastric emptying, bacterial overgrowth, vomiting, renal insufficiency, myxedema, ascites

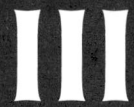

INFLAMMATORY BOWEL DISEASE

3.01 CROHN'S DISEASE

(Aliment Pharmacol Ther. 2003;18:263-77. Am J Gastroenterol. 2001;96:635-43. N Engl J Med 2002; 347:417-29)

DEFINITION:
- Idiopathic or nonspecific *transmural* inflammation of the *any segment* of the GI tract with *skip* areas of ulceration (aphthous or serpiginous)
- In 5-10% of patients with chronic colitis a clear distinction between UC and CD cannot be made even with mucosal biopsy ("indeterminate colitis")

DDX:
- Infectious: bacterial *(E. coli, Salmonella, Shigella, Yersina, Campylobacter, Mycobacterium, C. difficile)*, amebic, CMV/HSV, STDs
- Ischemic colitis, Diverticulitis, Colorectal cancer
- Intestinal lymphoma, Collagenous/Lymphocytic colitis (Microscopic colitis), Celiac sprue, Radiation enteropathy
- IBS, Appendicitis, Solitary rectal ulcer syndrome
- Drugs (NSAID enteropathy, OCP, allopurinol)

EPIDEMIOLOGY:
- Prevalence 1:3000 (high because often presents in younger population initially); ♂ = ♀
- *Bimodal* with peaks in 20's and 50-70's; ↑ incidence in Caucasians, Jews, and smokers

ETIOLOGIES:
- The cause is unknown; one theory is cow's milk containing *Mycobacteria Tuberculosis*
- Mutation of the NOD2/CARD 15 gene found in 20% of patients and is associated with ileal and fibrostenosing disease
  - In 20% of cases, Crohn's occurs in more than one first or second degree family member (i.e. familial CD)
- Three genetic syndromes associated: Turner's, Glycogen storage disease 1B, Hermansky-Pudlak (albinism, platelet defect)

PATHOPHYSIOLOGY:
- Extent: can affect any portion of GI tract from mouth to anus, with *skip* lesions
  - **Distribution:** 25% ileitis, 50% ileocolitis, and 20% colitis; Isolated upper tract disease is rare (5%)
- Appearance: non-friable mucosa, *cobblestoning*, deep & long fissures
- Microscopy: *transmural inflammation* with mononuclear cell infiltrate, **non-caseating granulomas** (Only seen in 10-30% of biopsies), fissures

CLINICAL MANIFESTATIONS/PHYSICAL EXAM:
- **Smoldering disease with abdominal pain (RLQ) ± abdominal mass;** Mucus-containing **non-grossly bloody diarrhea**
- Fevers, malaise, **weight loss/malnutrition**
- **Perianal disease:** fissures, fistulas
- Crohn's Disease Activity Index (CDAI): used in clinical trials; weighted score of clinical/laboratory values: <150 = Remission, >450 = Severe disease
- **Extracolonic:**
  - Seronegative (RF −) **arthritis** is most common, 25% of patients: large joint, unilateral, non-deforming (coincides with colitis activity)
    - Ankylosing spondylitis (CD > UC), Osteoporosis, Sacroiliitis: (most don't coincide with colitis activity)

    Osteopenia/Osteoporosis: risks: steroid use, malabsorbed Ca/D, ↓ BMI, tobacco; generally treated like any other patient (i.e. Bisphosphonates)

  - Derm:
    - **Erythema nodosum:** painful pretibial erythematous subcutaneous nodules (coincides with colitis activity)
    - Pyoderma gangrenosum: pustular lesions that ulcerate and exhibit pathergy (doesn't coincide with colitis activity)
    - Aphthous ulcers

CHAPTER 3.01 CROHN'S DISEASE

- Ocular: anterior uveitis (iritis), episcleritis (if HLA-B27 + doesn't coincide with colitis activity; If HLA-B27 −, it does coincide with colitis activity)
  - Any ocular symptom in an IBD patient should prompt a referral to an ophthalmologist
- Vascular: Hypercoagulable states/Thromboembolic events (after search for hypercoagulable state, use standard therapy for treatment)
- Liver: Chronic hepatitis, cirrhosis, PSC has ↑ risk cholangiocarcinoma (risk: UC >> CD, doesn't respond to bowel therapy)
- **Gallstones** (due to malabsorption of bile salts)
- **Kidney stones** (Ca oxalate stones due to binding of intraluminal Ca to unabsorbed bile salts allowing increased oxalate absorption)

■ **Smoking makes it worse**! (These patients must absolutely stop smoking)

Classification of type of Crohn's:
■ **Inflammatory:** Intestinal ulcerations with diarrhea, abdominal pain, inflammatory mass, ± fever & weight loss
  - Responds best to anti-inflammatory therapy but recurrence is the rule rather than exception
  - Natural history is aggressive with early recurrence

■ **Stricturing:** All Crohn's begins with inflammation, but predominant pathology in some is extensive fibrosis in lamina propria
  - Surgery is best therapeutic option: resection or strictureplasty
  - Natural history is a more indolent course but doesn't respond to anti-inflammatory therapy

■ **Fistulizing:** characterized by enterocutaneous and/or enteroenteric fistulas
  - Fistulas occur in areas of inflammation yet often originate in segment of bowel proximal to stricture
  - Most patients benefit from maintenance anti-inflammatory medical therapy to minimize risk of recurrence
  - If perianal or any septic processes: drainage, antibiotics, and Seton rings placement can facilitate continued drainage and promote healing
  - Natural history is recurrence after medical or surgical therapy

LABORATORY STUDIES:
- ↓ Hct due to Fe, B12, folate deficiency or chronic disease; ↑ WBC from active disease or abscess; ↑ ESR, p-ANCA only 10% sensitivity
- Diarrheal wasting: hypoalbuminemia, hypokalemia
- Serologies: Anti-saccharomyces cerevisiae antibodies **(ASCA)** 60-70% of CD (Seen <10% of other GI diseases, including UC & IBS)
  - Positive serology warrants confirmatory tests (e.g. endoscopy)
  - These serologies are included in: Prometheus IBD serology 7
- Acute flare: always consider infection compromise: *C. diff*, Stool culture, O&P, CMV serology/biopsy

DIAGNOSTIC STUDIES:
- Endoscopy:
  - Ulcers: Aphthoid, deep ("rake") and serpiginous along the longitudinal axis of the bowel
  - Skip areas, cobblestoning, pseudopolyps, rectal sparing
  - Biopsies: noncaseating granulomatous inflammation (unfortunately found in only 10-30% of cases) is diagnostic
  - Note: oral sodium phosphate colonic preps can cause small aphthous-type erosions in colon that may mimic CD
- Small Bowel Series or CT enterography:
  - String sign: narrowed terminal ileum
- Barium Enema:
  - Sharp lesions, long ulcers, fissures and strictures (not pseudopolyps like UC)
- Capsule Endoscopy:
  - May be useful for evaluating extent of disease in small bowel, but its precise role is yet to be defined
- DEXA scan for bone loss

SECTION III INFLAMMATORY BOWEL DISEASE

TREATMENTS:
- *See also IBD- Treatment Crohn's and UC (Chapter 3.03)*
- Must avoid smoking and NSAIDs

Postoperative Treatment: (Am J Gastroenterol. 2000;95:1139–1146)
- Recurrence postoperative most likely with:
  - Resections with anastomosis (as opposed to end-ileostomy), Second (or more) surgical resection
  - Tobacco use, Young age
  - Extensive small bowel disease
- Prophylaxis of postoperative recurrence: Antibiotics, Probiotics, 6 MP/Azathioprine (further studies still needed)
  - How to treat? Start early; 6 MP/Azathioprine ± short term Metronidazole; Assess with Cscope in 1 year
  - If can't tolerate 6 MP, consider Mesalamine 4 gm/day, ? other biologics (Infliximab/Adalimumab); Assess with Cscope in 1 year

COMPLICATIONS:
- **Perianal fissures, perirectal abscesses**
- **Stricture:** postprandial bloating, distention, borborygmi
- **Fistulas:** abscesses, bacterial overgrowth & malabsorption; If refractory to therapy, consider other diagnosis such as common variable immunodeficiency
- **Abscesses:** fever, chills, tender abdominal mass, high WBC
- Cancer:
  - Colon: risk is slightly higher than general population
  - Small bowel: much higher risk; Distribution is ileum > jejunum > duodenum (exact opposite of sporadic small bowel cancer)
- Surveillance: yearly C-scope with random biopsy after 8 yrs of pancolitis or 15 yrs of left-sided colitis to look for dysplasia » colectomy
  - Similar surveillance to UC; *See also IBD- Ulcerative Colitis (Chapter 3.04)*
- **Crohn's treatment resistance (not in remission):**
  - DDX: Incorrect diagnosis, Progression of disease, Super-infection, Under-dosing/Non-compliance, IBS, Smoking, NSAIDs

PROGNOSIS:
- Recurrence risk:
  - Smokers have twice the recurrence rate as non-smokers, additive effect with oral contraceptive use
  - Intestinal infection and NSAIDs may increase risk
- Pregnancy:
  - Fertility is normal in inactive UC and CD; it is decreased with active IBD but most are still able to conceive
  - Sulfasalazine causes reversible infertility in men as a result of abnormal spermatogenesis and decreased motility
  - For women in remission before pregnancy, 2/3 stay in remission during pregnancy and postpartum
  - Controversy about offspring birth defects, most studies *do not* show increased risk, one showed risk with males on 6 MP (but evidence is weak)
    - Preterm delivery and decreased birth weight are reported

NOTES

3.02 MICROSCOPIC & RADIATION COLITIS

MICROSCOPIC COLITIS (Am J Gastroenterol 2004, 94:451-65)

Definition:
- Idiopathic colitides with mild inflammatory changes diagnosed only by colorectal biopsy and thus only microscopically
- Microscopic colitis is an umbrella term encompassing both Collagenous and Lymphocytic Colitis

	Collagenous Colitis:	Lymphocytic Colitis:
Gender incidence (F:M)	5:1	1:1
HLA B27 Positive	No	Yes
Histology:		
-Increased intraepithelial lymphocytes	Yes	Yes
-Increased lymphocyte lamina propria	Yes	Yes
-Surface epithelial flattening	Yes	Yes
-Thickened subepithelial collagen band	Yes	No

Epidemiology:
- Collagenous Colitis: 1/100,000; Most common with females, age 50-60
- Lymphocytic Colitis: 3/100,000; Equal in both male/female
  - Both are far less common than IBD

Pathophysiology:
- Collagenous Colitis
  - Diagnostic triad: increased **intraepithelial lymphocytes,** flattened surface epithelium, **thickened subepithelial collagen band**
- Lymphocytic Colitis
  - Increased **intraepithelial lymphocytes,** flattened surface epithelium but without subepithelial collagen band
- Biopsies also show *no* crypt architecture distortion (IBD has distortion of crypt architecture)
- Can affect any part of colon; Patchy in nature
- MOA (theory): Autoimmune (both) and NSAIDs (Collagenous only); Other theories: bile acid malabsorption, unidentified infection

Clinical Manifestations/Physical Exam:
- Diarrhea (watery, non-bloody)
- May have associated cramping, abdominal pain, weight loss, urgency, incontinence
- Reported associated conditions: Rheumatoid arthritis, Polyarthritis, Thyroid disease, Sicca syndrome, DM, SLE, PBC
- Dehydration, high fevers, nausea, vomiting, or hematochezia should raise the possibility of another diagnosis

Laboratory Studies:
- Celiac serology (up to 1/3 of celiac patients have colon biopsies consistent with microscopic colitis - hence they often co-exist)

Diagnostic Studies:
- Colonoscopy: mucosa appears normal, should take multiple random biopsies; EGD to rule out Celiac sprue with small bowel biopsies

Treatments:
- Natural history is unknown; spontaneous resolution may occur; No treatment is uniformly effective: Lots of options: Stop NSAIDs is a must
  - Loperamide: 2-16 mg/day, Lomotil 1-8 tabs/day
  - Bismuth subsalicylate (Pepto-Bismol): 2 tabs (262 mg) 3-4 times/day
  - Cholestyramine 4 gm 1-4 times/day
  - Sulfasalazine 2-4 g/day, Asacol 1.4-4.8 g/day, Pentasa 2-4 g/day
  - Azathioprine (Imuran) 2 mg/kg/day, Mercaptopurine (Purinethol) 1-1.5 mg/kg/day
  - Budesonide: 9 mg/day, Prednisone 30-60 mg/day tapered

CHAPTER 3.02 MICROSCOPIC & RADIATION COLITIS

- **Algorithm for Microscopic:** exclude celiac, stop NSAIDs, Trial (in order): Loperamide » Bismuth » Budesonide; ? 5ASA, ? Cholestyramine
- Treatment is generally continued for 8-12 weeks and then attempt to taper therapy can be considered
  - For those with recurrent symptoms, chronic maintenance can be used (except steroids/Budesonide)

Complications:
- Can be easily missed on pathology and miss classified as Diarrhea Predominant IBS

Prognosis:
- Course can be waxing and waning and spontaneous resolution has been reported
- There does not appear to be a risk for progression to more overt forms of IBD or cancer

RADIATION COLITIS

Definition:
- Inflammation of the colon due to the effects of radiation

Epidemiology:
- 5-20 % incidence with radiation therapy

Pathophysiology:
- Rectosigmoid is highly susceptible because it is immobile
- Microscopic: connective tissue fibrosis (stricturing) and obliterative endarteritis with local tissue ischemia
- Prevention: limit dosage and area of exposure if possible
  - Implant radiation causes less severe damage because of the smaller field of radiation

Clinical Manifestations/Physical Exam:
- Diarrhea and Tenesmus usually occurring within 6 weeks
- Rectal bleeding is usually a symptom of chronic radiation colitis

Diagnostic Studies:
- Endoscopy: may be normal or may show pallor, erythema, prominent telangiectasias, ulcerated or friable mucosa
- Barium enema: mucosal ulcerations, poor distensibility, increased presacral space, rectal narrowing, strictures, fistulae

Treatments:
- Enemas: steroids, sucralfate (20 cc of 10% or 2 grams in water, BID)
- PO: Prednisone, 5ASA
- Endoscopic: APC, Heater probe, Bipolar for bleeding telangiectasias (multiple sessions often needed ~every 4 weeks)
- Surgery: for refractory symptoms

Complications:
- Strictures that may need: endoscopic dilation, surgery

3.03 TREATMENT: CROHN'S DISEASE & ULCERATIVE COLITIS

Goals of therapy for IBD: Induction and maintenance of remission (Gastroenterology. 2006;130:935-987)

CATEGORY: 5ASA (5 AMINO SALICYLIC ACID) Induction/maintenance for UC; Induction/maintenance for very mild CD only

Sulfasalazine (5ASA + sulfa); **Mesalamine** (5ASA in pH-sensitive or time-dependant capsules)
- Topical/Local delivery: Induction/Maintenance; Either is best for mild to moderate proctitis and proctosigmoiditis
    Suppository (effective to 10-15 cm): Canasa; Enema (effective to splenic flexure): Rowasa
- Oral: **FDA approved for induction/maintenance of UC,** not Crohn's

Generic	Proprietary	Strength	Sulfasalazine Equivalent	Bond	Action Site
Sulfasalazine	Azulfadine	500 mg	8 qd: 4 g	Sulfa (diazo) 5ASA	Cleaved by bacteria in *Colon*
Mesalamine Compounds:					
—	Pentasa	250 mg 500 mg	16 qd: 4 g 8 qd: 4 g	Coated 5ASA	Time released *duodenum to colon*
—	Asacol	400 mg	12 qd: 4.8 g	Coated 5ASA	pH released in *TI and colon* (pH >7.0)
—	Lialda	1.2 mg	4 qd: 4.8 g	Coated 5ASA	MMX technology, pH released *TI and Colon*
Balsalazide	Colazal	750 mg	9 qd: 6.75 g	PABA (diazo) 5ASA	Cleaved in *Colon*
Olsalazine	Dipentum	250 mg	Not Used	5ASA (diazo) 5ASA	Cleaved in *Colon*

- Goal of 5ASA is 4-gram equivalent of Sulfasalazine, typically given in BID or TID dosing (Olsalazine rarely used due to ↑ secretary diarrheal side effect); PABA is an inert carrier
- Drugs are dose dependant (i.e. more you give, the more they work; No plateau ever demonstrated)
- Major side effects: idiosyncratic reaction (i.e. worsening of initial symptoms 5%), N/V, Fever, AIN, Sulfa allergy (except Olsalazine)

CATEGORY: STEROIDS Induction of UC and Crohn's
Not for maintenance; Not for stricturing and fistulizing type Crohn's
- Topical: Cortifoam/Cortenema (Best for mild to moderate proctitis and proctosigmoiditis, not for maintenance)
    Budesonide (Entocort): oral, but pH released in *TI and right colon* and acts as a topical steroid, with low systemic absorption
- Oral: Goal is prednisone equivalent of 40-60 mg (no evidence for >60 mg); Taper should be over 1-2 months or longer
- IV: Solumedrol 20 q 8 hr, Hydrocortisone 100 q 8 hr (In acute setting, if no response after 3-5 days of steroids, consider next step or a different diagnosis)
- Problems include steroid dependence & resistance; Side effects: diabetes, cataracts, osteoporosis, etc. Get baseline DEXA; give Vit Ca/D at same time

CATEGORY: ANTIBIOTICS Mild effect of Induction/maintenance for CD
The use of antibiotics for CD is controversial (No benefit with UC)
- Metronidazole (Flagyl) 750-1000 mg/day and Cipro 1000 mg/day: useful in perianal, fistulizing and active colonic CD (caution with pregnancy)
- Rifaximin used by some clinicians (no studies yet)

CATEGORY: NUTRITION (J Parenter Enteral Nutr. 2005;29:S179 & 2002;26:73SA. Clinical Gastro & Hep 2005;3:358-69.)
- Used as primary or adjuvant therapy mostly with inflammatory CD; Enteral nutrition can help induce remission (not quite as effective as steroids) or be used with resistance or intolerance to meds and/or replete and maintain nutrition status
- Data more limited with UC; Enteral nutrition enriched with fish oils, soluble fiber, and antioxidants can reduce steroid use
- More studies needed

CHAPTER 3.03 TREATMENT: CROHN'S DISEASE & ULCERATIVE COLITIS

CATEGORY: OTHER
- Bowel rest, stop antidiarrheals, low residue diet
- Serial abdominal exams and radiographs/CT to rule out dilation, perforation or abscess

CATEGORY: IMMUNOMODULATORS/BIOLOGICS
These are mostly immunosuppressive. Must rule out infection first!

	Ulcerative Colitis		Crohn's Disease I: Inflammatory S: Stricturing F: Fistulizing		Side Effects	Cautions
	Induce	Maintenance	Induce	Maintenance		
6MP (Purinethol) **Azathioprine** (Imuran)	OK	Yes	Yes (I, F)	Yes (I, F)	Pancreatitis (2-5%), Hepatitis, Allergy/flu like syndrome, BM toxicity	√ WBC, LFTs; Supplement Folate

-CD & UC: steroid dependant, refractory disease, intolerance/non-response to other meds; CD specific: fistulizing, prevent postop recurrence
-MOA: Purine analogs: interfere with DNA synthesis of rapidly dividing cells, such as lymphocytes (T > B) & macrophages; Takes weeks/months to work
-Dosage: *(See diagram and text on next page)*

| **Infliximab**
(Remicade) | Yes | Yes
(FDA Approved 2005) | Yes
(I, F) | Yes
(I, F) | Infusion reaction,
↑ Lymphoma risk,
long term, +AMA | √ TB and
HBV before
starting |

-CD & UC: refractory/intolerant steroids & 6 MP/Azathioprine, prominent joint sx; CD specific: significant perianal and/or extensive small bowel disease
-MOA: IgG mouse antibody to TNF (binds to soluble and surface membrane TNF), causing lysis
-Dosage: Induction 5 mg/kg IV (round to closest 100 mg) 3 doses at 0, 2, 6 wks; Maintenance: 5 mg/kg q 8 wks *(See also text on next page)*

| **Adalimumab**
(Humira) | ? | ? | Yes
(I,F) | Yes
(I,F)
(FDA approved 2007) | | √ TB and
HBV before
starting |

-MOA: Fully human antibody to TNF (no mouse component)
-Dosage: 160 mg sq at day 1; then 80 mg sq at day 15; then 40 mg sq every other week; then reassess after several weeks

| **Cyclosporine**
(Neoral) | Yes | Unlikely | Yes,
High
doses | ? | Hirsutism, Gingival
hyperplasia,
HTN, CRF,
Opportunistic
infections;
↓ Lipids =
↑Seizure risk | √ Lipids, renal
function;
Bridge to
other
therapies;
There are
better
options |

-MOA: Inhibits IL-2 release and activation of T lymphocytes
-Dosage: 2 mg/kg IV (some use 4 mg/kg); po doses 8 mg/kg/day *(See also text on next page)*

| **Methotrexate**
(MTX) | No | ? | OK | Yes | Liver toxicity,
infections,
teratogenic | Supplement
folate |

-MOA: Inhibits dihydrofolate reductase (folate antagonist); Inhibits lymphocyte proliferation
-Dosage: 25 mg q wk × 16 wks (give IM as it confirms absorption); reassess and continue 15 mg po or 25 mg IM q wk

SECTION III INFLAMMATORY BOWEL DISEASE

6MP (Purinethol)/Azathiprine (Imuran): (Clinical Gastroenterol Hepatol. 2004;2:731-743)
- TPMT (thiopurine methyltransferase) genetics (Phenotype): high, normal, intermediate, lacking
    - High: ↑ 6MMP leads to liver toxicity; Check LFTs regularly
    - Normal (90% of patients): start full dose
    - Intermediate: best
    - Lacking or block xo (Allopurinol), then shunt more to 6-TGN, risking toxicity (BM suppression)
- Check level of 6 TGN: should be in range of 200-400
    (levels have been shown to correlate with clinical response)
- Check level of 6-MMP: should be <5700

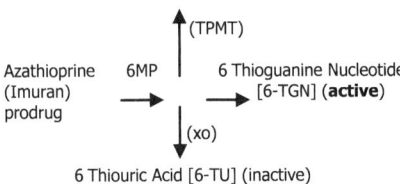

- Side effects: takes weeks/months to work! Follow CBC (For low WBC), LFTs
    - 6-MMP: hepatotoxicity, myalgias, headaches
    - 6-TGN: bone marrow suppression, allergic/flu like reaction (occurs ~2 weeks, re-challenge occurs in hours), pancreatitis, GI upset
    - Small ↑ risk of lymphoma (B-cell)
    - Inhibits folate absorption (prescribe folate at same time); Likewise, Methotrexate inhibits folate metabolism
- Approach to po dosing: start with low dose (12% have low TPMT); follow labs; slowly ↑ dose based on relative leucopenia & weight based

    Check baseline TPMT activity: EnzAct (other alternative is checking phenotype as above):
    Normal (>23.6 EU) » **6MP (Purinethol)** 1.0-1.5 mg/kg; **Azathioprine (Imuran)** 2.0-2.5 mg/kg
    Intermediate (<6.7-23.6 EU) » **6MP (Purinethol)** <1.0 mg/kg; **Azathioprine (Imuran)** <2.0 mg/kg
    Low/Absent (<6.7 EU) » Avoid

    Lab monitoring: CBC/Diff q week × 4; q 2 weeks × 4; q month × 3; then q 3 months indefinitely
    LFT at 1 month and then q 3 months

- Assess response ~2-3 months: **Responding** » follow clinically
    Not responding or low baseline TPMT » check metabolite levels:

	6-TGN (Active)	6-MMP (Inactive)	
Inadequate dose	↓	↓	
Non-adherence	↓↓↓	0	
6-MMP shunting	↓	↑↑↑	(unproven: block TPMT with 5ASAs for ↑ shunting to 6TGN)
Drug resistance	↑↑↑	↑	

Infliximab: (N Engl J Med. 2005;353:2462-2476. Am J Gastroenterol. 2002;97:2962-2972)
- Anti-infliximab Ab's association: ↑ risk for infusion reactions and ↓ response
    Rate of antibody formation ↓ with maintenance therapy (rather than giving episodic therapy)
    Concomitant use of immunosuppressant may reduce the risk for development of antibodies, especially in episodic treatments

CHAPTER 3.03 TREATMENT: CROHN'S DISEASE & ULCERATIVE COLITIS

- Approach to dosing:
  - Things to do before starting Infliximab:
    Explain that therapy will last at least 1 year with regular dosing intervals; Concomitant immuno-suppressive agent often used (i.e. 6 MP)
    Check for TB & Hepatitis B **(black box warnings):** baseline PPD (?anergy issues), CXR if prior TB exposure; Hepatitis serology
    Ensure adequate draining of infection in patients with perianal disease; rule out superimposed CMV in immunosuppressed
  - Premedicate: Diphenhydramine 25–50 mg po/IV 2 days before/1 day after, Acetaminophen 650 mg po same day, ? IV steroids
  - If maintenance dosing breakthrough:? higher dose at 10 mg/kg and more frequent dosing

Cyclosporine: (Am J Gastroenterol. 1997;92:1424–1428)
- Check for contraindications: creatine clearance with >30% GFR decrease, total cholesterol <120 mg/dl, low magnesium
- Use: check daily levels, electrolytes; Start prophylactic Bactrim at same time; If HTN develops, CCB are best used for therapy

INDICATIONS FOR SURGERY:
- U/C (30–40% of patients): failed medical treatment or neoplasm
  - Complications: hemorrhage, perforation, stricture, toxic megacolon without responding to 48-72 hrs of medical therapy
  - Dysplasia or carcinoma; *See also Complications in IBD- Ulcerative Colitis (Chapter 3.04)*
- CD (70–80% of patients): failed medical treatment or neoplasm
  - Complications: fistula, abscess, stricturing type disease, chronic steroid dependency
  - Dysplasia or carcinoma; *See also Complications in IBD- Ulcerative Colitis (Chapter 3.04)*
  - Surgery is not a cure; Wide margins are not associated with decreased recurrence

GENERAL IBD TREATMENT GUIDELINES:
- **Mild:** 5ASAs, budesonide, rectal 5ASAs, flagyl/cipro
- **Moderate:** Oral steroids, immunomodulators/biologics (See also table above on page 151)
- **Severe:** IV steroids, immunomodulators/biologics, other (bowel rest, TPN, IV antibiotics, serial exams, radiographs/CT, etc)

TREATMENT OF IBD IN PREGNANCY:
"The greatest risk to pregnancy is active disease – not active medications!" I.e. continue Mesalamine during pregnancy and breastfeeding

Summary of IBD Medications During Pregnancy			Summary of IBD Medications During Breastfeeding		
Safe	Limited Data	Contraindicated	Safe	Limited Data	Contraindicated
Oral Mesalamine	Corticosteroids	Methotrexate	Oral Mesalamine	Azathioprine	Methotrexate
Local Mesalamine	Olsalazine	Thalidomide	Local Mesalamine	6MP	Metronidazole
Sulfasalazine	Azathioprine/6MP	Sulfa	Sulfasalazine	Infiximab	Ciprofloxacin
Ciprofloxacin Metronidazole	Cyclosporine Infiximab	Tetracycline	Corticosteroids		Cyclosporine

3.04 ULCERATIVE COLITIS

(Am J Gastroenterol. 2004;99:1371-1385.; Gastroenterology. 2004;126:1582-1592.; N Engl J Med. 2002; 347:417-429)

DEFINITION:
- Idiopathic inflammation of the *colonic mucosa* (as opposed to Crohn's which is transmural and any segment of the GI tract)
  - Distinction between UC and CD is important, as surgery is a 'cure' via total colectomy for UC
- Backwash Ileitis: Unusual cases of ulcerative colitis involving the terminal ileum
  - Endoscopic/Radiologic appearance same as UC; If deeper linear ulcers/strictures seen in ileum, Crohn's Disease is most likely diagnosis
- Intermediate Colitis:
  - In 5-10% of patients with chronic colitis a clear distinction between UC and CD cannot be made even with mucosal biopsy
  - Many Crohn's Disease cases diagnosed after 'curative surgery for UC'; Recurrent ileitis of ileostomy or ileoanal pouch leads to diagnosis of Crohn's
- Cuffitis and Pouchitis: See end of this section

DDX:
- Infectious: bacterial (*E. coli, Salmonella, Shigella, Yersinia, Campylobacter, Mycobacterium, C. difficile*), amebic, CMV/HSV, STDs
- Ischemic colitis, Diverticulitis, Colorectal cancer
- Intestinal lymphoma, Collagenous/Lymphocytic colitis (Microscopic colitis), Celiac sprue, Radiation enteropathy
- IBS, Appendicitis, Solitary rectal ulcer syndrome
- Drugs (NSAID enteropathy, OCP, allopurinol)

EPIDEMIOLOGY:
- Prevalence 1:1000 (high because often presents in younger population initially); ♂ = ♀
- *Bimodal* with peaks in 20's and 50-70's; ↑ incidence in Caucasians, Jews, and non-smokers
- Appendicitis prior to age 20 and tobacco use have been reported to be protective against the development of UC
  - Prophylactic appendectomy for a normal appendix has no protective value

ETIOLOGIES:
- The cause is unknown
- Greatest risk is positive family history (10-15% have a family history); Genetic link has not been identified
  - Less familial association than Crohn's
- Three genetic syndromes associated: Turner's, Glycogen storage disease 1B, Hermansky-Pudlak (albinism, platelet defect)

PATHOPHYSIOLOGY:
- Extent: Involves *rectum* (95%) and extends proximally and *contiguously*
  - **Distribution:** 50% proctosigmoiditis, 30% left-sided colitis, and 20% extensive colitis
- Appearance: granular, friable mucosa with diffuse ulceration confined to only colon (not small bowel)
- Microscopy: superficial microulcerations; crypt abscesses (PMNs); goblet cell depletion; basal plasmacytosis

CLINICAL MANIFESTATIONS/PHYSICAL EXAM:
- **Rectal disease with grossly bloody diarrhea,** left lower abdominal cramps with tenesmus and urgency; Perianal disease is rare
- **Fulminant colitis:**
  - Progresses rapidly over 1-2 wks: ↓ Hct, ↑ ESR, fever, hypotension, >6 bloody BMs per day, distended abdomen/no bowel sounds
- **Megacolon** (6-13% of patients): colon dilation (Transverse ≥6 cm on KUB), colonic atony, and systemic toxicity
  - **Toxic Megacolon** (2 or more): HR >100/min, Temp >101.5°F (38.6°C), WBC >10,000, Hypoalbuminemia <3.0 gm/dl

CHAPTER 3.04 ULCERATIVE COLITIS

- Perforation: pneumoperitoneum, peritonitis
- **Extracolonic** (25%): most mimic disease activity:
  - Seronegative (RF−) **arthritis** is most common, 25% of patients: large joint, unilateral, non-deforming (coincides with colitis activity)
    - Ankylosing spondylitis 30-fold increase: 50% are HLA-B27 positive (doesn't coincide with colitis activity)
  - Osteopenia/Osteoporosis: risks: steroid use, malabsorbed Ca/D, ↓ BMI, tobacco; generally treated like any other patient (i.e. Bisphosphonates)
  - Derm:
    - **Erythema nodosum:** painful pretibial erythematous subcutaneous nodules (coincides with colitis activity)
    - **Pyoderma gangrenosum:** pustular lesions that ulcerate and exhibit pathergy (doesn't coincide with colitis activity)
  - Ocular: **anterior uveitis (iritis), episcleritis** (if HLA-B27 + doesn't coincide with colitis activity; If HLA-B27−, it does coincide with colitis activity)
    - Any ocular symptom in an IBD patient should prompt a referral to an ophthalmologist
  - Vascular: Hypercoagulable states/ Thromboembolic events (after search for hypercoagulable state, use standard therapy for treatment)
  - Liver:
    - **PSC** has ↑ risk cholangiocarcinoma (risk: U/C >> CD, doesn't coincide with colitis activity); Only 'cure' is transplant
    - Chronic hepatitis, cirrhosis, fatty liver
  - CD sees more Gallstones and Kidney stones due to ileum involvement
- **Smoking helps/protective!** (Patients are reluctant to stop smoking)

Classification of severity of Ulcerative Colitis:
- **Mild:** Fewer than 4 stools/day, with or without blood; No systemic disturbance and a normal ESR
- **Moderate:** More than 4 stools/day, but with minimal systemic disturbance
- **Severe:** More than 6 stools/day with blood and systemic disturbance (fever >37.5°C, tachycardia >90 bpm, Hb <7.5, ESR >30)

LABORATORY STUDIES:
- ↓ Hct due to Fe; ↑ WBC from active disease or abscess; Diarrheal wasting: hypoalbuminemia, hypokalemia
- Serologies: **p-ANCA** 60-70% sensitivity for UC (also associated with pancolitis and PSC); Less likely in CD (10%)
  - More common with UC & Pouchitis; Not related to disease activity
  - These serologies are included in: Prometheus IBD serology 7
- Acute flare: always consider infection compromise: *C. diff*, Stool culture, O&P, CMV serology/biopsy

DIAGNOSTIC STUDIES:
- Endoscopy: loss of vascular pattern, mucosal granularity, friability, mucous exudates, focal ulcerations
  - Rectal involvement with continuous disease (no skip areas or cobblestoning)
  - Biopsies: No granulomas (granulomas are generally diagnostic of CD, but only found in 10-30% of the cases)
  - Can have inflammation around appendix, called Cecal patch, and this should not be confused with segmental colitis due to CD
  - Note: phosphosoda enemas can cause changes in distal colon similar to UC (loss of vascular pattern, granularity, friability)
- Small Bowel Series or CT enterography:
  - Normal TI
- Barium Enema:
  - *Pseudopolyps* » hazy margins, loss of haustra ('lead pipes'); most typical radiographic finding of UC
- KUB (flat and upright):
  - Rule out toxic megacolon
- Capsule Endoscopy:
  - May be useful for evaluating extent of disease in small bowel, but its precise role is yet to be defined
- DEXA scan for bone loss
- **Note:** With UC patients, strictures should heighten suspicion for cancer

SECTION III INFLAMMATORY BOWEL DISEASE

TREATMENTS:
- *See also IBD- Treatment Crohn's and UC (Chapter 3.03)*
- Toxic Megacolon: *see also Bowel- Megacolon (Chapter 2.20)*
- Refractory Pyoderma Gangrenosum may require Tacrolimus or Cyclosporin therapy
- Must avoid NSAIDs and Narcotics
- Hospitalization: daily abdomen exam and KUB, IV steroids, avoid narcotics/anticholinergics, consider checking C. *diff*, stool culture, CMV
  - Partial response: change to po steroids and consider 5ASA, 6MP/Azathiprine as outpatient
  - No response after 3-5 days: consider flex sig with biopsy, stool studies; further considerations: infliximab, cyclosporine, surgery

COMPLICATIONS:
- Strictures (rarely occurs in rectosigmoid)
- **Colon Cancer:** -Patients with *pancolitis* are at greatest risk (8-10% cumulative risk at 20 years, as high as 35% at 30 years)
  -Patients with left-sided colitis, family history of CRC and PSC are also at increased risk (difficult to quantify exact risk)
  -No increased risk with ulcerative proctitis (rectal involvement), hence no surveillance recommended
  -Remember: in addition these patients are at the same general population risk for developing sporadic adenomas

Surveillance: with colonoscopy (recommended timelines are not universally agreed upon by all major GI societies)

Who: looking for dysplasia in pancolitis of at least 8 yrs or 15 yrs of left-sided colitis (some start surveillance at 8 yrs for left side colitis)

When: q2-3 yrs up to 15 yrs of disease, every other year for next 10 yrs (15-25 yrs of disease), yearly thereafter; PSC: q1 yr starting at diagnosis

How: Flat mucosa (biopsy 10 cm intervals in 4 quadrant fashion; minimum 33 biopsies detects dysplasia with 90% confidence)
Raised/polypoid lesions (biopsy placed in separate bottles)
All biopsy histology confirmed by expert GI pathologist

Endoscopy Finding	Recommendation
DALM or Flat mucosa with LGD, HGD, or CA	Colectomy (Colectomy for LGD is controversial to some clinicians)
ALM with dysplasia anywhere in colon	Colectomy
ALM without dysplasia anywhere in colon	Polypectomy and UC surveillance with ↑ frequency (Ideal frequency not defined)
Sporadic Adenoma	Polypectomy and routine UC surveillance
No dysplasia on random biopsy or "Indefinite dysplasia"	Continued UC surveillance or Repeat Cscope in 3-6 months respectively

Dysplasia Associated Lesion/Mass (DALM): dysplasia of polypoid lesion, mass, plaque or stricture (within the colitis; not removable via scope)
Adenoma-like mass (ALM): well-circumscribed, sessile or pedunculated, resembling a sporadic adenoma (but occurs within the colitis)
Sporadic adenoma: occurs proximal (outside) of any colitis; i.e. right-sided polyp in a patient with left-sided colitis
  -Need to distinguish because DALM = colectomy, Sporadic adenoma = routine CRC surveillance (i.e. the treatments vary vastly)
  -Clues: DALM more likely to occur in younger, longer duration and more extensive disease, larger lesions (i.e. >1.5 cm)
  -Clues: Sporadic adenomas appear like others (pedunculated, sessile) rather than having flat, ulcerated, plaque-like appearance; They are not associated with dysplastic changes in flat mucosa elsewhere in the colon! (Chromoendoscopy may help differentiate in future)

CHAPTER 3.04 ULCERATIVE COLITIS

PROGNOSIS:
- Disease activity
  - Intermittent exacerbations in 75-85% (Medication required for remission)
  - Continual active disease in 10-15%
  - Severe initial attack requiring urgent colectomy in 5-10% (If perforation prior, 50% mortality)
- Mortality rate for severe attack of UC is <2% (usually due to Toxic Megacolon)
- Life expectancy is the same as those without UC
- Pregnancy (See Prognosis under **IBD- Crohn's disease Chapter 3.01**)

CUFFITIS:
- Disease (i.e. UC) is still present at the surgical remnant!
- Treatment: Canasa PR 500 mg BID; Second line, Annusol PR

POUCHITIS: (Gastroenterology. 2003;124:1636-1650)
- Inflammation of pouch likely from infection; Symptoms of diarrhea, urgency, and fecal incontinence
- Occurs in 50% within 5 years; Chronic pouchitis is 5-10% at 5 years
- Risk factors: Extensive UC, Backwash Ileitis, PSC, P-ANCA, Ex-smoker, NSAID use
- Treatment: Antibiotics: Flagyl, Cipro, Xifaxan; Alternative: Belladona/Opiate (B&O) suppositories PR 30 mg BID
  - Mesalamine can be tried if fail antibiotics; Rarely need steroids/immunomodulators

3.05 POTPOURRI

IBD PEARLS
Outpatient:
Always confirm the diagnosis: how was IBD diagnosed, particular bowel location involved (colon vs. small bowel), response to any prior therapy, medication use (NSAIDs), tobacco use, etc

Preventive therapy: dysplasia screening performed, DEXA bone scan (Treatments: Ca/VitD and/or Bisphosphonates), labs: CBC/LFTs, B12/Folate, trace elements, etc

Inpatient:
Don't forget to check stool for *C. difficile* and O&P; Serology and biopsy for CMV (especially if on immunomodulators or immunosuppressed)
Empiric bacterial overgrowth? Treat with Cipro 250 bid or Flagyl 250 TID for 7days

IBD MIMICKERS
Infections: *strongyloidosis, TB, Amebiasis, Campy,* HIV, CMV
Ischemia
Diverticular disease

SMALL BOWEL RESECTION AND MALABSORPTION (With Colon Intact):
>100 cm Ileum resected (Fatty Acid Diarrhea)
Most of bile salts not absorbed due to increased loss of ileum resulting in massive loss of bile salts into the colon; Loss exceeds the capacity of liver to compensate: therefore total circulation of bile acid pool is diminished; Get low effective postprandial bile salt concentration and hence fat malabsorption and steatorrhea; Diarrhea now consists of malabsorbed fatty acids (steatorrhea) from limited bile salts
Treatment: low fat diet (med-chain FFA), calcium supplements, antidiarrheal agents; Cholestyramine may worsen the steatorrhea

<100 cm Ileum resected (Bile Salt Diarrhea)
Some bile salts not absorbed in resected ileum, but liver revs up production/secretion to help digestion of fats; However the malabsorbed bile salts stimulate the secretion of electrolytes/water from the colon and cause diarrhea; Suspect post-op in patient with diarrhea after ileal resection and normal diet is started
Treatment: cholestyramine binds bile salts and prevents wastage in the colon; Cholestyramine can bind medications too!

KIDNEY STONES
Why Ca Oxalate Stones in IBD (and Short Bowel Syndrome)?
Because of increased concentration of FFAs in lumen of small bowel (malabsorption), calcium is complexed to malabsorbed neg-charged FFAs (normally, calcium and oxalate bind each other); The reduction in concentration of calcium results in unopposed colonic absorption of dietary oxalates, resulting in increased excretion of oxalate in urine and formation of calcium-oxalate stones; Excessive luminal FFAs and bile acids appear to increase colonic permeability to oxalate, further increasing its absorption: hence hyperoxaluria appears to depend on the presence of an intact colon
Treatment: high calcium, low-fat, low-oxalate diet

IV

LIVER

4.01 α1-ANTITRYPSIN DEFICIENCY

DEFINITION:
- Deficiency in alpha-1-antitrypsin (α1-AT) characterized by liver and/or lung injury
- Other inheritable forms of liver disease: Hemochromatosis, Wilson's

EPIDEMIOLOGY:
- 1 in 2,000 is homozygous and 1 in 30 is a heterozygous carrier (Z allele)
- Causes neonatal hepatitis in 15-30% of children with ZZ phenotype

ETIOLOGIES:
- Autosomal recessive
- Gene is located on chromosome 14 (replacement of glutamic acid by lysine at 342 position), leading to deficiency in sialic acid
- Abnormal α1-AT » polymerization in liver (cirrhosis) & uninhibited protease activity in lung (emphysema)

PATHOPHYSIOLOGY:
- α1-AT is a protease inhibitor (enzyme) made in liver that helps to break down trypsin and other tissue proteases
  - Responsible for inhibiting trypsin, collagenase, and elastase; With α1-AT deficiency, these are left unopposed
  - Lungs: can lead to progressive decrease in elastin and development of premature emphysema (not same MOA as liver disease)
  - Liver: failure to secrete α1-AT, aggregates of the defective protein found (i.e. not true 'deficiency')
    - Unclear means to the development of cirrhosis
- Over 75 different protease inhibitor (Pi) alleles have been identified:
  - M/M is normal (95% of population)
  - Z/Z results in lowest levels of α1-AT and this phenotype confirms the diagnosis

CLINICAL MANIFESTATIONS/PHYSICAL EXAM:
- Adults and children with liver involvement have no symptoms until they develop signs and symptoms of chronic liver disease
- Symptoms, other than liver, Emphysema: lower lung blebs (exacerbated markedly by smoking)
- Consider α1-AT in any adult who presents with chronic hepatitis, cirrhosis, portal HTN, or HCC of unknown etiology

LABORATORY STUDIES:
- α1-AT phenotype; Designates the allelic protein type in the serum – **Primary test**
  - Order in the workup of all chronic liver patients, since there is no presenting symptoms
  - Abnormal protease inhibitor (Pi) type (Phenotype):
    - Z/Z = cirrhosis; M/Z = usually don't develop cirrhosis unless another chronic liver condition present; M/M = normal
    - If Z protein is trapped in hepatocytes, can be seen in liver with + PAS inclusion bodies on liver biopsy
- α1-AT serum level should NOT be used because it is falsely increased with any inflammatory disorder, pregnancy, or malignancy
  - Additionally, unlike lung disease, liver damage does not correlate with serum levels
- PAS-D (Periodic acid-Schiff-diastase) stains both glycogen and α1-AT globules dark, reddish-purple; Diastase digests glycogen
  - Therefore when PAS-D used, only positive staining globules are due to α1-AT
- SPEP: blood proteins separated on basis of electrical migration in gel, several bands form, one of these is α1-AT
  - Therefore α1-AT deficiency results in flattening of the α1-AT band on SPEP
- Direct assay that uses monoclonal antibody against α1-AT
  - Degree of binding can be measured in a spectrophotometer

DIAGNOSTIC STUDIES:
- Biopsy shows:
  - Classic **PAS-positive,** diastase-resistant globules with periportal hepatocytes
    - These globules may be present in heterozygotes and homozygotes without liver disease
    - Globules presence does not imply liver disease; Since globules have variable distribution their absence does not exclude α1-AT
  - Portal fibrosis and chronic hepatitis may also be present which does imply liver disease

TREATMENTS:
- Symptomatic management of complications and liver transplant (for cirrhosis)
- With transplant the phenotype becomes that of the transplanted graft; Must transplant before advanced lung disease develops
- α1-AT replacement (used for emphysema) does not work for liver disease
- Avoid tobacco (risk of emphysema) and ETOH
- Genetic counseling/screening for family members (see Complications below)

COMPLICATIONS:
- This is an inheritable disease; Once patient is diagnosed, all first-degree relatives should be screened for α1-AT phenotypes
  - Screening is largely for prognostication, as definitive therapy for liver disease, other than transplant, is not available
- Older (>50 yrs) patients, especially men, are at risk for developing hepatocellular carcinoma
  - Screen for HCC with U/S and AFP

PROGNOSIS:
- Depends on underlying severity of disease; Typically those with liver disease don't have lung disease, and vise versa
- Patients with transplant usually do fine (α1-AT, like Wilson's disease does not reoccur as it is inherent to the organ itself, which is unlike Hemochromatosis and can recur)

4.02 ABSCESS OF LIVER

DEFINITION:
- Two types of liver abscess; Areas affected by either: Right lobe only (65%), Both lobes (30%), Left lobe only (5%)
  - Pyogenic, usually arise from intraabdominal infections
  - Amebic, usually arise from colonic infections with invasive *Entamoeba histolytica*

EPIDEMIOLOGY:
- Pyogenic: middle to older age (median age 51), affects ♂ = ♀
- Amebic: younger population (30-40 years), ♂ > ♀

ETIOLOGIES:
- Pyogenic: Majority of causes unknown (Cryptogenic)
  - Biliary tract diseases are the **most common known source** (35% of cases); Most cases result from cholangitis or acute cholecystitis
  - Another 30% of cases caused by: Diverticulitis, Crohn's, Ulcerative Colitis, Bowel perforation
  - Another 15% occur via direct extension from a contiguous source, such as subphrenic abscess or empyema of the gallbladder
  - Intraabdominal infections with bacterial seeding via portal vein can occur, i.e. dental disease, endocarditis
  - Other causes: Malignancy of pancreas, common bile duct, ampulla; Endoscopic and surgical intervention of the biliary tree
- Amebic:
  - Bile is lethal to amebas, thus infections of gallbladder and bile ducts do not occur

PATHOPHYSIOLOGY:
- Pyogenic
  - Organisms: gram(−) organisms 50-70% of cases *(E. coli)*, gram(+) 25% of cases, Anaerobes 50% of cases
  - Abscesses from biliary origin tend to be multiple and small size, involving both lobes of the liver
  - Septic emboli via portal vein tend to be solitary; Contiguous sources tend to be solitary
- Amebic:
  - Usually arise from colonic infections with invasive *Entamoeba histolytica*
  - Tend to be solitary and large, most common in right lobe

CLINICAL MANIFESTATIONS/PHYSICAL EXAM:
- Pyogenic: nonspecific, but include fever (absent in 30%), chills, RUQ pain (only present in 45%), malaise, weight loss
  - Clinical picture may be dominated by the underlying cause: appendicitis, diverticulitis, biliary disease
  - Comorbidities common: diabetes, malignancy, alcoholism, cardiovascular disease, chronic renal failure
- Amebic: more severe right upper quadrant pain and febrile in 90% of cases
  - Clinical picture may be associated with recent travel to endemic areas, although may be remote
  - Prior symptoms suggestive of previous colonic amebiasis are present in only 5-15%
  - Concurrent hepatic abscess and amebic dysentery are unusual

LABORATORY STUDIES:
- Routine labs are not diagnostic for either Pyogenic or Amebic abscess: WBC (high), Anemia (normocytic/normochromic), Sed Rate (high)
  - Eosinophilia is characteristically absent in amebic cysts
  - LFTs nonspecific: 90% of patients have high Aφ; AST/ALT are elevated, but to a lesser degree
    - If high bili, the biliary tree is the likely sources of the abscess; Low albumin (<2 gm/dl) is a poor prognosticator
- Pyogenic: Blood cultures: positive in 50%; Aspirates from abscesses are positive for bacteria in 75-90%
  - Negative aspirates do not necessarily indicate nonpyogenic abscess: ensure proper collection (esp. with anaerobes)

CHAPTER 4.02 ABSCESS OF LIVER

- Amebic: Most aspiration does not yield an organism; Trophozoites found in <20% of aspirates; most abscesses are odorless
  - Serologic tests are positive only in patients with invasive amebiasis, typically negative in asymptomatic carriers
  - Gel diffusion precipitin tests are generally best, titers usually become negative after 6 months, high titers suggest abscess

DIAGNOSTIC STUDIES:
- CXR: may be abnormal in 50-80% of patients with liver abscesses: RLL atelectasis, R pleural effusion, R hemidiaphragm elevation
- KUB: air in abcess cavities 10-20% of cases, gastric displacement due to enlargement of liver may be seen
- U/S: **initial test of choice;** noninvasive and highly sensitive (80-90%): preferred modality to distinguish cystic from solid lesions
  - Usually U/S is more accurate for visualizing biliary tree; However, operator-dependent and may be affected by body habitus
- CT (IV contrast): aids in diagnosis of smaller abscesses, assesses entire peritoneal cavity which may provide info about primary lesions
- MRI: does not add much to the sensitivity of CT scanning; useful in patients who cannot tolerate contrast
- Aspirate when thought to be Pyogenic (multiple abscess, coexistent biliary disease, intraabdominal inflammatory process) and non-Amebic
  - Amebic aspiration if Pyogenic can't be ruled out, or when patient doesn't respond to amebic therapy, or abscess is large and painful
  - Surgical drainage of amebic abscess when located in left lobe or response to therapy is not dramatic within 24-48 hours

TREATMENTS:
- Pyogenic: Antibiotics and percutaneous (preferred) drainage result in 76% cure rate (60% for either alone)
  - Antibiotics: aminoglycoside/cephalosporin (gram −), clindamycin/metronidazole (anaerobes), penicillin/ampicillin (enterococci)
  - Surgical drainage if more conservative measures fail in complete resolution or if needed to treat primary intraabdominal lesion
- Amebic: Metronidazole is only drug active against extraintestinal form of amebiasis: 750 mg TID × 10 days
  - Eradicate intestinal form too: Iodoquinol 650 mg TID × 20 days; Consider aspiration if failing therapy

COMPLICATIONS:
- Pyogenic: untreated 100% mortality
  - Rupture into peritoneal cavity: subphrenic, perihepatic, subhepatic abscesses or peritonitis; Metastatic septic emboli: lung, brain
  - Left lobe abscesses can be complicated by cardiac tamponade, pericarditis
- Amebic: similar to Pyogenic; Abscesses in dome of liver or complicated by bronchopleural fistula are typically amebic in origin

PROGNOSIS:
- Pyogenic: depends on rapidity of diagnosis and underlying illness:
  - Morbidity is generally high (50%) due to complexity of therapy and need for prolonged drainage
  - Mortality is 5-10% with prompt recognition and adequate antibiotic therapy; higher in patients with multiple abscesses
- Amebic generally do well with treatment, morbidity (4.5%), mortality (2.2%)

4.03 ACUTE LIVER FAILURE (FULMINANT HEPATIC FAILURE)

(Hepatology 2005;41:1179-97)

DEFINITION:
- Acute hepatic disease + coagulopathy (INR >1.5) + encephalopathy (without a history of prior liver disease, except Wilson's & AIH)
  - Fulminant = develops within 8 weeks
  - Subfulminant (late-onset hepatic failure) = develops between 8 weeks and 6 months
- Proposed other definitions: (Lancet 1993;342:273-275)
  - Hyperacute = encephalopathy develops within 7 days of the onset of jaundice
  - Acute = encephalopathy develops between 8-28 days of the onset of jaundice
  - Subacute = encephalopathy develops between 29 days and 12 weeks of the onset of jaundice

EPIDEMIOLOGY:
- Rare: ~2000 cases/year; Prior to transplant, survival was 15%

PATHOPHYSIOLOGY:
- Outpouring of cytokines by a dying liver
- See also Clinical Manifestations/Complications below

ETIOLOGIES: *See also Liver- Drug Induced Liver Disease (Chapter 4.11)*
ABC's: Acetaminophen, HAV, AIH- HBV- HCV, CMV, Crypto- HDV, Drugs- E (esoteric): Wilson's, Budd Chiari - Fatty: NASH, AFLP
- **Viral:**
  - HAV, **HBV,** HCV (rare), HDV + HBV, HEV (especially if travel history or pregnant)
  - HSV (immunocompromised hosts), EBV, CMV, Adenovirus, Paramyxovirus, Parvovirus B19
- **Drugs/Toxins:**
  General rule of thumb, new drugs started within 6 months of FHF
  - Acetaminophen **(most common cause: ~40-50% of all cases),** accidental or suicidal
  - Other drugs (15-20%, 3rd most common cause): phenytoin, INH, rifampin, sulfonamides, tetracycline, valproate, amiodarone, PTU
  - Toxins: fluorinated hydrocarbons, CCL_4, *Amanita phalloides*
  - Alternative remedies: black cohosh, kava, ma huang, gum thistle, he shon wu, comfrey, sunnhemp, bai-fang
- **Vascular:**
  Should see global ischemia if this is the cause (i.e. ischemic pancreas); Liver has two blood supplies (Portal Vein, Hepatic Artery)
  - Ischemic hepatitis, Budd-Chiari syndrome, Hepatic veno-occlusive disease, Malignant infiltration
- **Malignancy:**
  - Infiltrative types (i.e. HSM on exam): metastatic breast, melanoma (check LDH and get biopsy!), lymphoma/leukemia, small cell lung
- **Autoimmune Hepatitis** (check ASMA, consider transjugular biopsy): Need to confirm because patients are likely to respond to steroids
- Miscellaneous:
  - Wilson's (always rule out in young person; ↑ unconjugated bili/hemolysis, urine copper; ↓ Aφ, ceruloplasmin) needs transplant urgently!
  - α1-AT deficiency, hemochromatosis, PBC, acute fatty liver of pregnancy, HELLP syndrome, Reye's syndrome
- Idiopathic (second most common cause ~20-30%)
  - No markers of acute or chronic viral hepatitis, autoimmune hepatitis, or Wilson's disease; No evidence of malignancy or pregnancy
  - No history of drug, toxin, alternative remedies or mushroom ingestion; No evidence of vascular etiology
  - Possible etiologies: viral hepatitis without markers, non A-E viral hepatitis, atypical non-hepatitis virus infection, unrecognized metabolic disorder or exposure to hepatotoxin

CHAPTER 4.03   ACUTE LIVER FAILURE (FULMINANT HEPATIC FAILURE)

CLINICAL MANIFESTATIONS/COMPLICATIONS:
Most sequela are a combination of vasogenic edema, cytotoxicity via ammonia, systemic/intrarenal pressure changes, and immune derangements
- Neurologic
  - **Encephalopathy:** Stage I: mental status change; Stage II: lethargy, confusion
    Stage III: stupor, but arousable; Stage IV: coma
      Asterixis: stages II & III, sometimes I; EEG abnormal: stages II,III, IV
      Intubate patient: stages III, IV (use Propofol)
  - **Cerebral Edema:** *Most common cause of death (40%): ICP/Herniation;* Etiology unclear; 75% occurrence in stage IV PSE
      Late stages: Cushing's triad (HTN + bradycardia + irregular respiration), pupillary dilation, decerebrate posturing, apnea

- Cardiovascular: **Hypotension** (vasodilators, likely NO) with low SVR and high cardiac output; Most are resistant to vasopressors

- Pulmonary: Pulmonary edema and infection 30%; **Respiratory Alkalosis,** impaired peripheral 02 uptake, ARDS

- GI: GI bleeding (**25% of patients** cause of death), Pancreatitis

- Renal: **Hepatorenal syndrome,** *See also Liver- Hepatorenal Syndrome (Chapter 4.18)*
  - Others: ATN 30-50%, 75% with Tylenol overdose (seen early); hyponatremia (↑ADH), hypokalemia, hypophosphatemia (K,po^4: intracellular shift)
  - Clinical: Una ↓ without diuretics/tubular injury; BUN unreliable due to ↓ urea production; Alkalosis, followed by Metabolic Acidosis & Respiratory Alkalosis

- Hematology: **Coagulopathy** (due to ↓ synthesis of clotting factors, ± DIC); ↑ PT, PTT and ↓ Plt's are seen in both FHF and DIC
  - Factor 8 (only factor synthesized in vascular endothelium, not in liver): Therefore it is normal in FHF! Consumed/Low in DIC!

- **Infection: 90% of patients**, due to suppressed immune function, impaired neutrophil function, and deficiency of opsonins
  - Especially gram + organisms and fungi; SBP in 32% of patients; fever and leukocytosis may be absent

- Endocrine: **Hypoglycemia** (↓ stores and gluconeogenesis via the liver, ↑ circulating insulin) - monitor closely

LABORATORY STUDIES/DIAGNOSTIC STUIDES/WORK UP:
- Liver Bx: Essentially no role for liver biopsy, unless ? malignancy (If precluded by coagulopathy consider transjugular)

- Studies: CT brain (rule out bleed and for ICP monitoring)
    Liver Vascular/Doppler ultrasound, CT or MRI abdomen, DEXA scan
    TTE, EKG, CXR, Spirometry

- Labs: PT/PTT, CMP/LFT, CBC/Diff, Type/Screen, ABG, CMV IgG, Vitamin: A,E,D25, TSH, HIV, RPR, VZV titer, AFP, CA19-9
    Hepatitis Panel (Acute and Remote), HCV Quant (viral load) & genotype, HBV DNA, Amylase/Lipase, Lactate, Ammonia
    Urine/Blood toxicology (acetaminophen levels q 1-2 hr until peak determined), Random cortisol, Blood/Urine cultures
    Possibly needed: Iron studies, ANA, AMA, ASMA, Ceruloplasmin/serum copper, α1-AT, HCG (♀), CK/Troponin

- Consults: Cardiology/Anesthesia, Psychiatry, Social Service, Chemical dependency if appropriate

SECTION IV LIVER

TREATMENTS:
ICU-Level care at liver transplant center potentially including invasive monitoring and treating ICP, hemodynamic and ventilatory support, reversing coagulopathies, aggressive monitoring for and treatment of infection, D10 drip for hypoglycemia, etc.

- Neurologic
  - Encephalopathy: See above under Clinical Manifestations/Complications for definitions
    Lactulose: po or enema; Neomycin or Flagyl may be needed
  - Cerebral Edema: ICP invasive monitoring: **Brain CT first (rule out bleed/mass),** Correct platelets and coags (FFP)
    -Indication: when you can't monitor mental status anymore, i.e. intubation, coma
    -Complications: hemorrhage and infection
    -Goal: ICP <20–40 mmHg; Arterial NH_3 >200 correlates with ↑ ICP
    -Goal: CPP (cerebral perfusion pressure) = mean arterial pressure – ICP; Goal 60–100 mmHg, via ↑ MAP, ↓ ICP
    -↓ agitation (hypoxia, cough, vomiting, fever, suctioning while off ventilator), No IVF (or use hypertonic NS), HOB ≥ 20–45°
    -Hyperventilate to $PaCO_2$ <30 mmHg (for acute treatment only; can be detrimental if used chronically)
    -Mannitol 0.5–1 g/kg IV bolus (pOsm: 310–325), use with ICP >25 mmHg
    -Other more rare methods: cooling blankets (to temp 32–34°C), ? phenobarb or barbiturate induced coma
    -Note: prolonged ↑ ICP may indicate brain death (generally a contraindication to transplant); sudden ↓ may indicate brain herniation

- Cardiovascular: If patient deteriorating, check wedge pressure: if low consider GIB; if normal consider pneumonia, tamponade, sepsis
  Use **vasoactive pressors** and IVF if needed

- Pulmonary: Mechanical ventilate: careful with PEEP as can worsen ICP

- GI Bleed: **PPI** via IV for prophylaxis

- Renal: Supportive/Preventive: avoid hypotension, treat infection, avoid nephrotoxic drugs
  If HD needed, best is **CVVHD**; Treat hypokalemia (↓ k promotes ammonia and PSE)

- Hematology: Coagulopathy: No prophylactic FFP
  FFP indicated for active bleed or invasive procedures (placement of ICP monitor); **Vitamin K** 5 mg sq TID × 3 doses; Platelets prn

- Infection: Resp, UTI, Blood: most common; Clues: worsening PSE and renal function; If patient is infected, not a transplant candidate!
  Broad spectrum antibiotics (Zosyn) and antifungals (Fluconazole) (avoid aminoglycosides): ↓ risk of infection, but not ↑ survival

- Endocrine:
  - Hypoglycemia: Keep BS >65; **Use dextrose-based IVF**
  - Adrenal insufficiency: **Hydrocortisone** may be needed (determined based on random cortisol levels)

- Nutrition: Encephalopathy stage I & II: **Enteral feeds;** Encephalopathy stage III & IV: **TPN/PPN**

- **Treat specific causes:** (see also each corresponding topic)
  - Acetaminophen: **N-acetylcysteine IV**
  - AIH: Corticosteroids
  - Wilson's: Chelation therapy
  - Pregnancy: Delivery
  - Budd Chiari: Anticoagulation, TIPS, Surgical decompression
  - *Amanita phalloides:* Forced diuresis, charcoal, Penicillin + Silibinin
  - HSV: **IV Acyclovir** (consider in patients who might have HSV hepatitis)

- In General: Do NOT use steroids, charcoal hemoperfusion, prostaglandins

CHAPTER 4.03 ACUTE LIVER FAILURE (FULMINANT HEPATIC FAILURE)

PROGNOSIS:
- Survival 10–70% without liver transplant
- Extracorporeal liver assist devices now under evaluation as 'bridge' to transplant
- **King's College Criteria** for rapid liver transplantation in FHF
  Patients fulfilling the following criteria have a mortality range of 80 to 95% and will benefit from liver transplant:

Acetaminophen-Induced Disease:	Specific Disease:	All Other Causes:
Arterial pH <7.3	Wilson's disease	PT >100 (irrespective of PSE grade)
OR	Budd Chiari	**OR any 3 of the following**
Grade III/IV PSE, *and*		Age: <10 or >40 yrs
PT >100 sec, *and*		Etiology: Non-HAV, Non-HBV, halothane, idiosyncratic drug rxn
Creatinine >3.4 mg/dL		Jaundice onset >7 days before PSE
		PT >50 sec
		Bili >18 mg/dL

- **Liver transplantation:** only proven treatment, 1-year survival rate >80%; ***See also Liver- Transplantation (Chapter 4.28)***

4.04 ALCOHOLIC LIVER DISEASE

(Am J Gastro 1998;93:2022-36)

DEFINITION:
- Clinical spectrum includes fatty liver (occurs in days & is reversible), alcoholic hepatitis and alcoholic cirrhosis; Only 20% of alcoholics develop the later two
- Dependency: impairment or distress, as manifested by three or more of the following within 12 months:
  - Tolerance, Withdrawal, Desire to cut down, Giving up important social activities, Continued use despite knowing of adverse effects
- Abuse: impairment or distress, as manifested by one or more of the following within 12 months:
  - Not fulfilling obligation at work/school, Recurrent substance-related legal problems, Continuing situations when physically hazardous
- Acute Alcohol Toxicity: large quantities of alcohol consumed over a short period can result in acute liver toxicity (acute alcohol poisoning)
- Alcoholic Hepatitis: usually associated with heavy alcohol consumption for more than 10 years

EPIDEMIOLOGY:
- Prevalence of alcohol abuse in general population: 9.4%; Alcohol is implicated in >50% of liver-related deaths in the U.S.
- Incidence of progressive liver injury or cirrhosis is significantly increased in those who consume >40-60 gm alcohol/day
  - Approximately 20% of men drinking >8-12 beers/day develop cirrhosis in 10 years

ETIOLOGIES:
- Beer (12 oz), Wine (5 oz), Hard liquor (1.5 oz/80 proof) = 10-14 grams of ethanol
  The percentage of alcohol in each of the above is Beer: 6%, Wine: 10-20%, Hard liquor: 45%
  "Proof" refers to the percentage multiplied by 2
  - Moderate alcohol consumption: <20 gm/day ♀ and <40 gm/day ♂; Heavy alcohol consumption: >20 gm/day ♀ and >80 gm/day ♂
  - 60-80 gm/day of ethanol (or 6-8 drinks/day) for 10 years will likely develop cirrhosis in ♂; half as much required in ♀
  - An average alcoholic beverage raises blood alcohol concentration by 15-20 mg/dl, the amount metabolized by the liver in 1 hour

Blood Level (mg/dl)	Expected Symptoms
20-99	Impaired coordination, euphoria
100-199	Ataxia, decreased mentation, poor judgment, anxiety
200-299	Marked ataxia, slurred speech, anxiety, nausea and vomiting
300-399	Sedation, memory lapse, labile mood
>400	Respiratory failure, coma, death

PATHOPHYSIOLOGY:
- Ultimately, the total amount of alcohol consumed per weight determines who is at risk for alcohol-related disease
- Alcohol is metabolized mainly via the liver: alcohol dehydrogenase metabolizes to acetaldehyde, which in turn is oxidized by the liver via hepatic aldehyde dehydrogenase and the microsomal ethanol-oxidizing system cytochrome P450 (CYP2E1) to acetate
  - Aldehyde dehydrogenase (ALDH) is responsible for variable rates of alcohol clearance based on genetic inheritance
    - Certain Asian populations carry impaired ALDH activity = accumulating acetaldehyde = symptoms of flushing, tachycardia, N/V: N/V, Flushing
    - Disulfiram (Antabuse) takes advantage of this mechanism, inhibiting ALDH, and deters alcohol use because of symptoms: N/V, Flushing
- **Most common form of alcoholic liver disease: Fatty liver or hepatic steatosis;** Reversible with abstinence from alcohol intake
  - As a consequence of preferential alcohol oxidation, the liver develops fatty deposition

CHAPTER 4.04 ALCOHOLIC LIVER DISEASE

- **Alcoholic Hepatitis:** usually associated with heavy alcohol consumption for more than 10 years
  - Related to toxic effects of acetaldehyde production from hepatic metabolism of alcohol, resulting in micronodular fibrosis
  - Biopsy: hepatocellular disarray, PMNs, Mallory's hyaline bodies, some cholestasis, fibrosis/necrosis

CLINICAL MANIFESTATIONS/PHYSICAL EXAM:
- Identify those at risk using CAGE (a positive answer to any question helps identify those at risk for alcohol abuse)
  - Ever felt the need to **C**ut down on your drinking?
  - Ever get **A**ngry when someone asked about your drinking?
  - Ever feel **G**uilty about your drinking habits?
  - Ever have **E**ye-opener in the morning to steady your nerves or get rid of a hangover?
- Extrahepatic manifestations of alcoholic liver disease:
  - Ascites, Spider angiomata, Hypogonadism, Gynecomastia, Korsakoff's/Wernicke's encephalopathy, Palmer Erythema, Asterixis
- **Fatty liver or hepatic steatosis:**
  - First clinical manifestation is asymptomatic hepatomegaly
- **Alcoholic Hepatitis:** range of presentation is anicteric hepatomegaly to fulminant/acute liver failure
  - Jaundice, fever, hepatomegaly, high WBC (25% present with infection and manifestations of portal hypertension, i.e. ascites)
  - Up to 30% of patients are infected with HCV as well

LABORATORY STUDIES:
- **Fatty liver or hepatic steatosis:** AST:ALT >2:1 (however totals **usually <300-500**); Bili usually acutely out of proportion (high)
  - ALT production depends on B6, which is depleted with ETOH, hence the reason for the AST: ALT ratio
  - This transaminitis usually resolves after several days of abstinence
- **Alcoholic Hepatitis:** moderate elevation of AST to 2-5 times the upper limits of normal (rarely >300-500)

DIAGNOSTIC STUDIES:
- RUQ to exclude: cholecystitis, biliary obstruction, hepatic vein thrombosis (all may present in similar manner to alcoholic hepatitis)
- Liver biopsy: often not needed due to advances in non-invasive studies; indicated if diagnosis is uncertain (transjugular approach is best)
  See also Liver- Histopathology of Liver (Chapter 4.19)
  - Helps differentiate Hemochromatosis, Wilson's, AIH, HCV
  - Demonstrates: centrilobular PMNs and hepatocyte swelling, ballooning degeneration, macrovesicular steatosis and Mallory bodies
    - Characteristic: hepatocytes containing PMNs and Mallory bodies, and Megamitochondria (giant mitochondria)

TREATMENTS:
- Abstinence is key for short- and long-term survival: 5 year survival is 60% and that drops to 30% if drinking continues
- **Alcoholic Hepatitis:** Steroids are used, but pathophysiology to explain efficacy is not well understood; May decrease cytokines
  - Treatment indicated when discriminate function **>32** OR encephalopathy (without GIB or infection)
    Maddrey Discriminate Function = [4.6 × (PT-control)]+ total bilirubin (mg/dL)
    Score is not linear, for example a score of 33 is the same as 48 (i.e. both above 32); Scores >32 have 50% mortality at 1 month!
  - **Prednisone** or prednisolone 40 mg qd × 1 month then taper over 4-6 weeks
    (mortality 12% prednisolone vs. 55% placebo at day 66)
  - **Pentoxifylline** (Trental), nonselective phosphodiesterase inhibitor of TNF production (i.e. ↓ immunity), 400 mg po tid × 1 month
    (mortality: 25% pentoxifylline vs. 46% placebo at 4 wks; Use may decrease development of hepatorenal syndrome)
    (especially good if suspicious of infection and do not want to use prednisone)
  - Nutrition is key (start tube feeds if necessary): alcoholic patients are malnourished, ↓ vitamin stores and hepatic glutathione levels
  - Infection is a common cause of death due to malnutrition, cirrhosis, iatrogenic complications; evaluate for SBP, pneumonia, etc

SECTION IV LIVER

- Liver transplantation: alcohol related disease is second most common indication for transplant (after HCV); *See also Liver- Transplantation (Chapter 4.28)*
  - However, only 20% get a transplant due to continued drinking
  - Up to 10-30% recurrence requiring abstinence from alcohol

COMPLICATIONS:
- Tylenol ingestion: Alcohol induces P450 and results in depleted glutathione stores
  - Hepatic metabolism of Tylenol results in toxic intermediates, normally conjugated with glutathione

PROGNOSIS:
- Cirrhosis: accounts for 75% of deaths due to alcoholism

NOTES

4.05 ASCITES & PORTAL HYPERTENSION

(Hepatology 2004;39:1-16)

DEFINITION:
- Accumulation of fluid within the peritoneal cavity

EPIDEMIOLOGY:
- More than 30% of patients with ascites have an ascitic fluid infection at the time of admission or during hospitalization; Therefore tap 'em!

ETIOLOGIES:
- More than 80% of patients with ascites have decompensated chronic liver disease (cirrhosis)
- Peritoneal carcinomatosis is the second most common cause (10%)
- Other causes: heart failure (5%), acute alcoholic hepatitis, fulminant or subacute hepatic failure, pancreatic disease, dialysis ascites, nephrotic syndrome, hepatic vein obstruction, chylous ascites, bile ascites

PATHOPHYSIOLOGY:
- **Bottom line is sodium retention!**
- Cirrhosis:
    - Portal/Sinusoidal HTN » Lymph formation >> Absorption = Ascites (i.e. movement of extra fluid into the peritoneal space)
    - Systemic vasodilation via nitric oxide (probably) » Arterial underfilling » Release of hormones:
        - Aldosterone: **Na/Water retention** » Expanded plasma volume leads to Portal/Sinusoidal HTN (See above)
        - Antidiuretic hormone: Free water retention » Hyponatremia
        - Norepinephrine/Angiotensin: Renal vasoconstriction » Hepatorenal syndrome
- Cirrhotics have low protein ascites because the now *fibrotic* sinusoids no longer allow proteins (albumin, compliment) to escape to space of disse

CLINICAL MANIFESTATIONS/PHYSICAL EXAM:
- Shifting dullness and Fluid wave has 60% sensitivity

LABORATORY STUDIES:
- Paracentesis technique: Am J Gastroenterol 2006;101:1954-55
- Send fluid for: albumin, total protein, cell count, gram stain & culture; Others: amylase, cytology, LDH
- **Serum-ascites albumin gradient (SAAG);** 95% accuracy
Subtract albumin concentration of ascites from albumin concentration of serum (obtained on same day)
Physiologically based on oncotic-hydrostatic balance and is related directly to portal pressure

    - ≥1.1 g/dl : Portal HTN "Transudate"
        - Pre Sinusoidal
            - Portal or Splenic vein thrombosis
            - Schistosomiasis (*pHTN without cirrhosis*)
        - Sinusoidal
            - **Cirrhosis** (81%), including **SBP**
              Note: most SBP occurs with pHTN & Cirrhosis
              Reason: Ascites with dilute proteins have ↓ concentration of opsonins and ↑ SBP risk
            - Acute hepatitis
            - Extensive malignancy (HCC or mets)
            - Congenital hepatic fibrosis (*pHTN without cirrhosis*)
            - Partial nodular transformation (Nodular regenerative hyperplasia)
            - Sarcoidosis (pHTN if large enough granulomatous burden, *pHTN without cirrhosis*)
            - Idiopathic (thought to be arsenic toxicity as one of the causes)
        - Post Sinusoidal
            - Right-sided heart failure (including RV dysfunction, constrictive pericarditis and tricuspid regurgitation)
            - Budd-Chiari syndrome, Veno-occlusive disease

CHAPTER 4.05 ASCITES & PORTAL HYPERTENSION

- ≤1.1 g/dl: Non-portal HTN related "Exudate"
    * Non-portal HTN related
        * **Peritonitis**: TB, Ruptured viscus (↑ amylase), Fungal (granuloma on biopsy)
        * **Peritoneal carcinomatosis**
        * **Pancreatitis** (↑ amylase >1000 U/L, total protein >3 gm;
            High amylase also with gut perforation, disrupted pancreatic duct)
        * Sarcoidosis (granuloma on biopsy)
        * Vasculitis
        * SBP is NOT here with other 'infections' or 'exudates' (Non-portal HTN) for reason stated above
    * Miscellaneous- Hypoalbuminemic states: nephrotic syndrome, protein-losing enteropathy; Meigs' syndrome
    * Chylous (TG level higher in ascites than serum or presence of chylomicrons): lymphoma, TB, Trauma
- **Ascites fluid total protein (AFTP):**
    * Useful when SAAG ≥1.1 to distinguish cirrhosis (AFTP <2.5 g/dl) from cardiac ascites (AFTP >2.5 g/dl)
- **Urine Sodium:** <10 mEq/day = 20% 2-year survival; >10 mEq/day = 60% 2-year survival
- If portal hypertensive etiology, consider standard cirrhosis workup; *See also Liver- Cirrhosis and Encephalopathy (Chapter 4.08)*
- Rule out infection: cell count with diff, gram stain & culture (± AFB) & *bedside inoculation* of blood culture bottles (yield 90%)
- Other tests as indicated (i.e. amylase; triglycerides; cytology; adenosine deaminase for TB)

DIAGNOSTIC STUDIES:
- U/S detects if >100 cc ascitic fluid
- Hepatic Venous Wedge Pressure Gradient **[HVWPG]** = ~6 mmHg normally
    * HVWPG represents the pressure difference between the wedged hepatic vein (which reflects the portal vein pressure) and the direct measurement of the abdominal IVC (or the free hepatic vein pressure)
    * Similar concept to a right heart catheterization (Swan-Ganz), in other words:
    HVWPG = Wedge Pressure (balloon up)-Free Hepatic Vein (balloon down)

Type of Portal HTN	Wedge Pressure	Free Hepatic Vein	HVWPG
Pre-Sinusoidal	Low	Low	Normal
Sinusoidal	High	Low	High
Post-Sinusoidal	High	High	Normal

Varices do not form until HVWPG >10 mmHg
Ascites does not form and varices do not bleed until HVWPG >12 mmHg
Strongest risk of variceal re-bleeding with HVWPG >20 mmHg
Goal: reduce HVWPG to <12 mmHg or by 20% of pre-treatment value

TREATMENTS: Goal: create a net negative balance of sodium and hence mobilize the ascitic fluid
- **Low Na intake** (1-2 gm/day or 50-88 mEq/day) Normal kidneys excrete ~2 gm/day or 120 mEq/day on a 90 mEq/d diet
    * 1 teaspoon of salt has 5.2 g of sodium chloride or 2 g of sodium! This also means no normal saline (large salt load) in hospital!
    * Free H_2O restriction if hyponatremic (<120 mEq/L), i.e. 1–2 liters per day maximum
- **Diuretics** (effective in 80% of cases); Lasix:Aldactone ratio is usually 2:5, so Lasix 40, Aldactone 100 (ratio helps maintain K+)
Aldactone (start 100 mg qd) ± Furosemide (start 40 mg qd); ↑ in proportion if weight does not ↓ or UNa does not ↑ after 2–3 days
    * Lasix: inhibits loop Na resorption, forcing more Na to be seen by DCT, which has been blocked by Aldactone
    * Aldactone: antagonizes DCT aldosterone receptors: pee out Na, hold K
    * Ceiling doses are Aldactone 400 mg and Furosemide 160 mg per day; **No effect = definition of 'Refractory Ascites'**
    * Goals: diurese ~1 L/day, steady weight loss, urinary Na/K ratio >1 (indicating effective blockade of endogenous aldosterone)

SECTION IV LIVER

- Options for **Refractory Ascites** (ensure diet & medicine compliance (no NSAIDS), rule out bacterial infections, GIB)
  - Large Volume Paracentesis. remove 4-6 L
    - <5 L removed: low risk of post-paracentesis circulatory dysfunction
    - >5 L removed: Can get post-paracentesis circulatory dysfunction via activation of sympathetics and Renin-angiotensinogen activation (hypotension, hyponatremia, azotemia)

    Albumin replacement controversial ($\downarrow$ asymptomatic chemical abnormalities i.e. hyponatremia, azotemia; but no change in mortality)

    Albumin 5% [plasma isotonicity] 1 liter = 50 grams; Albumin 25% [concentrated] 100 cc = 25 grams
    Generally, 8-10 gm per liter removed; Hence, 100 cc (25 g) for every 3 liters removed

  - TIPS: (Hepatology 2005;41:1-15)
    $\downarrow\downarrow$ ascites in 75%, $\uparrow$ CrCl, $\uparrow$ transplantation-free survival
    However, $\uparrow$ encephalopathy risk, 40% need TIPS revision for stent stenosis
    No change in quality of life/mortality; Consider if refractory ascites, Child's class A or B, Patient has minimal encephalopathy
    Contraindications: Bili >3-5 mg/dl, PT >20 sec, Cr >2 mg/dl, Recurrent encephalopathy

  - Liver transplantation if patient is a candidate; only therapy that increases long-term survival

COMPLICATIONS:
- Hepatorenal syndrome *See also Liver- Hepatorenal Syndrome (Chapter 4.18)*
- Pleural effusions (Hepatohydrothorax)
- Bacterial Peritonitis *See also Liver- Bacterial Peritonitis (Chapter 4.07)*

NOTES

4.06 AUTOIMMUNE HEPATITIS

(Hepatology 2002;36:479-97)

DEFINITION:
- Autoimmune Hepatitis (AIH) is an unresolving inflammation of liver, unknown cause:
  - Characterized by interface hepatitis (histology), autoantibodies & hypergammaglobulinemia (serum)
- Types of AIH:

Features	Type 1 (Classic)	Type 2	Type 3 (Least Established Form)
Predominant age	Adult (some children)	Child (girls > boys)	All ages ? if really a variant of Type 1 AIH
Auto Antibodies	ASMA* ANA, pANCA Anti-Actin	LKM1^ Liver cytosol 1	anti-SLA*^ ANA
Organ-specific Ab	± (thyroid)	± (thyroid, parietal cells)	?
Autoantigen	Unknown	P450 2D6 (CYP2D6)	tRNP
HLA phenotype	B8, DR3, DR4	DR3, DR7	DR3
Fulminant onset	Possible (but rare)	Possible	Unknown
Concurrent disease	40% (see below)	32% (see below)	60% (see below)
Gamma globulin ↑	Yes	Slight	Moderate
Progress Cirrhosis	35%	80%	Probably
Steroid responsive	Yes	Yes	Yes

*anti-smooth muscle antibody, ^anti-liver/kidney microsome type 1, *^anti-soluble liver antigen

- Overlap or Variant Syndrome:
  - Autoimmune Hepatitis & PBC or PSC; Has high titers of AMA and cholestasis; *See also Liver- PBC (Chapter 4.23)*

EPIDEMIOLOGY:
- F:M = 5:1, can occur at any age but typically before 4th decade; Represents <10% of all chronic hepatitis in the U.S. but 6% of transplants
- Concurrent immunologic diseases can be present in patients, **most common:** autoimmune thyroiditis, ulcerative colitis, Graves, synovitis, RA

Others:	Celiac sprue	Erythema	ITP	Myasthenia	Pernicious	Sjogren's
	Coomb's +	nodosum	Insulin DM	gravis	anemia	SLE
	hemolytic anemia	Focal myositis	Iritis	Neutropenia	Pleuritis	Urticaria
	Cyroglobulinemia	Gingivitis	Lichen planus	Pericarditis	Pyoderma	Vitiligo
	Dermatitis herpetiformis	Glomerulonephritis		Peripheral neuropathy	gangrenosum	

ETIOLOGIES:

Differential diagnosis	Diagnostic tests (See each corresponding diagnosis/chapter for details)
Wilson's	Copper studies: ↓ ceruloplasmin, ↓ serum copper, ↑ urinary copper
PSC	Cholangiography: Focal biliary strictures; Liver biopsy: fibrous obliterate changes
PBC	Auto Antibodies: AMA >1:40; Liver biopsy: florid duct lesion, ↑ hepatic copper
Autoimmune cholangitis	Liver biopsy: cholangitis, ductopenia
Chronic Hepatitis C	Viral labs: anti-HCV/RIBA positive, HCV RNA present
Drug-induced Hepatitis	Clinical history: exposure to minocycline, nitrofurantoin, propylthiouracil, isoniazide, methyldopa
Hemochromatosis	Genetics: C282Y, H63D mutations; Labs: ↑ Iron/Ferritin; Liver biopsy: iron overload, HII >1.9
α1-AT	Phenotype: ZZ or MZ; Liver biopsy: hepatic inclusions, PAS+
NASH	Clinical: obesity, DM, hyperlipidemia; Liver biopsy: macrosteatosis; U/S: hyperechogenicity

CHAPTER 4.06 AUTOIMMUNE HEPATITIS

PATHOPHYSIOLOGY:
- Pathogenic mechanisms unknown; Two theories: 1. Antibody-dependent cell-mediated form of cytotoxicity & 2. Cellular form of cytotoxicity
    1. Defect in modulation of B-cell production of IgG, creating an antigen-antibody complex on hepatocyte surface
    2. Autoantigen displayed on surface of antigen-presenting cells in association with HLA class II antigens
- Multiple viruses thought to trigger AIH, including HAV, HBV, HCV; Currently, the definite diagnosis requires the exclusion of viral infections
- Drugs can produce clinical syndromes of AIH and must be excluded at time of presentation; Usually discontinuing drug ameliorates disease
    - Implicated meds: **minocycline, nitrofurantoin,** isoniazid, propylthiouracil, methyldopa
- Histology: **Interface hepatitis (piecemeal necrosis** or periportal hepatitis); Not pathognomonic: also with viral, drugs, ETOH, toxins
    - Lobular hepatitis (prominent cellular infiltrates lining sinusoidal spaces); Not pathognomonic
    - Marked plasma cell infiltration of portal tracts
    - More specific for AIH: centrilobular (zone 3) necrosis and hepatocytic giant cells, relative sparing of bile ducts

CLINICAL MANIFESTATIONS/PHYSICAL EXAM:
- Many are asymptomatic (still need therapy) or present with fatigue, jaundice, myalgias; Cirrhosis present in 25–35% of patients at presentation
- An acute, even fulminant presentation is possible (up to 40%) and the disease may be mistaken for acute viral or toxic hepatitis
- Caution: pruritus, weight loss and hyperpigmentation are incompatible and suggest other diseases (i.e. biliary obstruction, HCC)

LABORATORY STUDIES:
- See Types above: ASMA and ANA are most common serologic markers; Most transaminase levels are <500 U/L at presentation
    - Patterns of seropositivity also change during the disease: one disappears and one appears; Titers >1:80 ↑ diagnostic confidence
- Hypergammaglobulinemia, especially IgG, is a **hallmark** of the disease and the diagnosis is suspect without it (i.e. order SPEP)
- Caution: Cholestatic features are incompatible; ↑ Aφ and/or bile duct lesions (histology) suggest other diseases, i.e. PBC, PSC, cholangitis
- Caution: serologic evidence of active infection: HAV, HBV, HCV, EBV, CMV argues against the diagnosis

DIAGNOSTIC STUDIES:
- **Definite diagnosis:**
    - Histological evidence of **interface hepatitis** with or without lobular hepatitis or bridging necrosis is a hallmark
      Histology typically shows an absence of biliary lesions, granulomas, copper deposits, or changes suggestive of a different etiology
      Hence, liver biopsy should be performed at presentation to establish the diagnosis and stage the disease or anytime of deterioration
    - ALT/AST abnormally increased and dominate biochemical profile
    - Total serum globulin, gamma globulin, or immunoglobulin G must be greater than 1.5 times ULN
    - Serum titers SMA, ANA, anti-LKM1 >1:80 (diagnosis is in question with lower titers)
    - Ruled out: active viral infection; Wilson's, Hemochromatosis, α1-AT (i.e. inherited liver diseases); any drug-induced hepatitis

SECTION IV LIVER

- **Probable diagnosis:** made when similar findings are less pronounced
- Scoring system for Definite vs. Probable diagnosis; Balances clinical, laboratory, and histological manifestations*.
(Proposed by International Autoimmune Hepatitis Group; J Hepatol 1999;31:929-38) (Nl = Normal)

Female	+2	Hepatitis markers		Histological findings		**Aggregate score**
Aφ:AST <1.5	+2	Positive	−3	Interface	+3	**before treatment:**
1.5–3.0	0	Negative	+3	Lymphoplasmacytic	+2	Definite AIH: >15
>3.0	−2	Hepatotoxic Drugs		Rosette formation	+1	Probable AIH: 10–15
IgG × Nl >2.0	+3	Positive	−4	None of above	−5	**Aggregate score after**
1.5–2.0	+2	Negative	+1	Biliary changes	−3	**treatment:**
1.0–1.5	+1	Average ETOH		Other changes	−3	Definite AIH: >17
<1.0	0	<25 g/d	+2	Response to steroids		Probable AIH: 12–17
ANA/SMA >1:80	+3	>60 g/d	−2	Complete	+2	
1:80	+2	Concurrent disease	+2	Relapse	+3	*Scoring system often
1:40	+1	Novel auto-abs	+2			not used clinically
<1:40	0	HLA DR3 or DR4	+1			(Used as a research tool)
AMA +	−4					

TREATMENTS:
- Indications:

Absolute:	Relative:	None:
AST ≥10 × Nl	AST 3–9 × Nl	AST <3 × Nl
AST ≥5 × Nl & IgG ≥2 × Nl	AST ≥5 × Nl & IgG <2 × Nl	Severe cytopenia
Histology: bridging necrosis	Histology: interface hepatitis	Histology: inactive or minimally active cirrhosis
Symptoms: incapacitating (Tx even with cirrhosis, PSE)	Persistent symptoms	Liver failure with minimal inflammatory activity (Decompensated inactive cirrhosis)

- AIH and Viral Markers:
  - Treat the predominant disorder; Corticosteroids if AIH, Antiviral if viral predominant emerge with steroid withdrawal
    - Remote viral infection (HBsAg−/anti-HBs+, IgM anti-HBc−, IgM anti-HAV−) = Steroids for AIH
    - False-positive viral markers (Anti-HCV+/RIBA−, Anti-HCV+/HCV RNA−) = Steroids for AIH
    - Uncertain viral infection (Anti-HCV+/RIBA±) = Steroids for AIH
    - True viral infection: Biopsy consistent with viral and ANA or ASMA titer <1:320 = Treat viral infection
      Biopsy consistent with AIH and ANA or ASMA titer ≥1:320 = Steroids for AIH
      Biopsy consistent with viral and Anti-LKM1 = Treat viral infection

- Medical Therapy (most treated for 12-24 months with goal being remission):
  -Treatment schedules established only for Type 1, but the same regimen is used in all types
  -Combination drug candidates (*preferred*): Postmenopausal ♀, HTN, Emotional instability, Obesity, Acne, Osteoporosis, Long-term trial (>6 months)
  -Single drug candidates: Pregnant, Active neoplasia/malignancy, Severe cytopenia, Short-term trial (<6 months)

Interval	Prednisone (mg/day)	Prednisone (mg/day)	& Azathioprine/Imuran* (mg/day)
Week 1	60	30	50 (alternatively: 1mg/kg)
Week 2	40	20	50
Week 3	30	15	50
Week 4	30	15	50
Daily maintenance	10–20	10	50
Treatment failure	60	30	150
			*see IBD Treatment for specifics

-Other: Urosodiol 300 mg po TID

CHAPTER 4.06 AUTOIMMUNE HEPATITIS

- End points of therapy: remission, drug toxicity, clinical deterioration (treatment failure) or confirmation of an incomplete response; Liver biopsy must be done before drug withdrawal; Histological improvement lags behind clinical/biochemical 3–6 months
  - Remission: symptom resolution, labs <2 × Nl, histological improvement: normal (ideal), inactive cirrhosis or portal hepatitis
    - 65% remission within 3 years; however
    - 50% relapse on withdrawal of meds at 6 months; Up to 90% by 3 years; Therefore most will require long-term treatment
    - Biopsy predicting relapse: Normal biopsy: 20% relapse, Portal hepatitis: 50%, Interface hepatitis: 80%

    Relapses justify re-treatment with original drug schedule or alternative treatment strategy after >2 relapses

    28% of those who relapse and get re-treated will ultimately develop inactive disease/medication withdrawn (don't give up on therapy)
  - Treatment failure: worsening of labs, persistent symptoms, ascites formation, PSE despite compliance with medication; See above for treatment; Results in laboratory remission: 75%, but only 20% achieve histological remission
- Liver transplant: 5 year survival 92%, and autoantibodies disappear within 2 years; Disease recurs in up to 15–30% (most are mild)
  - De novo AIH in a graft (transplanted for non-AIH reasons) can occur in up to 3%; Treatment as above is usually successful
- Future therapies?: Budesonide, Cyclosporine, Tacrolimus

COMPLICATIONS:
- Up to 13% of patients may lack a confident etiologic diagnosis and most are diagnosed with **cryptogenic cirrhosis** but may have AIH
  - They escaped diagnosis by conventional serologic testing; The scoring system is best way of securing diagnosis
- Cirrhosis in 36% of patients within 6 years despite steroid therapy
- Hepatocellular carcinoma may develop in patients with AIH who have cirrhosis, but it is rare
- Portal hypertension, liver failure and death are other possible consequences

PROGNOSIS:
- Labs: Sustained AST of 10 × normal *or* 5 × normal with hypergammaglobulinemia of at least 2 × normal: 3 yr survival 50%, 10 yr survival 10%
- Histology: inflammation between portal tracts *or* bridging necrosis: 5 yr survival 45% and frequency of cirrhosis of 82%
- Histology: interface hepatitis: 5 yr survival normal and frequency of cirrhosis 17%; Unpredictable spontaneous resolution in 13–20%

4.07 BACTERIAL PERITONITIS

(Hepatology 2000;32:142-53)

Type	Ascites Cell Count/mm^3	Ascites Culture
Sterile	<250 polys	–
SBP	>250 polys	+ (one organism)
(CNNA) Culture-neg Neutrocytic ascites	>250 polys	–
(NNBA) Non-neutrocytic bacterascites	<250 polys	+ (one organism)
Secondary	>250 polys	+ (polymicrobial)
Peritoneal dialysis-associated	>100 (mostly PMNs).	+

SPONTANEOUS BACTERIAL PERITONITIS (SBP)

Epidemiology:
- Occurs in 10-30% of inpatient cirrhotics and <4% of outpatient cirrhotics

Etiologies:
- Risk factors:
  - Cirrhotic patients with GI bleed
  - Ascites fluid total protein (AFTP) <1.0 g/dl (i.e. Low AFTP)
  - Serum bilirubin >2.5 mg/dl or Platelets <98 K
  - Prior SBP
  - Fulminant hepatic failure

Pathophysiology:
- 70% GNR (*E. coli, Klebsiella*)
  - Suspected bacterial translocation via gut, which is supported by bacterial overgrowth in cirrhotics (↓ immune & complement function)
- 30% GPC (*S. pneumococcus,* other streptococci - *viridans, Enterococcus*); GPCs seen with ↑ frequency probably because of prophylactic antibiotics

Clinical Manifestations/Physical Exam:
- Ascites (100%), fever (50-75%), abdominal pain (50-75%), mental status change (30-75%), rebound tenderness (40%), ileus (20%)
  - Clinical signs may be unreliable/asymptomatic; therefore have a low threshold for diagnostic paracentesis

Laboratory Studies:
- See table above (PMN's >250); Takes only minutes to get result back
- Gram stain positive in only 5-10%, and culture takes at least 12 hours

Diagnostic Studies:
- Paracentesis!
- Correction for 'bloody tap' (250RBC:1WBC); So RBC/250 = X, WBC - X = real WBCs; Then look at Neut % of the real WBCs

Treatments:
- Third generation cephalosporins: Cefotaxime 2 gm IV q 8 hr × 5 d (Other options Ceftriaxone or Zosyn); Repeat tap in 48 hrs to confirm ↓ WBC
- IV Albumin 1.5 g/kg at diagnosis and 1 g/kg on day 3 results in survival benefit, especially those with renal failure
- **Prophylaxis:** Norfloxacin 400 qd *or* Bactrim DS qd *or* Cipro 750 qwk
  - Definite prophylaxis needed: history of SBP (70% chance of recurrence), current GIB ± ascites, fulminant hepatic failure
  - Questionable prophylaxis needed: those while being hospitalized or AFTP <1.0 g/dl
  - No prophylaxis needed: ascites due to cardiac and non-portal hypertensive causes (low risk due to intact opsonic and compliment activity)

Complications:
- Secondary Bacterial Peritonitis or Superinfection; Re-culture 48 hours after initial treatment if no clinical improvement:
  - Same organism, likely Secondary Bacterial Peritonitis: see below (emergent CT and surgical consultation)
  - New organism, likely superinfection: choose new antibiotic

Prognosis:
- 2 year mortality: 50%

CULTURE-NEGATIVE NEUTROCYTIC ASCITES (CNNA):
- Variant of SBP with similar clinical course; also treated with antibiotics

NON-NEUTROCYTIC BACTERASCITES (NNBA):
- Asymptomatic patient: Often resolves without treatment; follow patient closely; Consider repeat tap to confirm resolution
- Symptomatic patient: Treat with antibiotics

SECONDARY: (Consider the cause to be intra-abdominal abscess or perforated viscus)
- Polymicrobial; Important to distinguish from SBP because many of secondary patients require surgery!
- Usually Ascites Fluid Total Protein (AFTP) >1.0 g/dl, ascitic fluid glucose <50 mg/dl, or ascitic fluid LDH >225 U/L
- Treatment: 3rd generation cephalosporin + metronidazole
- CT scan and likely exploratory laparotomy for definitive diagnosis and treatment; Confirm and localize possible visceral perforation

PERITONEAL DIALYSIS-ASSOCIATED:
- Pathogens: 70% GPC, 30% GNR
- Treatment: vancomycin + gentamicin (IV initially, but then may administer via peritoneal dialysis)

4.08 CIRRHOSIS & ENCEPHALOPATHY

DEFINITION:
- Fibrosis and nodular regeneration resulting from hepatocellular injury

EPIDEMIOLOGY:
- Cirrhosis and chronic liver disease accounted for more than 25,000 deaths and 375,000 hospitalizations in 1998

ETIOLOGIES: (See also corresponding chapters on each etiology for more detail)
- **Alcohol**
- **Viral Hepatitis:** (chronic HBV, HCV, HDV infection)
- **Autoimmune hepatitis:** (female, ↑ IgG, +ANA, +ASMA)
- **Congenital:** Hemochromatosis, Wilson's disease, α1-antitrypsin deficiency, Congenital hepatic fibrosis
- **Metabolic diseases:** NASH/NAFLD
- **Biliary tract disease:** PBC or PSC, Secondary biliary cirrhosis (calculus, neoplasm, post-op stricture, biliary atresia)
- **Vascular diseases:** Budd-Chiari syndrome, R-sided heart failure, Constrictive pericarditis
- **Cryptogenic:** may reflect terminal progression of NAFLD or some may be non/missed diagnosed AIH

PATHOPHYSIOLOGY:
- A late stage of progressive hepatic fibrosis characterized by distortion of the hepatic architecture and formation of regenerative nodules

CLINICAL MANIFESTATIONS/PHYSICAL EXAM:
- Subclinical or may present as progressive liver dysfunction (jaundice, coagulopathy, encephalopathy) and/or portal hypertension (ascites, varices)
- Liver:
  - Enlarged, palpable, firm, nodular » shrunken and nodular
- Signs of Liver Failure:
  - Jaundice, spider angiomata (marker of chronicity), palmar erythema, Dupuytren's contractures, white nail lines (Muehrcke's lines) & proximal nail beds (Terry's nails), ↑ parotid & lacrimal glands, gynecomastia, testicular atrophy, asterixis, encephalopathy, fetor hepaticus
  - Asterixis, seen with: Cirrhosis (PSE), Renal (Uremia), Lung (CO_2 retention)
- Signs of Portal HTN:
  - Splenomegaly, ascites, dilated superficial abdominal veins (caput medusae), epigastric 'Cruveilhier-Baumgarten' venous hum

LABORATORY STUDIES:
- ↑ bilirubin, ↑ PT, ↓ Albumin, ± ↑ aminotransferases and ↑ Aφ (variable)
- ↓ Na
- Anemia (marrow suppression, hypersplenism, iron and/or folate deficiencies)
  Neutropenia (hypersplenism)
  Thrombocytopenia (hypersplenism, ↓ Thrombopoietin production by liver)

DIAGNOSTIC STUDIES:
- ± Liver biopsy (percutaneous or transjugular); For indications and contraindications, *See also Liver-LFTs (Chapter 4.20)*
- Abdominal U/S doppler: liver size; rule out Hepatocellular cancer (HCC), ascites, assess patency of portal, splenic and hepatic veins
- Hepatic serologies (HBsAg, anti-HBs, anti-HCV)
- Autoimmune hepatitis studies (IgG, ANA, ASMA)
- Fe & Cu studies
- α1-AT phenotype
- AMA (PBC), p-anca (PSC)
- Echocardiogram (if concerned about right-sided heart failure)
- AFP to screen for HCC (with U/S)

CHAPTER 4.08 CIRRHOSIS & ENCEPHALOPATHY

TREATMENTS:
- All fevers and PSE get worked up: Blood Culture, Urine Culture, Paracentesis for SBP, UNa, RUQ U/S
- Ask about Tylenol (up to 2 g/day generally ok) and NSAIDs (stop along with other nephrotoxic drugs) and Low sodium diet
- Ask about GI bleeding: beta blocker use, variceal banding/EGD
- Ask about previous SBP and if they are on prophylaxis if diagnosed in the past
- Colloid solutions (albumin with D5, PRBC, FFP) are better replacements than crystalloids (normal saline)
- Monitor MELD and other labs
- Paracentesis prn ± albumin
- Consider the diagnosis of HRS early
- Vaccinate! Give HAV and HBV vaccines to chronic liver patients!

COMPLICATIONS:
- **Portal HTN**
  Hepatic Venous Wedge Pressure Gradient **[HVWPG]:** Normal ~6 or lower
  Explanation of HVWPG: *See also Liver- Ascites and Portal Hypertension (Chapter 4.05)*
  Causes of ↑ HVWPG:
  Cirrhosis, Acute Hepatitis, Metastasis, Congenital Hepatic Fibrosis, Sarcoid, Portal &/or Splenic vein thrombosis, Schistosomiasis; *See also Liver- Ascites and Portal Hypertension (Chapter 4.05)*

  - **Ascites:** (50% within 10 yrs) ± SBP (19%); *See also Liver- Ascites and Portal Hypertension (Chapter 4.05)*

  - Gastroesophageal Varices; *See also GI Bleed- Variceal Bleeding (Chapter 6.05)*
    Hepatic Venous Wedge Pressure Gradient [HVWPG] >12 mmHg is at high risk of bleeding
    In acute bleeds: Varices 50%; Nonvariceal source: Gastric erosions 50%, MWT 15%, Any PUD 14%, Erosive esophagitis 11%

  - Portal hypertensive gastropathy and Gastric antral vascular ectasias (GAVE): *See also GI Bleed- UGIB & LGIB (Chapter 6.04)*
    PHG: Mosaic mucosal pattern with or without submucosal hemorrhage, particularly in fundus (not in antrum); treated with TIPS
    Histology: Mucosal vasodilation, edema
    GAVE: linear aggregates of red spots in antrum (Watermelon stomach); treated with endoscopic electrocoagulation
    Histology: Vascular ectasia, Thrombi; Alternative treatment: daily mestranol 50 mg with norethindrone 1 mg

  - **Hepatohydrothorax:** diuretics, Na restriction, TIPS; Avoid chest tubes/pleurodesis (infections compromise OLT chance)

- **Coagulopathy:**
  A sick liver can produce a misbalance of clotting/anticlotting factors, hence a cirrhotic can form clots if more clotting factors produced
  - Vitamin K: Inpatient: 10 mg sq daily; Outpatient: 5 mg po daily
  - FFP when needed

- **Hepatic Encephalopathy:** failure of liver to detoxify noxious agents (NH_3 and others) (Am J Gastroenterol. 2001;96:1968-1976)
  - Stage I: mental status change; Stage II: lethargy, confusion
    Stage III: stupor, but arousable; Stage IV: coma
    Asterixis: stages II & III, sometimes I; EEG abnormal: stages II,III, IV
    Intubate patient: stages III, IV (use Propofol)
  - Precipitated by:
    - GI bleed, constipation, medication non-compliance, excess dietary protein (↑ gut *ammonia* (NH_3) *production*)
    - Hepatic failure, HCC, porto-systemic shunting, infection, fever (↓ *neurotoxin clearance*)
    - Dehydration, hypotension, azotemia, hyponatremia, hypokalemia, hypoglycemia, alkalosis (↓ *renal excretion of* NH_4^+)
    - Sedatives i.e. benzos (↑ *inhibitory neurotransmission/GABA*)
  - Treatment goal: decrease amount of ammonium that crosses into the blood-brain-barrier
    - Restrict dietary protein acutely, but only modestly (60-80 g/d) long term, Keep K+ high normal, Supplement Zinc
    - Lactulose po/PR (MOA #1: acidification of colon = NH_3 » NH_4^+; MOA #2: change gut flora » ↓ NH_3-producing organisms); Titrate 3 BM/day
    - Gut decontamination: Flagyl (250 po TID); Neomycin (1 g po BID, ↓ dose asap 2° renal toxicity); Rifaximin (200 mg po 2 tabs TID)

SECTION IV LIVER

- **Hepatorenal Syndrome:** *See also Liver- Hepatorenal Syndrome (Chapter 4.18)*

- **Hepatopulmonary Syndrome and Portopulmonary Hypertension:** *See also Liver Pulmonary Complications (Chapter 4.26)*

- **Liver Failure:** precipitated by progressive hepatic damage or stressors (infections, surgery): *See also Liver- Acute Liver Failure (Chapter 4.03)*

- **Infections:** SBP, *See also Liver- Bacterial Peritonitis (Chapter 4.07)*

- **Hepatocellular carcinoma (HCC):** *See also Liver- Hepatocellular Carcinoma (Chapter 4.17)*
  - Consider if ↑ liver size, ↑ ascites, abdominal pain, ↑ encephalopathy, ↓ weight, ↑ AFP, or hepatic mass on U/S, CT, MRI
  - Screening: Ultrasound and AFP level q 6 months (Risk 1-2% per year); AFP >400 has 95% predictability for HCC

PROGNOSIS:
- Correlates with **Child-Turcotte-Pugh class** (A > B > C)

	Points		
	1	2	3
Ascites	none	easy control	poor control
Encephalopathy	none	grade I or II	grade III or IV
Bilirubin (mg/dL)	<2.0	2.0-3.0	>3.0
Albumin (g/dL)	>3.5	2.8-3.5	<2.8
PT (sec > control)	<4	4-6	>6

	Classification		
	A	B	C
Total Points	5-6	7-9	10-15
1-year survival	100%	81%	45%
2-year survival	85%	57%	35%

- **Liver Transplantation and MELD (Model for End Stage Liver Disease),** *See also Liver- Transplantation (Chapter 4.28)*
  - Evaluate ± list when Child class >B7 or MELD ≥10

- **TIPS placement** (Hepatology. 2005;41:1-15)
  - Those with MELD >15 and/or Bili >5 are at ↑ risk of peri-TIPS complications
  - ↑ portal flow may disrupt few hepatocytes being fed by HA (i.e. ↓ pressure in hepatic artery 2° to ↑ portal vein flow with TIPS: local necrosis)
  - TIPS may ↑ platelet count in cirrhotics with counts <30 K; Consider before splenectomy (which is a big abdominal operation)

- **Pre-op Clearance of Cirrhotic Patient:** (Clin Gastroenterol & Hepatol. 2004;2:719-723. Am J Gastroenterol. 2005;100:2116-2127)
  - Those with CTP score ≥B8 or MELD ≥12 are at ↑ risk of peri-operative complications/mortality
  - Study is with cardiac patients; ≥30% mortality with cardiac surgery
  - Probably even higher risk/mortality with abdominal surgeries compared to chest surgeries

NOTES

4.09 CLOTS

VASCULAR ANATOMY OF LIVER
- Liver constitutes 5% of body weight and receives 20% of cardiac output via hepatic artery (Ha) and portal vein (Pv)
    - Hepatic artery is a branch of hepaticoduodenal artery from celiac axis and carries 30% of total flow, but >50% of needed oxygen; Under high pressure, highly variable, dependant upon systemic blood pressure, regulated by adenosine concentration
    - Portal vein is valveless (formed from splenic & SMV), carries 70-80% of total liver blood flow and delivers <50% of needed oxygen; Under low pressure, not affected by systemic circulation, not regulated
    - Both Ha and Pv defined into Right & Left branches and eventually become arterioles and venules that drain into the sinusoids
        - At this level, hepatic arteries and sinusoids have sphincters that dynamically regulate blood flow i.e. a reduction of Pv flow leads to an immediate increase in Ha flow (total sinusoidal blood flow maintained constant; However, Pv flow is relatively constant and is not influenced by Ha flow)
    - At the end of sinusoid, blood enters the central venule forming the hepatic venule; Three major hepatic veins(Hv): Right/Middle/Left
        - The veins have different blood distributions from Ha and Pv, influencing surgical intervention
    - The liver is divided into eight segments, each having own afferent and efferent blood supply
        - Note: the Caudate lobe is drained by small veins directly into the IVC, hence the compensatory hypertrophy in BCS
- Microarchitecture: *See also Liver- Histopathology of Liver (Chapter 4.19)*
    - Basic element of liver structure is liver cell plate, consisting of 15-20 hepatocytes lined up between the portal area and hepatic veins
    - Perivenular (Zone III) hepatocytes are subject to more hypoxia because they are at end of unidirectional sinusoidal blood flow
    - Zone II and III are involved in drug metabolism and are rich in cytochrome P450 enzymes

Pv (portal vein) Ha (hepatic artery) Hv (hepatic venules) E (fenestrated epithelium) (contain Kupffer cells) D (space of Disse) (contain Stellate cells) Bd (bile duct)	Blood from Pv and Ha, join and traverse sinusoids, leaving the liver from Hv; Low pressure circulation in sinusoids allows plasma to pass through E, and reach D, where via direct contact with hepatocytes, exchange of nutrients and metabolites takes place Note: Stellate cells when activated take on characteristics of fibroblasts and cause fibrosis or cirrhosis; Kupffer cells are phagocytic cells

- Note: a sick liver can produce a misbalance of clotting/anticlotting factors, hence a cirrhotic can form clots if more clotting factors produced

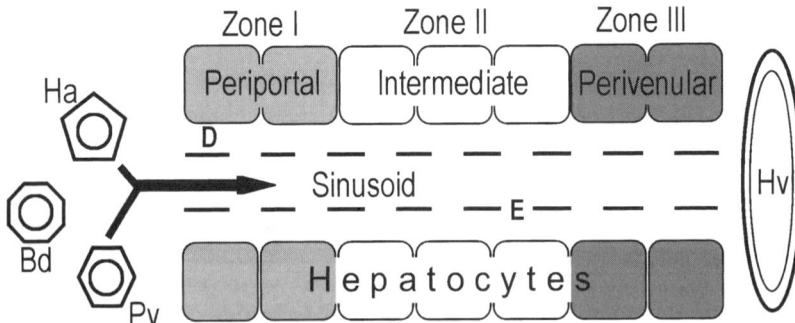

Modified with permission from McNally P. GI/Liver Secrets. 3rd ed. New York: Elsevier/Mosby, 2006:237.

CHAPTER 4.09 CLOTS

BUDD-CHIARI SYNDROME (BCS)

Definition:
- Thrombosis/occlusion of the hepatic veins (small venules, large hepatic veins), IVC or even the right atrium

Etiologies:
- Hypercoagulable: Myeloproliferative syndromes, Paroxysmal nocturnal hemoglobinuria, SLE, Protein C & S or antithrombin-III deficiency, Pregnancy/OCP
- Tumor invasion: HCC, Renal, Adrenal, Pancreas
- Inferior vena cava membranous web
- Trauma
- **Postpartum**
- Idiopathic (**Factor V Leiden** may be responsible for 25% of BCS considered 'idiopathic')

Pathophysiology:
- Increased sinusoidal pressure caused by obstructed hepatic venous outflow: hypoxic damage to hepatocytes and increased portal pressure
  - Continued obstruction leads to further hepatic necrosis and ultimately cirrhosis

Clinical Manifestations/Physical Exam:
- Ascites (>90% of patients) is cardinal feature
- RUQ pain (80% of patients)
- Hepatosplenomegaly, Jaundice (slight when present), PSE and Variceal bleeding are less common and late findings

Laboratory Studies:
- ± ↑ transaminases & Aφ (ischemic pattern)

Diagnostic Studies:
- Doppler U/S of hepatic veins (85% sensitive & specific): may show clot, decrease/absent flow, hyperechogenic cord replacing main HV
- CT or MRI/MRA: Caudate lobe hypertrophy
- Hepatic venography: 'spider web' pattern (gold standard)
- Liver bx: Acute: centrilobular congestion and dilation of the perivenular sinusoid
  - In severe cases: zone III necrosis; Centrilobular fibrosis develops in 4 weeks; Regenerative nodules and cirrhosis within 4 months

Treatments:
- Symptomatic treatments: Diuretics, Paracentesis
- Anticoagulation (heparin » warfarin) to prevent extension of thrombus and treat underlying cause
- Thrombolysis (tissue plasminogen and streptokinase) if acute thrombosis; However, inconclusive results; Risk of bleeding
- TIPS (possible bridge to OLT in fulminant BCS) if acute thrombosis or subacute thrombosis (if HVWPG <10); Risk occlusion
- Surgical shunt if subacute thrombosis (if HVWPG >10); Risk of procedure-related death
- Liver transplantation if: ESLD, or FHF, or deterioration of liver function after portosystemic shunting

Complications:
- Enlarged caudate lobe: compensatory (keeps liver functioning) hypertrophy due to separate hepatic veins that drain directly to IVC

Prognosis:
- Long-term prognosis is poor: >90% die within 3.5 years
- Transplantation can change this outcome: 5 year survival of 60% with 20% recurrence rate
- Leiden mutation is corrected once allograft is functioning

SECTION IV LIVER

PORTAL VEIN THROMBOSIS (PVT)

Definition:
- Occlusion of the portal vein

Etiologies:
- Most common of Children: infectious thrombosis due to omphalitis (infection of umbilical cord)
- Most common of Adults: low-flow states such as portal hypertension in cirrhosis, hypercoagulable states associated with BCS
- Others:
  - Neoplasm (pancreas, HCC), Hypercoagulable state
  - Intraabdominal inflammation/infection: pancreatitis
  - Surgery or Trauma: History of splenectomy is a risk factor by itself

Clinical Manifestations/Physical Exam:
- Acute phase: abdominal pain, fever, ileus, liver failure
- Chronic phase: ascites, splenomegaly, variceal bleeding

Laboratory Studies:
- LFTs usually normal

Diagnostic Studies:
- Venography is diagnostic test of choice; HVWPG may be normal or low (i.e. measuring free hepatic view to clot with the ↑ pressure is behind clot)
- CT: Chronic PVT shows cavernous transformation
- Others: U/S with Doppler, MRA

Treatments:
- Same as for portal HTN *See also Liver- Cirrhosis and Encephalopathy (Chapter 4.08)*
- Anticoagulation (heparin and thrombolytic agents have been tried with limited success)
- ? Surgery

Complications:
- If the PV thrombosis extends to the splenic or superior mesenteric veins, transplantation becomes technically impossible: Poor prognosis

VENO-OCCLUSIVE DISEASE (VOD)

Definition:
- Thrombotic occlusion of small/terminal hepatic venules and veins by connective tissue and collagen
- Associated with centrilobular congestion with or without hepatocellular necrosis
- Eventual progression into extensive perivenular fibrosis, central-to-central bridging, and eventually cirrhosis

Epidemiology:
- Incidence after **bone marrow transplant: 2-64%** depending on autologous or allogenic nature of transplant and chemotherapy
  - Presents with weight gain, ascites, jaundice, HSM, abdominal pain within **10–20 days after transplant**
  - Increased risk with chronic hepatitis and older age before transplantation

Etiologies:
- Bone marrow transplant
- Chemotherapy (vincristine, carmustine, doxorubicin, cyclophosphamide), Hepatic irradiation (XRT), Arsphenamine and Urethane therapy
- Azathioprine/6MP, Aflatoxin, Pyrrolizidine alkaloids (Jamaican bush tea)

Clinical Manifestations/Physical Exam:
- Hepatomegaly, ± Jaundice
- Ascites
- Weight gain, peripheral edema
- RUQ pain (capsular expansion)

Laboratory Studies:
- Elevated bilirubin, (↑ SAAG–post sinusoidal problem); Transaminases may be normal or elevated

Diagnostic Studies:
- U/S usually NOT helpful
- Diagnosis made clinically, or if necessary with liver biopsy and hepatic venography
  - HVWPG usually >10
  - Liver biopsy: perivenular sinusoidal dilatation with sclerosis/fibrosis, Zone III necrosis, central venular occlusion, phlebosclerosis
- For bone marrow transplant, Seattle criteria: bili >2 mg/dL, hepatomegaly, RUQ pain, weight gain >2%

Treatments:
- Mainly supportive: if ascites then maximize low Na diet, diuretics and paracentesis; If necessary, a TIPS may be done

Prognosis:
- Mortality is 20–40% (in those with bone marrow transplant)

HEPATIC ARTERY THROMBOSIS

Most happen in association with liver transplantation; Risk factors are technical ability for arterial anastomosis, clotting abnormalities, tobacco use, infection (CMV) or blood-type incompatible grafts; Presentation varies from mild pain to biliary strictures/intrahepatic abscess to FHF; Diagnosed with duplex U/S or angiography; Surgical correction is needed if detected early after transplant

4.10 CONGENITAL HEPATIC FIBROSIS

DEFINITION:
- Fibrous enlargement of the portal tracts with abnormally shaped bile ducts and no cirrhosis

EPIDEMIOLOGY:
- Autosomal recessive; Most commonly presents in childhood, but can be diagnosed at any age
- Incidence 1 in 10,000 to 1 in 20,000 births
- Often associated with Caroli's Syndrome; *See also Liver- Hepatobiliary Cystic Disease (Chapter 4.16)*
- Often associated with autosomal recessive polycystic kidney disease in children

ETIOLOGIES:
- Recent association with a mutation in polycystic kidney and hepatic disease 1 gene (PKHD1) gene
- Exact pathogenesis is unclear

PATHOPHYSIOLOGY:
- Histopathologic features:
  - Fibrous enlargement of the portal tracts, abnormally shaped bile ducts
  - No evidence of inflammation or cirrhosis

CLINICAL MANIFESTATIONS/PHYSICAL EXAM:
- Classically presents in one of three ways:
  - Variceal hemorrhage, Unexplained chronic and recurrent cholangitis, Asymptomatic hepatosplenomegaly

LABORATORY STUDIES:
- Typically normal liver function

DIAGNOSTIC STUDIES:
- SAAG >1.1; **Portal hypertension without cirrhosis!**
- Biopsy is generally diagnostic: Does not show cirrhosis
- Ultrasound: Hepatosplenomegaly, increased hepatic echogenicity, portal hypertension

TREATMENTS:
- Portosystemic shunting: Surgical shunts (distal splenorenal shunt) preferred over TIPS
  - Low incidence of postoperative complications
- May be a role for alternative approaches such as band ligation
- Ursodeoxycholic acid: ? role of treatment

COMPLICATIONS:
- Portal Hypertension: splenomegaly, varices/GIB
- Cholangitis: major complication that can lead to hepatic failure and death, often requires internal or external drainage or surgical therapy

PROGNOSIS:
- In general, the younger the presentation, the worse the prognosis
- Fatal hemorrhage and ascending cholangitis with sepsis is major cause of death

NOTES

4.11 DRUG & TOXIC INDUCED LIVER DISEASE

DEFINITION:
- More than 600 medicines have been reported to cause liver injury; Two most common: Acetaminophen and Alcohol; *See also Liver- Alcoholic Liver Disease (Chapter 4.04)*

EPIDEMIOLOGY:
- Drug-induced liver disease accounts for 2-5% of hospital admissions for jaundice in the U.S. and 10-20% of cases of fulminant liver failure

PATHOPHYSIOLOGY:
- Intrinsic injury (hepatotoxin with direct or indirect toxicity of hepatocytes): direct damage by covalently binding to cellular macromolecules
  - Example: Acetaminophen, Chloroform, Carbon Tetracholoride, Phosphorus
- Idiosyncratic injury (hyperimmune reaction): dose-dependent and hepatic injury cannot be reproduced in animal models
  - Clinical features of hypersensitivity common (rash, fever, eosinophilia)
  - Example: Phenytoin, Isoniazid, Ticrynafen, Halothane, Valproic Acid
- Patterns of injury: Cholestatic and Hepatocellular liver injury typically occurs 5-90 days after initial exposure
  - Drug stopped, biochemical improvement begins: Hepatocellular usually within 2 weeks, Cholestatic/ Mixed up to 4 weeks
  - Persistence beyond these intervals suggests coexistent or independent cause of liver disease: Viral, AIH, PBC, PSC, etc
- Drugs causing:
  - Chronic Hepatitis and Cirrhosis: Isoniazid, Methotrexate, Methyldopa, Nitrofurantoin, Oxyphenisatin, Trazodone
  - Mixed injury: Amitriptyline, Amoxicillin, Ampicillin, Captopril, Carbamazepine, Cimetidine, Flutamide, Imipramine, Nitrofurantoin, Phenylbutazone, Quinidine, Rantidine, Sulfonamides, Sulindac, Bactrim, NSAIDs
  - Cholestasis: Allopurinol, Amitriptyline, Azathioprine/6MP, Captopril, Carbamazepine, Phenytoin, OCP, Androgens/Anabolic Steroids
  - Granulomas causes: Allopurinol, Aspirin, Chlorpromazine, Diazepam, Diltiazem, Gold, Isoniazid, Mineral Oil, Nitrofurantoin, OCP, Oxacillin, Penicillin, Phenytoin, Phenylbutazone, Quinidine, Quinine, Tolbutamide
  - Drug-induced Steatosis (fatty liver):
    - Microvesicular Steatosis: Aspirin (Reye's), Ketoprofen, Tetracycline, Valproic Acid, Zidovudine (AZT), Valproic Acid
    - Macrovesicular Steatosis: ETOH, Acetaminophen, Cisplatin, Corticosteroids, Methotrexate, Tamoxifen
    - Phospholipidosis Steatosis: 4'4'-diethylamino ethyl hexestrol, Perhexiline maleate, Amiodarone, Bactrim, TPN
  - *See also Liver- Histopathology of Liver (Chapter 4.19)*

LABORATORY STUDIES/DIAGNOSTIC STUDIES:
- Patterns of drug-induced liver injury:

	ALT	Aφ	ALT:Aφ Ratio	
Hepatocellular	≥2-fold ↑	Normal	High (≥5)	**Aminotransferases**
Cholestatic	Normal	≥2-fold ↑	Low (≤2)	**>1000 and ↑↑↑ LDH:**
Mixed Injury	≥2-fold ↑	≥2-fold ↑	2-5	**'Shock Liver' (Ischemia)**

- Diagnosis of drug-induced liver injury requires exclusion of viral, toxic, cardiovascular, inheritable, and malignant causes
- Biopsy indications: medication stoppage not followed by improvement, cause still in question, severity necessitates intervention (i.e. OLT)

ETOH:
- *See also Liver- Alcoholic Liver Disease (Chapter 4.04)*

CHAPTER 4.11 DRUG & TOXIC INDUCED LIVER DISEASE

ACETAMINOPHEN HEPATOTOXICITY:
- Normal metabolism via glucuronidation and sulfation » non-toxic metabolites (protective detoxifying pathway); Pathway overwhelmed = problem
- Overdose (usually >7-10 g): N-hydroxylation by CYP2E1 (cytochrome p450) » reactive electrophilic compounds, such as N-acetyl-p-benzoquinone (NAPQI), that are scavenged by glutathione (an intracellular natural protectant) until reserves exhausted » result: hepatotoxicity
- Acetaminophen is toxic in nonalcoholic patients at doses >7.5 gm; Potential lethal dose: >140 mg/kg or 10 gm in 70 Kg man
    - Caution: Tylenol level may be normal if toxic dose taken 2-3 days previously and no further ingested since level drawn!
- CYP2E1 *induced* by fasting, alcohol, medication (i.e. INH) allowing 'therapeutic misadventure' in malnourished alcoholics taking even low-doses (2-6 g)
- Liver dysfunction may not be apparent for 2-6 days
- Treatment:
    - Ipecac given if time of ingestion can be verified to be <4 hours
    - Charcoal is controversial, may interfere with absorption of oral NAC
    - **N-acetylcysteine (NAC):**
      administer up to 36 hrs after ingestion if level above 'no-toxicity' zone
      or if time of ingestion unknown and decreasing levels (i.e. peak unknown)
      or if level unknown but reliable history of major poisoning (>10 g)
      (Rumack-Matthew Line helps predict the likelihood of liver injury)
      po dose: 140 mg/kg loading dose » 70 mg/kg q 4 hr × 17 additional doses
      IV dose (Acetadote): approved 2004, given for 48 hours with similar efficacy

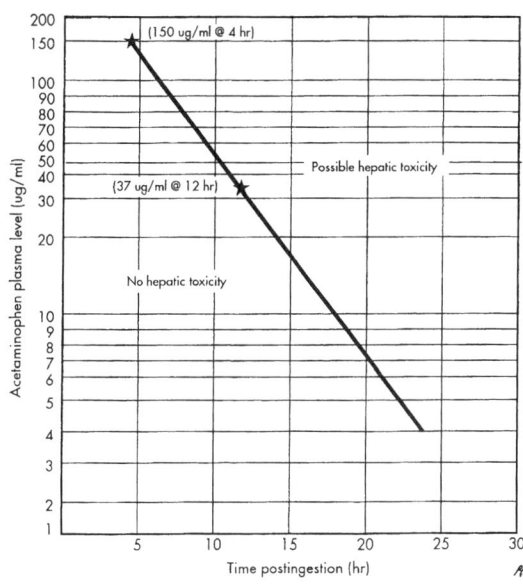

Rumack-Matthew nomogram.

Reprinted with permission from McNally P. GI/Liver Secrets. 2nd ed. Hanley & Belfus, Inc. PA; 2001:175.

RECREATIONAL: COCAINE, ECSTASY, MUSHROOMS
Cocaine:
- May present with jaundice, fatigue or malaise; Transaminase can be as high as 5000 IU/L; Mechanism is unclear
- Also may cause coagulopathy, rhabdomyolysis, DIC; Liver biopsy shows zone III injury, suggesting ischemia-related
- May be associated with viral hepatitis, acetaminophen and alcohol

SECTION IV LIVER

Ecstasy:
- Synthetic amphetamine; Makes users euphoric and more sociable and eliminates fatigue; Also causes arrhythmias, DIC, ARF, hyperthermia
- Suspect in young adult with acute hepatitis but no identifiable cause, can cause fulminant hepatitis

Toxic mushrooms *(Amanita phalloides):*
- Treatment: Penicillin 300,000–1,000,000 units/kg day (antagonist of amatoxin) AND Silibinin 20–50 mg/kg/day (prevents hepatocellular uptake of amatoxin)

ENDOCRINE:
Troglitazone: ↓ hepatic glucose output and ↑ skeletal muscle insulin sensitization; Fulminant cases have been reported; monitor monthly first 6 months
Sulfonylureas: Cholestatic: Chlorpropamide, Glipizide, Tolazamide, Tolbutamide; Hepatocellular/Mixed: remainder of the class
PTU/Methimazole: May cause hepatocellular or cholestatic injury
Steroids (Anabolic, OCP, Tamoxifen, Danazol, Glucocorticoids): Can cause cholestasis or canalicular type of injury
Lipid Lowering (Niacin, Statins): Niacin: mixed injury, more common with >3 gm/day (dose dependant)
Statins: low incidence, levels usually stabilize or return to normal spontaneously (most patients probably have NAFLD) or when discontinuing

ANTIBIOTICS & ANTIFUNGALS:
Isoniazid (INH):
- Presents insidiously from 4–6 months after starting therapy; Some experience influenza-like symptoms; risk hepatitis ↑ with age (2–3% >50 y/o)
- Transaminitis in up to 20% of patients, but usually subsides spontaneously
- Rifampin ↑ likelihood of INH toxicity; likewise acetaminophen toxicity is ↑ with use of INH (induces cytochrome P45)
- Those with history of liver disease need to be watched extremely closely with serial monitoring of ALT (level >100, consider alternate drug)

Nitrofurantoin:
- Cholestatic pattern usually seen; Symptoms of fever, rash and eosinophilia are common; Most cases are women taking ≥6 months
- Labs: high transaminases, gamma globulin, HLA-B8 histocompatibility markers, and often positive autoimmune markers (ANA)

Penicillin: Both Cholestatic and hepatitis-like patterns reported; Hypersensitivity is the mechanism of injury
Amoxicillin, clavulanic acid: Cholestatic hepatitis has been reported during or within weeks of administration
Sulfonamide: Mixed hepatocellular injury that is usually heralded by rash, fever and eosinophillia
Pyrimethamine-sulfadoxine: Hepatocellular injury is most common, but fulminant hepatitis and death have been reported
Tetracycline: Almost exclusively with parenteral form, more common in pregnant women; Microvesicular steatosis is common histological finding
Erythromycin estolate: Ethylsuccinate form is also known to cause Cholestatic hepatitis; Hypersensitivity picture seen days to weeks after exposure
Ketoconazole: Toxic hepatitis more common in older women (>40 yrs); Fulminant hepatitis has been reported; Periodic monitoring of LFTs recommended

ANESTHETIC AGENTS:
Note: post-operative non-anesthetic causes must be considered: viral, drug-induced, bile duct injury, TPN, sepsis, transfusion hepatitis, ischemia
Medications: Halothane, Enflurane, Methoxyflurane, Isoflurane

Halothane
- Risk increases with more exposure; Most patients present within 2 weeks: fever, nausea, rash, arthralgias, diffuse abdominal pain
- Labs: eosinophilia, AST/ALT range 500–1000 IU/L, Aφ usually <2 × normal
- Mechanism: appears to be related to development of sensitization to both oxidative metabolite (trifluoracetyl) and autoantigens (CYP2D6)
- Poor prognosis: short latent period from exposure to jaundice, obesity, age >40 yrs, PSE, high INR
- Steroids and exchange transfusions not helpful; Mortality of fulminant halothane hepatitis is 80% without OLT

CHAPTER 4.11 DRUG & TOXIC INDUCED LIVER DISEASE

ANTIARTHRITIC:

Ibuprofen: Relatively uncommon cause of liver injury

Sulindac (Clinoril): Cholestatic hepatitis; Symptoms: fever, rash, Steven-Johnson syndrome; Rarely 'trapped' CBD from sulindac-induced pancreatitis

Diclofenac (Voltaren): More common in women; Most hepatocellular injury; Fulminant hepatitis has been reported

Methotrexate (MTX):
- Reevaluation of MTX safety is advised with AST or ALT levels exceed 3 × baseline values
  - Liver biopsies are advised every 2 or 3 years (or every 1.5 gm of cumulative dose)
- Some advocate an index liver biopsy after 2-4 months of use, followed by serial repeat biopsies after every 1.0-1.5 gm of cumulative dose
- The American College of Rheumatology does not recommend pretreatment liver biopsy in absence of preexisting liver disease
- Histological grades and recommendations:

Grade	Fibrosis	Fatty Infiltration	Nuclear Variability	Portal Inflammation	Recommendations
1	None	Mild	Mild	Mild	Continue, repeat bx after 1-1.5 gm cumulative dose
2	None	Mod-Severe	Mod-Severe	Portal ↑/lobular necrosis	Continue, repeat bx after 1-1.5 gm cumulative dose
3A	Mild	Mod-Severe	Mod-Severe	Portal ↑/lobular necrosis	Continue, repeat bx in 6 months
3B	Moderate	Mod-Severe	Mod-Severe	Portal ↑/lobular necrosis	No further MTX, exceptional cases = close follow up
4	Cirrhosis				No further MTX, exceptional cases = close follow up

CARDIOVASCULAR:

Quinidine: Predominate injury is hepatocellular with focal necrosis, but granulomas can occur too; Has been reported after a single dose

Procainamide: Liver injury is rare, but hepatocellular, cholestatic and granulomatous injuries have been reported

Verapamil & Nifedipine: Cholestatic, hepatocellular, mixed injuries may occur within 2-3 weeks of use; Pseudoalcohol pattern of steatosis and Mallory's hyaline reported

Hydralazine: Hepatocellular and granulomatous injuries reported

Captopril: Hypersensitivity symptoms herald jaundice, cholestasis resolves with removal

Enalapril: Scattered cases of hepatitis and cholestasis have been reported

Amiodarone: A characteristic injury of phospholipidosis is seen

OTHER:

Phenytoin (Dilantin):
- Causes allergic hepatitis, cholestasis, granulomatous liver disease, and possibly fulminant hepatitis; Symptoms usually occur within 8 weeks
- Symptoms include pharyngitis, lymphadenopathy, atypical lymphocytosis (pseudolymphoma syndrome); Therapy may be steroids

Methyldopa (Aldomet):
- Liver injury usually occurs within 6-12 weeks of initiation of therapy; ALT should always be checked periodically during the first 4 months
- Women appear to be more susceptible to Methyldopa toxicity and clinical presentation may mimic autoimmune 'lupoid' hepatitis

Chlorzoxazone (Parafon Forte):
- Centrally-acting muscle relaxant; Hepatotoxic effects are rare, but fulminant failure has been reported; onset within 1 week
- Transaminase elevation may exceed 1000 IU/L; most exhibit hyperbilirubinemia; Discontinuation is usually suffice for recovery

HERBAL:

Milk thistle (silybum marianum): Safe substance that has been used for centuries to remedy liver disease; Many self medicate with it

Comfrey & Chaparral leaf: Known to be hepatotoxic

4.12 HEMOCHROMATOSIS & IRON OVERLOAD

(Hepatology 2001;33:1321-28)

DEFINITIONS:
- **Hereditary Hemochromatosis (HH):** Autosomal recessive inherited disorder of iron overload
  - Increased iron absorption from the gut, with preferential deposition of iron in liver parenchyma, heart, pancreas, and other endocrine glands (Wilson's disease is decreased copper secretion, not an increased absorptive process like HH)
- **Secondary iron overload:** some other stimulus causes the GI tract to absorb increased amounts of iron; There is an underlying disorder:
  - I.e. anemias due to ineffective erythropoiesis, chronic liver disease, and rarely, excessive intake of medical iron
- **Parenteral iron overload:** received excessive iron either as RBC transfusions or iron-dextran parenterally (always iatrogenic)
  - In patients requiring routine transfusions, a chelation program with deferoxamine should be initiated to prevent toxic iron overload
- **Neonatal iron overload:** Rare; Most likely related to intrauterine viral infection; Infants do very poorly and generally die without transplant
- **African iron overload (Bantu hemosiderosis):** previously thought to be related to excessive iron in ETOH due to brewing in iron drums
  - Recent studies suggest there may be a genetic component distinct from HH (i.e. not the HFE gene).
- Other inheritable forms of liver disease: α1-AT, Wilson's

EPIDEMIOLOGY:
- 1 in 300 is homozygous for the hemochromatosis mutation and 1 in 10 is a heterozygous carrier; Usually manifests in middle-age ♂
- HH is most common identified single-gene disorder in Caucasians

ETIOLOGIES:
- Gene responsible is HFE, which codes for MHC type-1 like protein; The mutation replaces a cysteine with a tyrosine at position 282 (C282Y)
  - The result is a problem with transferring receptor-mediated iron uptake into cells, leading to increased iron absorption = HH
- A second mutation, where histidine is replaced by aspartate at position 63 (H63D) is common but less important in cellular iron metabolism
- Hepcidin: a small polypeptide produced in the liver inhibits iron absorption in small intestines and prevents iron release from macrophages
  - May function as a iron regulator; increased in infectious/inflammatory diseases (may be responsible for anemia of chronic disease)
  - Levels are inappropriately low in HH; future studies may clarify pathophysiology or iron metabolism and HH

PATHOPHYSIOLOGY:
- Western diet consumes 10-20 mg iron/day; Absorption 1-2 mg/day, representing about 10% efficiency in absorption
  - Patients with iron deficiency, HH, or ineffective erythropoiesis absorb increased amounts of iron (up to 3-6 mg/day)
- Iron storage (normal 4 gm of total body iron): 2.5 gm hemoglobin, 1 gm reticuloendothelial (spleen, bone marrow, liver), 400 mg myoglobin
  - All cells contain some iron due to mitochondrial usage; Clinical manifestations occur when body iron levels reach 15-40 grams
- Iron is bound to transferrin in both the intra- and extravascular compartments
- Iron is stored as ferritin in cells, and as this amount increases it is found in hemosiderin
  - Serum ferritin equals total body iron stores in patients with iron deficiency and HH and is biochemically different from tissue ferritin

CHAPTER 4.12 HEMOCHROMATOSIS & IRON OVERLOAD

- Chronic iron overload = oxidant stress = lipid peroxidation of cells (such as the membranes) = organelle damage
  - Phagocytosis by Kupffer cells; These iron overloaded Kupffer cells become activated resulting in activated hepatic stellate cells:
    - Leads to increased collagen synthesis and fibrosis (hepatocellular injury)
- The DDX of increased hepatic iron is long, the pattern of iron distribution may help. *See also Liver-Histopathology of Liver (Chapter 4.19)*
  - Predominantly hepatocellular distribution: Genetic hemochromatosis, Alcoholic liver disease, Porphyria cutanea tarda
  - Predominantly in Kupffer cells: Multiple transfusions, Hemolytic anemias
  - Mixed hepatocellular and Kupffer cell distribution: Megaloblastic anemia, Anemia secondary to chronic infection

CLINICAL MANIFESTATIONS/PHYSICAL EXAM:
- Bronzing of the skin (melanin + iron), usually in sun exposed areas
- DM ("Bronze Diabetes")
- Hepatomegaly with or without cirrhosis
- Hypogonadism/Impotence
- Arthritis (2nd & 3rd MCPs) – See Complications below
- CHF/Heart Failure
- Infections *(Vibrio, Listeria, Yersinia)*
- Fatigue, malaise, lethargy

LABORATORY STUDIES:
- Serum Iron, TIBC (Total Iron Binding Capacity) or Transferrin, Serum Ferritin
- Suggestive: ↑ Fasting Transferrin Saturation (TS) [(Serum Iron/TIBC) × 100] = >45%,
  ↑ Ferritin (acute phase reactant and increased in various infections/inflammatory conditions; not an initial screening test)

- **Hepatic Iron Studies:**
  Hepatic Iron Concentration (HIC): used less due to genetic testing availability; Symptomatic pt >10,000; Threshold for fibrosis >22,000
  Hepatic Iron Index (HII); Progresses with homozygous HH, and no progression with secondary iron overload or heterozygous HH
  HII = HIC (umol/gm)/age (years); Homozygous ≥1.9; Genetic testing has seen up to 15% of HH with <1.9! HII is no longer gold standard

Condition	TS	Ferritin	Iron Index
Normal	≤45%	<200	<1.0
Alcoholic Liver Disease	≤60%	<500	<2.0
Hemochromatosis:			
Heterozygotes	variable	<500	<2.0
Asymptomatic Homozygotes	>50%	>500	>2.0
Symptomatic Homozygotes	>50%	>900	>2.0

NOTE: 30-50% of patients with viral hepatitis, ETOH liver disease, or NASH have abnormal iron studies
- Generally a fasting TS is more specific for HH; So if high ferritin and normal TS, another form of liver disease may be responsible
- Conversely, with a normal ferritin and a high TS, the likely diagnosis is HH (especially with young persons)

LABORATORY STUDIES, CONTINUED:
- **Genetic Testing:** If iron studies abnormal, then check for mutation analysis of HFE genes (C282Y and H63D) on chromosome 6
  The gene normally encodes for MHC class-I protein that complexes with the transferring receptor, decreasing its affinity for transferrin
  The mutation of HFE gene results in a protein that does not bind well to transferrin receptor and thus results in increased iron uptake
  (Note: 13% of patients can have a normal DNA panel (HFE genetic testing) and can still have hemochromatosis)

SECTION IV LIVER

Homozygote: C282Y/C282Y – 90% of Hereditary Hemochromatosis
Compound Heterozygote: C282Y/H63D–3% of Hereditary Hemochromatosis; Is also a risk factor for iron overload and needs treatment
C282 Heterozygote: Normal/C282Y
H63D Heterozygote: Normal/H63D

- If homozygous or compound heterozygote, under age 40, normal ALT/AST: no further tests, arrange therapeutic phlebotomy
- If older than 40, or abnormal ALT/AST, or markedly high ferritin (>1,000 ng/ml): liver biopsy
  - Biopsy should be sent for Prussian blue stain, hepatic iron concentration for Hepatic Iron Index calculation
  - Usually show iron found *in hepatocytes* and zone 1; In heavy overload, zone 1-3 is maintained but less distinct

DIAGNOSTIC STUDIES:

- Proposed algorithm:
  Fasting Transferrin saturation
  - More than 45%:
    » C282Y Homozygote:
      » Ferritin more than 1000 ng/ml: Liver biopsy
      » Ferritin less than 1000 ng/ml:
        » LFT abnormal: Liver biopsy
        » LFT normal: Ferritin elevated: begin phlebotomy or Ferritin normal: follow
    » C282Y/H63D Heterozygote:
      » Liver biopsy

- MRI: "black liver" from iron overload; In general, however, imaging is not very helpful; Genetic testing and Iron studies are best for diagnosis
- Biopsy: can tell you where iron is stored (hepatocytes vs. Kupffer cells), amount of iron can be graded, quantitative iron determination, and complications of iron storage (fibrosis, cirrhosis, hepatocellular carcinoma)
- Four stages of HH
  1. Genetic predisposition without iron overload
  2. Early iron overload: 2-5 gm Iron, up to 20 years of disease
  3. Moderate iron overload: 5-10 gm Iron, 20-40 years of disease
  4. Heavy iron overload: >10 gm Iron, >40 years of disease

TREATMENTS:

- Phlebotomy (500 cc) q week of whole blood until Fe parameters normal, then prn to keep in range
  - Each unit blood contains 200-250 mg of iron; Therefore symptomatic HH with 20 gm excess, takes about 80 units over 2 yrs!
  - Goal: decrease tissue stores, not create iron deficiency
  - Once ferritin <50 ng/ml and TS <50%, majority of excessive iron stores have been successfully depleted
  - Maintenance phlebotomy regime ~1 unit every 2-3 months (4-8 phlebotomies annually)
- Deferoxamine if can't undergo phlebotomy; cumbersome because they are subcutaneous infusions, expensive and much less effective
  - Complexes with trivalent ions (ferric ions) to form ferrioxamine which is excreted in the kidneys If necessary, renal dosage is required
- Genetic counseling/screening for family members; 25% of siblings and 5% of children will have the disease!
- Avoid iron or iron containing supplements; Zinc supplements may be beneficial; Red meat only in moderation; Avoid ETOH

COMPLICATIONS:

- This is an inheritable disease; Once patient is diagnosed, all first-degree relatives should be screened for HFE mutations and iron studies!
- Hepatocellular cancer occurs with HH and cirrhosis
- Rheumatological Manifestations:
  - Arthritis 40-75%; non-inflammatory, but degenerative: 2nd & 3rd metacarpophalangeal joints (MCP) or proximal interphalangeal joints
    - Phlebotomy does not stop the progression of arthropathy; No correlation between severity of arthropathy and liver disease

- May be presenting complaint of hemochromatosis! and frequently diagnosed as seronegative (RF negative) rheumatoid arthritis!
- Calcium Pyrophosphate Disease (CPPD)/Pseudo Gout: occurs in wrist and knees of 20–50% of those with hemochromatosis
- Osteoporosis: due to gonadal dysfunction from pituitary insufficiency caused by the iron overload state
- Osteomalacia: due to vitamin D deficiency due to liver disease
- Hypertrophic Osteoarthropathy: cirrhosis of any cause, including hemochromatosis, can be associated with periosteal reactions of bones

PROGNOSIS:
- Pre-Cirrhosis & Diabetes- Phlebotomy: good outcome with improvement in fatigue, ALT, HSM, Cardiac, Diabetes, Impotence
  - Normal life span
- Risk factors for cirrhosis:
  - Age >40, Ferritin >1000 ng/ml, Hepatomegaly
  If cirrhosis has developed: Screen for complications: varices, HCC (i.e. U/S & AFP q 6 months): **high risk for HCC** even after iron normalizes
- Most common cause of death is complications of chronic liver disease and HCC
- Liver transplant (1%), must continue to follow periodically after OLT (unlike Wilson's Disease and α1-AT which is a cure since these are inherent to only liver)

4.13 HEPATITIS A, D, E

HEPATITIS A
Definition:
- A hepatotrophic virus; the liver is the primary site of infection, replication and cellular damage

Epidemiology:
- Undeveloped countries: Africa, Asia, etc. In U.S., most are predominant in western states (especially American Indians)
- Causes 40% of cases of acute viral hepatitis in the U.S.

Etiologies:
- Transmission: fecal-oral route; contaminated food, water, shellfish; day-care center outbreaks
  - HAV is the most infectious and transmittable viral hepatitis of all viral hepatitis
- Incubation: 2-6 weeks

Pathophysiology:
- Virus: RNA, linear gene shape, no envelope, 28 nm in size

Clinical Manifestations/Physical Exam:
- Natural History: anorexia, nausea, vomiting, fatigue, abdominal pain, mild fever, jaundice, dark urine, light stools
- Children, especially under age 14, rarely have symptoms

Laboratory Studies:
- Acute hepatitis: +IgM anti-HAV; Persist for 3-6 months
- Past exposure or vaccination: +IgG anti-HAV (−IgM); Note: 'Total' tests are both IgM and IgG

Treatments:
- Treatment of acute HAV is supportive
- Vaccine: Children 1-18 yrs (daycare), travelers to endemic areas, military, male-male sex, IVDA, cirrhosis any cause (50% mortality with HAV)
  - VAQTA or HAVRIX: Adults, 1 ml (50 U) at time 0 and 6 months
                    Children, 0.5 ml (25 U) at time 0 and 6-18 months
    - Sufficient serum level post immunization (not established, only advised): >20 mIU/ml; Vaccine doesn't compromise other vaccines given at same time; If given 1st dose, 2nd dose can be given any time within 5 years and still achieve immunity; 100% show immunity at 12 years
- IVIG: No role for pre-exposure prophylaxis, just start vaccination processes; Ok for short-term immunity or children who can't take vaccine
  IVIG dose: Dose 0.02 ml/kg for <3 months protection, 0.06 ml/kg q 5 months for longer

Complications:
- Chronicity: none; Cleared within 6 months (IgM becomes negative and IgG persists for life); 50 fulminant cases per year

Prognosis:
- Most recover without any problems (rarely a transplant is needed); Recovery infers lifelong immunity

HEPATITIS D (DELTA)
Definition:
- A hepatotrophic virus; the liver is the primary site of infection, replication and cellular damage (requires the presence of HBsAg to replicate)

Epidemiology:
- For unknown reasons, Hepatitis D is almost never seen anymore (without HBV, it is non-pathogenic)
  - Have high suspicion if a patient has acute HBV or acute exacerbation of chronic HBV

Etiologies:
- Transmission: percutaneous or sexual (IV drug users are the group of HBV patients with highest risk for HDV)

Pathophysiology:
- Virus: RNA, circular gene shape, envelope, 43 nm in size
- Requires HBV: co-infection (AntiD IgM, HDV RNA+, Ig**M** anti-HBc+, HBsAg+) or superimposed infection (Same except Ig**G** anti-HBc+)

Clinical Manifestations/Physical Exam:
- Natural History: more severe hepatitis, faster progression to cirrhosis

Laboratory Studies:
- anti-HDV (ELISA)

Treatments:
- IFN-α; Follow during treatment, HDV RNA (by PCR) has high relapse rate

Complications:
- Can lead to chronic infection, more likely to be associated with developing cirrhosis; Increased risk of primary hepatocellular carcinoma
  - Chronicity rates: occurs only with simultaneous hepatitis B infections, approaches 100% if chronic HBV superinfected with HDV

HEPATITIS E

Definition:
- A hepatotrophic virus; the liver is the primary site of infection, replication and cellular damage

Epidemiology:
- Affects mainly young adults; Pregnant females

Etiologies:
- Transmission: fecal-oral; travelers to Pakistan, India, South East Asia, Africa, Mexico; I.e. poor sewer systems; Animals may be reservoir
- Incubation: 6-7 weeks; Fecal shedding for 2-3 weeks before and after onset of illness

Pathophysiology:
- Virus: RNA, linear gene shape, no envelope, 32 nm in size

Clinical Manifestations/Physical Exam:
- Natural History: Acute hepatitis with increased mortality (10-20%) during **Pregnancy**

Laboratory Studies:
- IgM anti-HEV (test available at the CDC)

Treatments:
- Follow/Supportive

Complications:
- Chronicity: none; cleared within 6 months; Pregnancy complicated by HEV may progress to fulminant liver failure

Prognosis:
- Increased **fetal and maternal mortality** (20%) with HEV during pregnancy

4.14 HEPATITIS B

(Hepatology 2007;45:507-39. Clin Gastroenterol Hepatol. 2006;4:936-62; Hepatology. 2004;39:1-5)

DEFINITION:
- A hepatotrophic virus; the liver is the primary site of infection, replication and cellular damage
- Chronic hepatitis: presence of clinical, biochemical, and serologic abnormalities for up to 6 months

EPIDEMIOLOGY:
- 350 million cases worldwide; 1.25 million in US; most cases in Asia and Africa; causes 30% of acute and 15% of chronic hepatitis in the US
- 10th leading cause of death in the world, 5th leading infectious disease cause of death in the world
- Chronicity of HBV acquired during infancy: 90%; acquired during adulthood: 5%
  - In general, when a patient gets acute HBV: 95% recovery, 5% chronically infected, Fulminant hepatic failure (very rare)

ETIOLOGIES:
- Transmission: sexual (most common), percutaneous, perinatal
  - Household/intimate contacts need to be vaccinated since they are at most risk
- Incubation: 1-6 months
- Pregnant women/Vertical Transmission/Breastfeeding: Lamivudine for treatment; prophylaxis is available; *See also Liver- Pregnancy Pearls (Chapter 4.25)*
  - Hep B: Transmission 1st Trimester (10%), 3rd Trimester (90%); All women tested in 3rd trimester
    - Test mother for HBsAg, if +, Protect baby after delivery with HBIG (0.5 ml) and Vaccine (0.5 ml at birth and 1 & 6 months)
    - Test mother for HBsAg, If −, Baby should only get full dose of Hep B Vaccine (not HBIG) at delivery
    - Hep B Vaccine is safe in pregnant patients

PATHOPHYSIOLOGY:
- Virus: DNA, circular gene shape, envelope, 42 nm in size; Replicates at 10^{11} virions/day
- 8 genotypes identified: A-H; The future may tell us that certain genotypes are better treated with either Nucleosides analogues or PEG-INF
- Spilled blood contaminated with HBV can be infectious for up to one week (i.e. DNA viruses resist degradation)

CLINICAL MANIFESTATIONS/PHYSICAL EXAM:
- Natural History: anorexia, nausea, vomiting, fatigue, abdominal pain, mild fever, jaundice, dark urine, light colored stools
  - Acute: 70% subclinical, 30% jaundice, <1% fulminant hepatitis (100 cases/year)
  - Chronic: <5% (adult-acquired), >90% (perinatally-acquired); females are more likely to be chronic carriers
- Extra-hepatic: Polyarteritis Nodosa (<1%), Membranoproliferative Glomerulonephritis

LABORATORY STUDIES:
- Transaminitis (↑ ALT/AST); *See also Liver- LFTs (Chapter 4.20)*
- Serologic & Virologic:
  Surface: "Far & Away" (i.e. Ag & Ab separated by window)
  -**HBsAg:** appears before symptoms; used to screen blood donor; Neg = viral clearance
  -**anti-HBs:** indicates resolution of acute disease & immunity (sole marker after vaccination)

  Core: "In the middle" (i.e. Ab in the window)
  -**HBcAg** not found in blood tests
  -**IgM anti-HBc:** first Ab to appear; indicates acute infection
     Window Period = HBsAg become −, anti-HBs not yet +, anti-HBc only clue to infection
     Therefore, workup for suspected acute symptomatic HBV is HBsAg & IgM anti-HBc
  -**IgG anti-HBc:** indicates previous (HBsAg−) or chronic (HBsAg+) HBV infection
     'Total core tests' are both IgM and IgG and most labs use this as a screening; be careful!

CHAPTER 4.14 HEPATITIS B

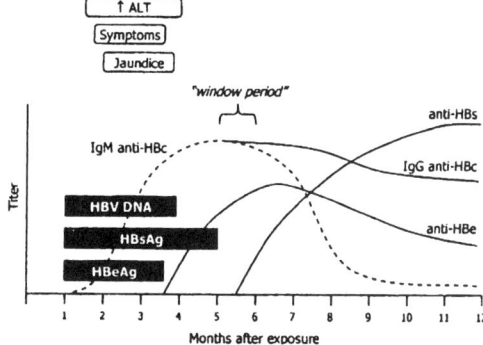

Reprinted with permission from Sabatine S: Pocket Medicine 2nd ed. Baltimore: Lippincott Williams & Wilkins, 2004:3–16.

E Particles: "Together" (i.e. Ag & Ab overlap)
-**HBeAg:** by product (evidence) of viral replication and defines ↑ infectivity/acute infection
  Precore Variant: eAg not generated with +DNA, but anti-HBe can develop due to cross-reactivity with cAg
  If HBeAg +, then HBV DNA must be +; If HBeAg −, then either Precore Variant (VL >100K), or Inactive Carrier (VL <100K)
-**anti-HBe:** indicates waning viral replication, ↓ infectivity/replication

DNA:
HBV DNA: presence in serum correlates with active viral replication in liver; Use hybridization, not PCR (too sensitive)

DIAGNOSTIC STUDIES:

- Biopsy: degree of inflammation (grade) & amount of fibrosis (stage); no other test makes this determination accurately
  - Stages (Fibrosis): 1. portal fibrosis, 2. periportal fibrosis, 3. septal fibrosis, 4. cirrhosis
  - Grade (Inflammation): 1. minimal lobular, 2. mild portal, 3. moderate piecemeal necrosis, 4. severe portal with piecemeal necrosis

	Surface:		Core:	E Particles:		DNA/ALT/Course of Action:
	HBsAg	anti-HBs	anti-HBc	HBeAg	anti-HBe	
-Acute hepatitis:	+	−	IgM	+	−	+DNA, Observe, resolution likely 90% to 95% of adults
-Window period:	−	−	IgM	±	±	+DNA
-Recovery (prior exposure):	−	+[a]	IgG	−	±	−DNA (protected from further infection)
-Immunization:	−	+	−	−	−	−DNA (protected from further infection)
-Chronic (*Replicative EAg+*):	+	−	IgG	+	−	+DNA, ↑ ALT: **EAg+/Wild Type**, Initiate tx w/goal » Inactive Carrier
Chronic (Immune Tolerant):	+	−	IgG	+	−	+DNA, nl ALT: **Immune Tolerant**, <5% respond to IFN, better with NA
Chronic (*Non-Replicative*):	+	−	IgG	−	+	− or ↓ DNA, nl ALT: Chronic **Inactive Carrier,** Observe
Chronic (Precore Variant):	+	−	IgG	−	±	+DNA, ↑ ALT: **EAg-/Precore Variant**, Initiate tx (likely lifelong)
-Isolated Core:	−	−	IgG	−	+	No significance, unless transplant patient*

[a] Notice only options with + anti-HBs
*Represents past infection with immunity, but loss anti-HBs; if transplanted, 50/50 chance the recipient will get HBV

SECTION IV LIVER

TREATMENTS:
- Acute: Supportive, HBIG (in nonvaccinated patients, given with first dose of vaccine), Self-limiting disease in 90% and resolves in 6 months
- Chronic: Best candidates for therapy:
    See table below, +HBsAg >6 months, Liver damage (↑ ALT or inflammation on biopsy)
    Treat even the cirrhotics and those with chronic HBV undergoing chemotherapy (since reactivation of HBV is a risk)
    HBV DNA level is the most important factor in the progression to cirrhosis or HCC

    No therapy indicated:
    Chronic Inactive Carrier (normal ALT), −eAg/+eAb (except Precore Variant), or non-detectable HBV DNA

Summary Treatment Table: *Think in terms of eAg (+) or (−)*

HBeAg	DNA(IU/ml)*	ALT	Recommendation
+	<20K	≤2 × ULN	No treatment, follow: 6–12 mon, some consider liver biopsy: ± treatment if histological disease
+	≥20K	≤2 × ULN	↓ HBeAg conversion rate (esp. young age), follow or consider biopsy and treat if disease with NA's
+	≥20K	>2 × ULN	Treatment with NA's (not Lamivudine) better than Peg-INF especially with high DNA levels
−	<2000	≤2 × ULN	No treatment (most inactive carriers), follow: 6–12 mon, some consider liver biopsy: ± treatment
−	≥2000	≤2 × ULN	Consider biopsy and treat with NA's if disease; If no biopsy then observe for rise in ALT
−	≥2000	>2 × ULN	Treat with long-term NA's (not Lamivudine)
±	<2000	compensated cirrhosis	May chose to treat with NA's (not Lamivudine) or observe
±	≥2000	compensated cirrhosis	Treat with NA's (not Lamivudine), long term therapy required, combination therapy may be preferred
±	<10^5	decompensated cirrhosis	Treat with combination NA's long term; refer to transplant center

*Note: 1IU/ml = 5.6 copies/ml; The historical ">10^5" (100K) copies/ml is arbitrarily and evidence suggest lowering to 20K (Gastro 2006;130:678-686)

- What to treat with: why and how (Note combination therapy of the medicines below is probably the future, much like HIV is treated)
  Nucleoside Analogues (NA): **Lamivudine** (100 mg qd) or **Adefovir** (10 mg qd) or **Entecavir** (0.5 mg qd)
  - Oral, rapid clearance, few side effects (Black box warning: lactic acidosis); No one really knows when to stop them if patient responds: ? 4 yrs of therapy
  - Efficacy of eAg conversion to eAb: 15% at 1 year; 50% at 5 years (Less with Lamivudine due to YMDD mutants)

  PEG-IFN-α-2a (more old school, but because of pegylation it is making a come back with some clinicians)
  - More durable after stopping therapy; however, it is an injection, multiple side effects ***See also Liver- Hepatitis C (Chapter 4.15)***
  - Never use to treat with HBV *Cirrhosis* as can make situation worse (precipitate decompensation)

  Goal of therapy: ↓ DNA (<10^5 copies/ml), Normalize LFTs, Seroconversion: −eAg/+eAb (i.e. Make Chronic Inactive Carrier); Occurs in 20–40%
  - Predictors of good response (eAg+): High ALT, Low DNA, Adult-acquired (esp. ♀), Active liver histology
  - Seroconversion (eAg−) does not preclude patients from ever experiencing a future complication from their liver disease
    - Depends on amount of liver disease prior to seroconversion

CHAPTER 4.14 HEPATITIS B

- YMDD mutant: the development of Lamivudine-resistant mutants; ~50% at 3 years
  - Typical course of YMDD is an initial response to Lamivudine, then a flare of hepatitis with minimal response
  - Adefovir-resistant mutants: ~5% at 3 years, ~30% at 5 years
  - Entecavir-resistant mutants not observed (yet?)
- Precore Variant: likely lifelong treatment, can't tell if eAb will ever develop; Some start Adefovir first, bypassing Lamivudine
- Counseling: Lifestyle modification (prevent transmission), decrease ETOH use
- Liver transplantation: 80–100% reinfection without therapy (goal ↓ DNA count low as possible prior to OLT)
  - Post transplant therapy begins immediately and lasts indefinitely: HBIG and NA (90% HBV recurrence prevented)

■ HBIG/Vaccines: 90% effective in long-term immunity after 3 doses even though 20–30% antibody titers can drop <10 mIU/ml within 5–9 years
- Boosters generally not needed for anyone, but give to immunocompromised (i.e. dialysis patients) if level <10 mIU/ml
- Who to vaccinate: Household/Intimate contacts, Adults at high risk, Children, Newborns; *See also Liver- Pregnancy Pearls (Chapter 4.25)*
HBIG: a high concentration of anti-HBs
  Perinatal: 0.5 ml IM within 12 hours of birth, followed by Vaccine (0.5 ml) at birth, and 1 & 6 months
  Sexual: 0.6 ml/kg IM within 14 days of sexual contact, followed by Vaccine at same time
Vaccine (RecombivaxHB, EngerixB; HeptavaxB no longer available in U.S.): Note: most given at 0,1, 6 months
- Recombivax: <u>Birth to 10 yr</u>: 0.5 ml at 0, 1, 6 months; <u>Adults</u>: 10 mg/1.0 ml at 0, 1, 6 months; <u>Dialysis</u>: 40 mg/1.0 ml at 0, 1, 6 months
- Engerix: <u>Birth to 10 yr</u>: 0.5 ml at 0, 1, 6 months; <u>Adults</u>: 20 mg/1.0 ml at 0, 1, 6 months; <u>Needlestick</u>: 20 mg/1.0 ml at 0, 1, 2 months; <u>Dialysis</u>: 40 mg/2.0 ml at 0, 1, 6 months
- Efficacy: Lasts at least 18 years (those given during infancy) and 22 years (those given during child/adulthood); probably lifelong
Screen for HAV (total antibody) and vaccinate if no immunity in HBV patients

COMPLICATIONS:
■ Can lead to chronic infection, more likely to be associated with developing cirrhosis
- Chronicity rates: neonates approaching 100%, children 70%, healthy adults: 1% (chronic illness are less likely to clear virus)
■ Increased risk of primary hepatocellular carcinoma; **Not all get cirrhosis before HCC,** therefore all get regularly screened (unlike Hepatitis C)
■ Rheumatological Manifestations
- Polyarteritis Nodosa (PAN): acute or chronic systemic necrotizing medium-vessel vasculitis without granuloma formation
  - Approximately 25% of PAN patients have HBsAg; ♂ > ♀; symptomatic hepatitis is usually not predominant feature
  - Symptoms: wt loss, fever, arthritis, fatigue/myalgias, livedo reticularis, coronary arteritis, abdominal pain and GI bleed/infarction
  - Dx: clinical suspicion, angiogram (typically mesenteric: 'corkscrewing'), biopsy (sural nerve or skin: medium-vessel vasculitis)
  - Tx: steroids, cyclophosphamide; Five-year survival 50–75%, most patients are extremely ill and need aggressive therapy
- Acute Polyarthritis-Dermatitis Syndrome: acute, severe, symmetric, involving both large and small joints, urticarial rash is usually present
  - MOA: due to deposition of circulating immune complexes; Improves with NSAIDs and resolved with onset of jaundice
- Cryoglobulinemia: most associated with hepatitis C, only 5% of essential mixed cryoglobulinemia is due to hepatitis B
■ Membranous Glomerulonephritis: nephrotic range proteinuria, worse prognosis in men

PROGNOSIS:
- Risk of hepatocellular carcinoma (HCC): 10–390 × increase risk even without cirrhosis (highest: perinatal acquired and HBeAg+/↑ viral load)
  All Hepatitis B patients get screening (even without cirrhosis)
  - Screen with serum AFP & hepatic U/S every 6 months

4.15 HEPATITIS C

(Gastro 2006;130:225-30 & 231-64. Hepatology 2004;39:1147-71. Hepatology 2002;36:S3-20)

DEFINITION:
- A hepatotrophic virus; the liver is the primary site of infection, replication and cellular damage
- Chronic hepatitis: presence of clinical, biochemical, and serologic abnormalities for up to 6 months

EPIDEMIOLOGY:
- Blood transfusion before 1985: 1/20 (5%) got HCV; After 1990: 1/200,000 (.0005%) got HCV! Has been and remains a very low risk
- The number of new cases of HCV has decreased dramatically over the last 10 years
- Acute Hepatitis C leads to: Chronicity of HCV 70-85%, Recovery of HCV 15-30% (HCV is a chronic disease)

ETIOLOGIES:
- Transmission: percutaneous >>> sexual; ~20% without a clear precipitant
  - Needle stick risk: HBV > HCV > HIV
- Incubation: 1-4 months
- Pregnant women/Vertical Transmission/Breastfeeding: No prophylaxis/vaccine available; *See also Liver- Pregnancy Pearls (Chapter 4.25)*
  - Generally don't treat, low risk of vertical transmission (5%); HIV co-infection or viral load >2 million (can be 50% transmission)
  - According to CDC, breastfeeding is not contraindicated; No transmission via breastfeeding has been documented

PATHOPHYSIOLOGY:
- Virus: RNA, linear gene shape, envelope, 50 nm in size; Several genotypes identified, most common: 1-3

CLINICAL MANIFESTATIONS/PHYSICAL EXAM:
- Natural History: anorexia, nausea, vomiting, fatigue, abdominal pain, mild fever; jaundice is much less common compared to HAV/HBV
  - Acute HCV leads to: 75% being subclinical and 25% leading to jaundice; 15-30% lead to full recovery
    Fulminant HCV hepatitis very rare (i.e. rarely do you come across and treat acute Hep C)
  - Chronic HCV leads to: 70-85% continuing to be chronic, 20-30% of whom develop cirrhosis (after ~20 yrs)
    i.e. Most will not develop cirrhosis, ? who is at risk-suggestions are: ♂, ETOH use, steatosis, coinfection with HBV or HIV
  - Chronic: hepatocellular carcinoma develops in 2-5% of HCV cirrhotics/year (usually after 20-30 yrs)
- **Extra-hepatic** (38% have at least one extra-hepatic symptom): cryoglobulinemia, porphyria cutanea tarda (PCT), MPGN, lymphoma, aplastic anemia

LABORATORY STUDIES:
- Transaminitis (↑ ALT/AST); *See also Liver- LFTs (Chapter 4.20)*
- Serologic (ELISA/RIBA) & Virologic (HCV RNA/Genotypes): 4 antigens on HCV virus, body makes antibodies to all 4

  - **anti-HCV (ELISA):** + in 6weeks; The antibody does *not* imply recovery; May become negative (~10%) after recovery
    Some skip ELISA and get Qualitative as first test
    Positive (6 wks) = acute infection OR **resolving infection** OR **false positive**
    Need to confirm positive anti-HCV (ELISA) with HCV Qualitative

  - **HCV RIBA:** used to confirm +anti-HCV ELISA with −HCV Qualitative RNA
    Need at least 2 of 4 antibodies for HCV to be positive, ↑ specificity compared to ELISA for antibodies
    RIBA is generally not used anymore due to Qualitative/Quantitative tests that have largely replaced it
    Positive = infection (ELISA +, but Qualitative doesn't detect, i.e. <50 IU/ml) OR **remote/resolved infection**
    Negative = false positive anti-HCV

- **HCV *Qualitative* RNA (PCR):** ↑ sensitivity, gives a yes/no answer, detection is as low as 50 IU/ml
  Positive (2 wks) = **Marker of active infection**
  Always order with HIV (immunodeficient patients) and hemodialysis patients (they don't make antibodies, don't depend on ELISA)

- **HCV *Quantitative* RNA (PCR) "Viral load":** gives a numerical answer, detection range 600 IU/ml–800,000 IU/ml
  Used only for guiding therapy; if not going to treat then no point ordering; >800,000 IU/ml: high; <800,000 IU/ml: low

- **Genotype (1–6):** Type 1 is 70% of U.S. infections

■ Biopsy: degree of inflammation (grade) & amount of fibrosis (stage); No other test makes this determination accurately
  - Stages (Fibrosis): 1. portal fibrosis, 2. periportal fibrosis, 3. septal fibrosis, 4. cirrhosis
  - Grade (Inflammation): 1. minimal lobular, 2. mild portal, 3. moderate piecemeal necrosis, 4. severe portal with piecemeal necrosis

DIAGNOSTIC STUDIES:
■ See Laboratory Studies above

TREATMENTS:
■ Acute HCV: supportive; No vaccine available

■ Treat if ↑ ALT & active inflammation and fibrosis (stages 2 and 3) on biopsy
  Goal of treatment: achieve SVR
   ? who progresses to cirrhosis, so all should at least be evaluated for treatment

■ What to treat with: why and how
Pretreatment labs: HCV RNA & genotype, Albumin/Bili/PT, Iron studies, ANA/ASMA, α1-AT, Ceruloplasmin, HBsAg, HIV, Liver Biopsy; Overview:

- IFN-a-2b » ~20% sustained response rate
- IFN & Ribavirin » ~44% sustained response rate (non-PEG interferons are not used now)
- PEG-INF-α-2a » 29% sustained response rate (PEG adds polyethylene glycol moiety, resulting ↑ $T_{1/2}$, ↑ potency, ↓ side effects)
- **PEG-INF-α-2a & Ribavirin** » ~56% sustained response rate (~90% SVR if treated in acute phase)

  - **Genotype 2 & 3:** (PEG/Ribavirin) 16–24 wk (4–6 month) therapy
    Note: Genotype 2 & 3: In reality, some don't check RVR/EVR and just treat for 24 weeks (since >80% will achieve SVR)

  - **Genotype 1:** (PEG/Ribavirin) 48 wk (12 month) therapy if EVR
    Note: Genotype 1: 1st wk: begin therapy; 4 wk: RVR?; 12 wk: EVR?; 24 wk: repeat viral load; 48 wk: EOT?; 72 wk: SVR or Relapse?

    RVR [Rapid viral response]: at 4 weeks of therapy: ≥2 log drop in viral load; >90% go on to SVR; Continue Rx regardless
    EVR [Early viral response]: at 12 weeks of therapy: ≥2 log drop in viral load; If no EVR stop therapy as they will not respond
    EOT [End-of-Treatment Response]: virus undetectable at completion of therapy
    SVR [Sustained viral response]: viral detection remains negative for 6 months after therapy completed
    Relapsers: negative during therapy (i.e. EVR at 12 weeks), but become viremic after stopping therapy
    Non-Responders: did not respond, or didn't have a chance to respond (i.e. medication side effects, non-compliance)

- **Medication Dosage/Side Effect Specifics:**
  PEG-INF-α-2a (Pegasys): Standard dosing for all: 180 mcg sq given on same day once per week
  PEG-INF-α-2b (Peg-Intron): Weight-based dosing: 1.5 mcg/kg sq given on same day once per week
  Ribavirin: <75 Kg: 1000 mg/day po (400 am/600 pm)
  >75 Kg: 1200 mg/day po (600 am/600 pm)

  Side effects: *Anemia/Neutropenia* (cause of most dose reductions); decompensated patients should not be treated
  INF: Flu-like symptoms (often 2nd day post shot), BM suppression, **Depression**/Mania/Confusion/Irritability, Insomnia
  RBV: Teratogenic (must agree to contraception for therapy & 6 months post therapy), **Hemolysis/anemia,** Rash, Bronchospasm
  Other: May need procrit/epogen, Thyroid abnormalities may be permanent in 5%, No effect with ETOH use (patients must stop drinking)!

  Contraindications: Most important is decompensated cirrhosis
  Others: BM suppression (low platelets), Mental illness, Alcohol use, Autoimmune disease, Pregnancy, Advanced co-morbid conditions

- **Consensus Interferon (Infergen):** Used for non-responders to PEG-INF therapy; ↑ BM suppression; ? 40% response rate
  15 mcg/day given 3 or 7 days/week (Not FDA approved for 7 days/week)

- **Liver Transplant** » 100% reinfection rate; some with rapidly progressive disease; See Post-Transplant Issues below

■ Positive predictors of response:
  - Viral genotype other than 1 (for genotypes 2 & 3, sustained response rates with PEG-INF-α-2a & Ribavirin are ~80%)
  - HCV RNA <2 million copies, absence of cirrhosis/fibrosis, female gender, age <40 yrs
■ Negative predictors of response:
  - Genotype 1, ↑ viral load, African American, Cirrhosis (or advanced fibrosis), Intolerability of meds, Obesity (BMI >30), ETOH use
■ Vaccines for HCV do not exist: It is problematic to design because of the multiple viral genotypes
  - Vaccines for HAV and HBV should be given

COMPLICATIONS:
■ Can lead to chronic infection, more likely to be associated with developing cirrhosis as noted above under Clinical Manifestations
■ Increased risk of primary hepatocellular carcinoma and cholangiocarcinoma; **Most get cirrhosis before HCC** (unlike Hepatitis B) (Hepatology 2005;42:1208–36)
■ Rheumatological Manifestations
  - Cryoglobulinemia: 10–60% of HCV patients
    - Immunoglobulins that precipitate at cold temps as they flow through vessels: small vessel vasculitis (leukocytoclastic vasculitis)
    - Symptoms: fever, arthritis, renal disease (MPGN), paresthesias, petechial rash/palp purpura, HSM, lymphadenopathy, Raynaud's
    - Labs: ↑ RF, ↓ C3/4, + cryoglobulins; Hepatitis is not a predominant feature
    - Treat with PEG/INF, if failure, pheresis/steroids; Cryoglubulins improve with treatment of HCV
  - Nonerosive Polyarthritis: 5–10% of HCV patients; intermittent, mono- or oligoarthritis affecting large and medium joints
  - Autoantibody production: RF, ANA, Anticardiolipin antibody, ASMA, Antithyroid, Anti-LKM1 (seen in children with Type II AIH)
  - Porphyria Cutanea Tarda (blister formation/scarring): metabolic disorder, ↓ hepatic activity of uroporphyrinogen decarboxylase (phlebotomy)
■ Membranoproliferative Glomerulonephritis: nephrotic range proteinuria, worse prognosis in men

CHAPTER 4.15 HEPATITIS C

PROGNOSIS:
- Risk of hepatocellular carcinoma (HCC) with chronicity develops in 2–5% of cirrhotics/year (usually after 20–30 yrs)
  - Screening ultrasound and AFP every 6 months
- The risk of relapse after successful treatment is low (<5%); should still recheck HCV-RNA a year after completed therapy
  - Still need screening for HCC if they were cirrhotic, for how long to keep screening is currently not known (i.e. 5 years?)
- If co-infected: With HIV, start HAART first, then HCV treatment; With HBV coinfection, treat for HCV (HBV is usually quiescent)
  - If CD4 count >500 can treat HCV first

POST-TRANSPLANT ISSUES:
- Should we treat HCV while waiting for re-transplant? MELD ≤18 should be considered for treatment (especially with non type-1 genotype)
  - However, must be administered via experienced clinicians at tertiary care center
- How to treat recurrent HCV in transplanted patient (Occurs in 100% of OLT)? Goal: eradicate HCV and prevent liver disease progression
  - No standard approach and no universally accepted treatment
  - Two approaches: Pre-emptive and Histologically confirmed recurrence: generally the latter is more tolerated
  - Therapy: PEG-INF/Ribavirin: average SVR 23%; This suboptimal response rate is currently undergoing trials
- Is re-transplant an option? Difficult clinical dilemma; Not contraindicated, but poorer outcome; No accepted criteria for selection
  - Lower 1-yr survival (60%) and even worse with high bili, INR, Cr; Four-times higher cost of transplant

4.16 HEPATOBILIARY CYSTIC DISEASE

BILE DUCT CYSTS: major classes and subtypes
- **Ia:** choledochal cyst
- **Ib:** segmental choledochal dilation
- **Ic:** diffuse or cylindrical duct dilation
  - **II:** extrahepatic duct diverticula
- **III:** choledochocele
  - **IVa:** multiple intra- and extrahepatic duct cysts
  - **IVb:** multiple extrahepatic duct cysts
- **V:** intrahepatic duct cysts

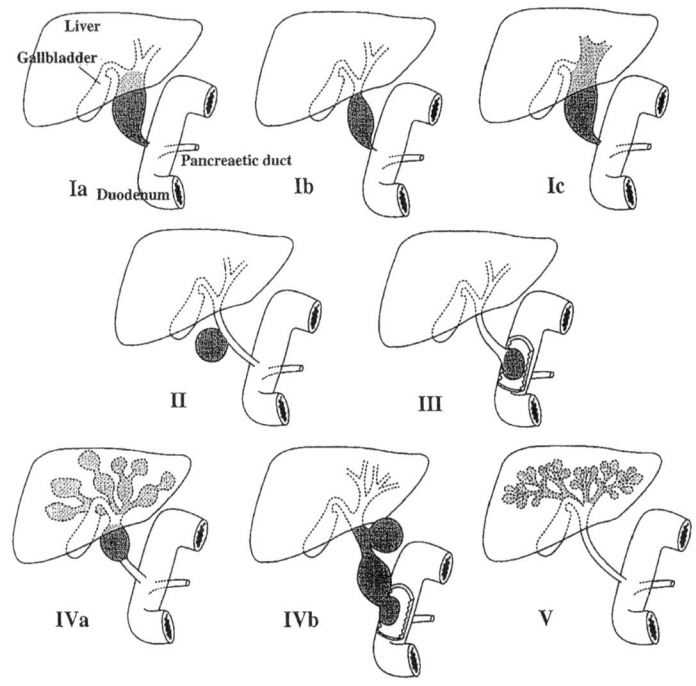

Reprinted with permission from McNally P. GI/Liver Secrets. 3rd ed. New York: Elsevier/Mosby, 2006:310.

- Female predominance
- Most bile duct cysts are diagnosed in childhood via U/S; Incidence of cancer with bile duct cysts is 2-15% **(i.e. not a benign process!)**
- Triad of abdominal pain, jaundice, and abdominal mass; Typically, only one or two present at any one time; Fever is common
- Cholangiopancreatography: percutaneously, endoscopically, interoperatively: critical for planning excision
  - Caution with Caroli's due to increased risk of recurrent cholangitis and sepsis
  - MRCP may be the preferred imaging modality, but most found via U/S
- Preferred treatment is complete surgical resection of the cyst, rather than internal drainage
  - Complications 8%: stricture, recurrent jaundice, cholangitis; Corresponding complications with internal drainage: 50%
  - Risk of bile duct cancer is reduced, but not eliminated with surgery (i.e. can develop in other parts of biliary tree)
  - Recurrent symptoms may be candidates for transplant if no evidence of cholangiocarcinoma

CHAPTER 4.16 HEPATOBILIARY CYSTIC DISEASE

CAROLI'S: congenital dilations of intrahepatic bile ducts; Usually symptomatic as children with abdominal pain and HSM
- Caroli's Disease: have cystic dilations limited to the larger intrahepatic bile ducts, predisposing to recurrent calculi and cholangitis
- Caroli's Syndrome: cystic dilations along portal tract, believed to result from a ductal plate malformation that affects bile ducts at all levels
  - More common, autosomal recessive. Also called Caroli's Disease Type 2
  - Associated with congenital hepatic fibrosis, hence patients have portal hypertension: splenomegaly, varices

POLYCYSTIC LIVER DISEASE (PLD): characterized by numerous cysts scattered throughout the liver parenchyma
- Most commonly associated with autosomal dominant polycystic kidney disease (ADPKD); Can rarely occur as autosomal recessive
- Presence and severity of PLD with ADPKD ↑ with age, female gender, number/frequency of pregnancies, severe renal disease
- Common complications include mass effect and cyst infection; Suspicion for infection should prompt CT or U/S guided FNA
- Hepatic function usually not affected by liver cyst; If no complications, AST/ALT, Bili, Aφ typically within normal range
- Treatment of symptomatic cysts percutaneously or surgically
  - Sclerosing agent decreases recurrence (used only if no communication with biliary system or peritoneal cavity)
  - Infected cysts require both antibiotics and surgical intervention
  - Transplant for massive polycystic hepatomegaly ± combined liver/kidney transplant

SIMPLE HEPATIC CYSTS: often called solitary hepatic cysts, are benign fluid collections usually surrounded by a thin columnar epithelium
- Frequently noted as incidental finding on U/S or CT; Not associated with cystic diseases in other organs, no genetic transmission
  - Diagnosed with U/S: smooth margin with surrounding parenchyma, no appreciable wall, no internal echoes
    - CT appears as thin-walled lesion that does not enhance with IV contrast (density of water)
    - MRI appears homogeneous, very low-intensity on T1 scans and discrete high-intensity lesion on T2 scans
  - Most are asymptomatic; Treatment if symptoms develop: abdominal pain, increasing abdominal girth, obstructive jaundice

HYDATID CYST DISEASE: *Echinococcus granulosus* is a small tapeworm and the culprit
- Adult worm is 2–8 mm long, has a bulbous scolex with four suckers and hooklets
  - Lives in intestinal lumen of definitive host (dog, fox), eggs discharged in feces
  - Ingested via contaminated food/water with intermediate host (rabbit or sheep)
  - Humans usually infected as intermediate hosts when ingesting egg-contaminated food or water
    - Found throughout world, including Alaska, Canada, Western U.S.
    - Common in sheep and cattle raising areas where dogs assist in herding
- Cysts grow at a rate of 1–5 cm/year; Many unsuspectingly harbor the infection until they present with palpable abdominal mass
- Symptoms related to mass effect of the enlarging cyst:
  - Abdominal pain from hepatic capsule stretching, jaundice from bile duct compression, portal vein obstruction
  - 20% have cysts that communicate with biliary tree and have symptoms similar to those of choledocholithiasis
  - Leakage into peritoneal cavity can cause intense antigenic response, resulting in eosinophilia, bronchospasm, shock
- Diagnosed with CT: sharply defined, low density lesion with spoke-like septations; Calcified rim of daughter cysts
  - U/S: appears as complex mass with multiple internal echoes from debris and septations
  - ELISA for echinococcal antibodies are positive in 85–90% of patients
- Open surgical drainage is the preferred method of therapy
  - Albendazole with percutaneous drainage and hypertonic saline irrigation of cysts is as effective with fewer complications

4.17 HEPATOCELLULAR CARCINOMA

(Hepatology. 2005;42:1208-29)

DEFINITION:
- Hepatocellular carcinoma (HCC) or Hepatoma is a primary (as opposed to metastases) tumor of the liver

EPIDEMIOLOGY:
- Mortality: 4th most common cause of world cancer deaths (400,000-1 million) annually; Incidence remains on the rise worldwide: 3 per 100,000
- ♂ > ♀ (2-6 times more men affected); Mean age at presentation is 50-60 years with most being older than 55
- Approximately 80% of patients with HCC have cirrhosis

ETIOLOGIES:
- Can be seen in any chronic liver disease, but most often seen with:
  - Chronic hepatitis C (probably the most common); Chronic Hepatitis B; Hemochromatosis; α1-AT; Alcoholic cirrhosis
  - Environmental toxin exposure (i.e. alflatoxin)
  - Cirrhosis of any cause!

PATHOPHYSIOLOGY:
- Presenting forms: Nodular: most common, multiple nodules of varying size scattered throughout liver
  Solitary: occurs in younger patients; large, solitary mass, often right lobe
  Diffuse: rare; difficult to detect on imaging; widespread infiltration of minute tumor foci
- **Fibrolamellar carcinoma** (represents 7% of HCC): occurs in young people (mean age 26), ♂ = ♀, seldom have history of prior liver disease
  - Usually presents with abdominal pain due to large mass, most often left lobe (75%); AFP is normal
  - Histology includes deeply eosinophilic malignant cells interspersed between laminated strands of collagen
  - Imaging studies show fibrous central scar from bleed/necrosis; MRI T2 demonstrates hypointense (don't confuse with FNH)
  - Recognition is key as 50-80% are resectable at diagnosis; Liver transplant may be indication if not resectable

CLINICAL MANIFESTATIONS/PHYSICAL EXAM:
- Usually have no symptoms or may be manifestations of chronic liver disease
  - Rare: abdominal pain, early satiety, weight loss, jaundice, paraneoplastic syndromes, fever
  - In previously compensated cirrhotics, the development of decompensation should raise suspicion of HCC!
- Physical exam usually reflects the underlying liver disease:
  - Hepatomegaly/splenomegaly, ascites, jaundice; Less common: fever, palpable liver mass, hepatic bruit

LABORATORY STUDIES:
- Alpha-Fetoprotein (AFP) in a patient with chronic liver disease should raise concern that HCC has developed
  - Levels >500 ng/ml (normal 10-20) in a high risk patient is generally accepted to be diagnostic and further workup not required
    - AFP >200 ng/ml highly suggestive of HCC, less elevations may be 2° to chronic hepatitis; normalize with effective treatment
  - AFP is a glycoprotein normally produced during gestation via the fetal liver and yolk sac
  - Also elevated in pregnancy, tumors of gonadal origin, or in patients with acute/chronic liver disease without HCC
  - Limitations: usually normal in majority of patients with Fibrolamellar Carcinoma (as noted above is a variant of HCC) and 40% of small HCCs (<2 cm)

- Routine labs:
  - Sudden ↑ Aφ, Increase AST/ALT ratio; Paraneoplastic: hypoglycemia, hypercalcemia
- Ascites:
  - Cytology: 58–75% sensitive; Bloody ascites (>20K RBCs/ml) is found in 20% of patients

DIAGNOSTIC STUDIES:
- Ultrasound: poorly defined margins; irregular internal echoes; may be hypoechoic, isoechoic or hyperechoic
  - Advantages: widely available, noninvasive, assess vascular involvement at same time, sensitivity 65–80% and specific >90%
  - Disadvantages: operator dependent, visualization might be difficult: obese patients, overlying bowel gas
- CT scan with triple phase (i.e. scans taken before, during and after contrast bolus)
  - Advantages: sensitivity may be as high as 90%, improved detection of small lesions
  - Disadvantages: expensive, not widely available, requires IV contrast, can be difficult to distinguish regenerative nodules from HCC
- MRI: helpful in those who cannot have contrast; Helps distinguish HCC (T1:hypointense/T2:hyperintense) from regenerative nodule (opposite)
- Angiography: largely replaced by noninvasive techniques for diagnosis (HCC typically supplied by hepatic artery, not portal vein)
- Others: Technetium-99 m AFP imaging and PET scan; Neither are currently widely available
- Biopsy: Not all require biopsy, but helpful if diagnosis is uncertain; U/S or CT guided; Core biopsy better than FNA; Bleed risk ↑: 1.6–5%

  Mass on surveillance ultrasound in cirrhotic liver:
  Size <1 cm » Repeat U/S in 3–4 months:
  Stable over 18–24 months » Return to standard surveillance protocol (6–12 monthly)
  Enlarging » Proceed according to lesion size

  Size 1-2 cm » Two dynamic imaging studies:
  Coincidental typical vascular pattern on dynamic imaging » Treat as HCC
  Typical vascular pattern with one technique » Biopsy (see below)
  Atypical vascular pattern with both techniques » Biopsy (see below)

  Size >2 cm » One dynamic imaging technique:
  Atypical vascular pattern » Biopsy (see below)
  Typical vascular pattern on dynamic imaging or AFP >200 ng/ml » Treat as HCC

  The Biopsy:
  Diagnostic of HCC » Treat as HCC
  Other diagnosis » Treat accordingly
  Non-diagnostic » Repeat biopsy or imaging follow-up » Change in size/profile »
  Positive: Treat as HCC
  Negative: Repeat biopsy/imaging

- Staging: No system universally adopted
  - Several systems: TNM, Okuda, Barcelona-Clinic-Liver-Cancer (BCLC), Cancer of the Liver Italian Program (CLIP)
  Four features uniformly recognized as important:
  - Performance status, Severity of underlying disease, Size of tumor, Vascular invasion, Presence of metastases

SECTION IV LIVER

TREATMENTS:
- Surgery: only chance for cure; TACE > RFA for palliation or bridge to surgery

  Surgery:
  - Partial hepatectomy: candidates: solitary tumor amenable to resection, preserved liver function, no evidence of portal hypertension
    HVWPG <10 mmHg (portal hypertension can complicate surgery, but not an absolute contraindication)
    - Non-cirrhotic: up to 2/3 of liver can be removed; Cirrhotic: up to 1/4 of the liver can be removed
    - Outcome: Mortality variable and liver failure is leading cause, especially with cirrhotics
      Appropriate selection of patients and experienced surgeon are the keys; Five year survival as high as 70%

  - Orthotopic Liver Transplantaion (OLT)
    - Can cure both cirrhosis and HCC in same operation
    - Milan criteria (represents acceptable to transplant): 1 tumor <5 cm; 2 or 3 tumors <3 cm; No evidence of metastases
    - Milan criteria automatically raise MELD to 22 points; Preoperative therapies may be considered if waiting time >6 months
    - Outcome: Five year survival as high as 70% (Similar to partial hepatectomy, slightly worse than OLT for non-HCC)
      Yet to be determined: use of RFA/TACE prior to OLT or Living donor transplant

  Non-Surgery
  - Transarterial Chemoembolization (TACE): Injection of chemotherapeutic and embolic agents directly via the hepatic artery
    - Candidates: large or multifocal tumor not amenable to other treatments, patent portal vein, well-preserved liver function
    - Neither the optimal chemotherapeutic agent or embolization method has been established
    - Outcome: Primary treatment for unresectable tumors or prior to OLT
      Met-analysis has showed improved survival benefit
    - Complications: Hepatic decompensation (20%), Hepatic abscess or cholecystitis (14%)

  - Radiofrequency Ablation (RFA): Radiofrequency thermal energy applied directly to the HCC lesion
    - Candidates: Limited disease, well-preserved liver function; Performed percutaneously, laparoscopically, or via laparotomy
    - Outcome: Safe/effective means of disease control for those who cannot undergo therapy, recurrent disease, prior to OLT
      No survival benefit ever proven; Jury still out as large RCTs needed and role will be better delineated in future

  - Percutaneous Ethanol Injection (PEI): Injection of 95% ethanol directly into tumor
    - Similar effectiveness to RFA for tumors <2 cm, but RFA superior for tumors >2 cm

  Other:
  - Radiotherapy: High recurrence rates, may worsen liver function
  - Chemotherapy: Not recommended
  - Hormonal therapy (Tamoxifen, Anti-androgens): Not recommended

PROGNOSIS:
- Untreated the 5 year survival is less than 5%; Average survival is 10 months; In appropriate patients treatment drastically alters survival
- Screening for HCC: No survival advantage ever proven, unclear if cost effective; AASLD still recommends screening:
  - High-risk patients to screen:
    - Asian men >40 yrs or women >50 yrs with HBV (even without cirrhosis)
    - Hemochromatosis or ETOH *with* cirrhosis
    - Any patients with cirrhosis: Hemochromatosis or ETOH or HCV or HBV (even if treated)
    - Family history of HCC
    - Candidates for treatment of HCC
  - Strategy: Serial AFP and hepatic U/S every 6–12 months
  - AFP alone shouldn't be used for screening unless U/S not available

NOTES

4.18 HEPATORENAL SYNDROME

(Am J Gastroenterol. 2005;100:460-67)

DEFINITION:
- Renal failure (progressive azotemia) in patients with cirrhosis, liver failure, and portal hypertension

EPIDEMIOLOGY:
- 10% of hospitalized patients with cirrhosis and ascites
- 20% at 1 year, 40% at 5 years in patients with cirrhosis and ascites

ETIOLOGIES:
- Precipitants: GI Bleed, Overdiuresis, Paracentesis, Nephrotoxic drugs: aminoglycosides/NSAIDs
- Type 1 (see below) may be associated with SBP, Acute alcohol hepatitis, LVP without albumin expansion, GI bleed

PATHOPHYSIOLOGY:
- Hallmark is severe vasoconstriction of the renal circulation
- MOA progression and *[Treatment interventions at each stage]*:
    Cirrhosis *[OLT]* » Portal HTN » Splanchnic arterial vasodilation (mainly nitric oxide) *[Midodrine/Terlipressin]* » Arterial underfilling (↓ effective volume) *[Albumin]* » Stimulation systemic vasoconstrictors (Renin-angiotensinogen-aldosterone RAAS, Sympathetic nervous system SNS, Endothelin) *[TIPS]* » Renal vasoconstriction *[Avoid NSAIDs]* »
        Early stages of Cirrhosis » ↑ systemic and local vasodilators with preserved renal perfusion
        Late stages of Cirrhosis » ↓ in local vasodilators (overwhelmed) with increased local vasoconstrictors » HRS
    In other words, a vicious cycle ensues: hypoperfusion leads to more imbalance in intrarenal vasoactive systems, i.e. vasoconstrictors

CLINICAL MANIFESTATIONS/PHYSICAL EXAM:
- No specific clinical findings, most have features of advanced liver disease such as refractory ascites
- Low arterial blood pressure, reduced systemic vascular resistance, tachycardia, and increased cardiac output

LABORATORY STUDIES:
- No correlation with LFTs (bilirubin, albumin, PT) or Child-Pugh classification
- Severe **oliguria** (<500 ml/24 hrs) even with volume challenge
- Intense Na retention (**urine sodium <10 meq/L**), Dilutional **Na (serum sodium <130 meq/L)**, FENA <1
- Note: creatinine in HRS usually lower than values in non-liver patients due to reduced muscle mass and lower production of creatinine
- **Type 1:** *rapid* and progressive impairment of renal function within 2 weeks as defined by either:
    Doubling of initial serum creatinine to a level higher than 2.5 mg/dl OR
    50% reduction of the initial 24 hr creatinine clearance to a level lower than 20 ml/min
- **Type 2:** Impairment of renal function (creatinine >1.5 mg/dl) that does not meet the criteria of Type 1

DIAGNOSTIC STUDIES:
- Diagnosis of exclusion, depends mainly on level of creatinine
- Rule out other causes of ARF: Prerenal, Hypokalemia, ATN, Nephrotoxic drugs/dye, AGN in patients with Hep B/C
    Prerenal patients have improved renal function with IVF (i.e. NS 1500 cc ± albumin)
    Shock before ARF precluded HRS, likewise, HRS should only be diagnosed if ARF persists after complete resolution of an infection
    Proteinuria and ultrasound abnormalities indicate organic renal disease or obstructive uropathy
- **Diagnostic Criteria of HRS** (only Major criteria used for diagnosis)
    Major: -Low GFR (serum creatinine >1.5 mg/dl without diuretics) **Minor:** -U vol <500 ml/day
    -Exclude shock, infection, volume depletion, toxic drugs   -U Na <10 mEq/L
    -No improvement with stopping diuretics and NS infusion   -U Osm > Plasma Osm
    -No Proteinuria or U/S evidence of disease   -U RBCs <50/high-powered field
                                                                     -Serum Na <130 mEq/L

CHAPTER 4.18 HEPATORENAL SYNDROME

TREATMENTS:
- Low salt diets, Fluid restrict to 1 L/day, Avoid NSAIDs, Tap to rule out SBP, Stop diuretics, Assess for candidacy of liver transplantation
- **Vasoconstrictors:** Goal is to reduce serum creatinine below 1.5 mg/dl, Avoid in patients with CAD, PVD, CVA; Duration: 1–2 wks
  Terlipressin 0.5 mg IV q 4 hr; Can increase dose q 2–3 days to 1 mg IV q 4 hr, then 2 mg IV q 4 hr if no initial response (i.e. no drop in Cr)
  Midodrine 2.5–7.5 mg po TID (increase to 12.5 po TID PRN) *AND* Octreotide 100 mcg SQ TID (increase to 200 mcg TID PRN)
  Noradrenaline 0.5–3 mg/h continuous gtt
- Consider on all patients: Albumin gtt 1 g/kg on day 1, then 20–50 g/day
  Albumin 5% [plasma isotonicity] 1 liter = 50 grams; Albumin 25% [concentrated] 100 cc = 25 grams
- **TIPS:** ↓ portal pressure & ↑ return splanchnic blood to systemic, ↓ rennin-angiotensin-aldosterone, ↓ vasoconstrictor effect on kidneys
- **OLT:** Best treatment for suitable candidates: Cures diseased liver and circulatory/renal dysfunction
- **Dialysis:** Not routinely recommended, ineffective due to high side effects; Reasonable option as bridge to transplant in some patients
  - Future: ? extracorporeal albumin dialysis: enables the selective removal of albumin bound substances

PROGNOSIS:
- Worst prognosis of all complications of cirrhosis: without treatment median survival of Type 1 is <2 wks
- Main consequence of Type 2 HRS is diuretic-resistant ascites, but survival is longer than Type 1; Type 2 median survival is 6 months
- **Prevention** in two clinical settings:
  - SBP dx: give albumin with antibiotics (1.5 g/kg at dx and 1 g/kg 48 hr later): prevents circulatory dysfunction (Incidence 10%, vs 33% with no albumin)
  - Acute ETOH hepatitis dx: give Pentoxifylline (400 mg po TID × 28 days): TNF inhibitor (Reduces HRS/mortality 8% and 24%)

4.19 HISTOPATHOLOGY OF LIVER

LIVER MICROANATOMY AND INJURY PATTERNS
- Liver has three functional components: hepatocytes, central veins/sinusoids, portal tracts (triads)
  Basic architecture: cords of hepatocytes (one cell thick), separated by vascular sinusoids
  The sinusoids are lined with endothelial cells (E) and Kupffer cells (which have Mϕ capabilities)
  Central veins (aka, terminal hepatic venules, Hv) collect blood after it percolates through sinusoids and carry it back to larger hepatic veins (Hv)
  Distributed at regular intervals are portal tracts (bile ducts-Bd, hepatic arteries-Ha, portal veins-Pv)
  The row of hepatocytes immediately adjacent to portal tract is termed 'limiting plate'

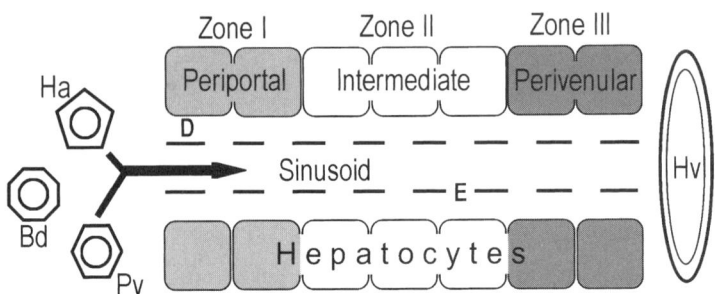

Modified with permission from McNally P. GI/Liver Secrets. 3rd ed. New York: Elsevier/Mosby, 2006:237.

- Functional unit of the liver is represented by Hepatic Acini: 3D units built around a central axis containing a portal tract and its blood vessels
  From the portal area, plates of hepatocytes radiate outward toward central veins, located at the periphery of the acinus
  The acinus is divided into three zones: 1 is closest to portal tracts, 3 is closest to the central vein; Zone 1 is best supplied by oxygen and nutrients

- Bridging fibrosis: portal tracts & central veins connected by scar tissue
- **Cirrhosis:** diffuse scarring altering the architecture into nodules of hepatocytes (must be diffuse by definition, not just focal nodular formation)
  - Micronodular: nodules ≤3 mm, most common with alcohol
  - Macronodular: nodules >3 mm, most common with viral hepatitis

- **Types of liver cell injury:**

Types of liver cell injury:	Causes:
Fatty change (Steatosis)	Ethanol, Obesity, Diabetes, Drugs
Councilman bodies (Acidophilic bodies)	Viral hepatitis, Drugs, Nonspecific reactions; Represents apoptosis
Mallory Hyaline	Ethanol, Obesity, Diabetes, Drugs, Wilson's, Biliary tract disease, Hepatocellular carcinoma
Hydropic change (Ballooning)	Viral hepatitis, Drugs, Cholestasis
Cholestasis	Duct obstruction or injury, Drugs, Viral hepatitis
Interlobular duct injury	PBC, PSC, Hepatitis C
Piecemeal necrosis	Viral hepatitis, PBC, Drugs, Wilson's disease
Increased iron stores	Hemochromatosis, Transfusions, Hemolysis
Granulomas	Tuberculosis, Sarcoid, Fungi, Drugs (complete list below); I.e. think infection, drug, sarcoid
"Reverse cirrhosis"	Central vein to central vein (not portal triad to portal triad), seen with cirrhosis 2° to Heart Failure

- *See also Liver- Drug Induced Liver Disease (Chapter 4.11)*

CHAPTER 4.19 HISTOPATHOLOGY OF LIVER

FATTY CHANGE AND STEATOHEPATITIS
- **Alcohol Liver Disease** can result in fatty liver, alcoholic hepatitis and alcoholic cirrhosis
  - Hepatocytes contain globules of fat, usually larger than & compressing the hepatocyte nucleus (referred to as **Macrovesicular** steatosis)
    - Initially the change is around the central veins, but may extend to involve the entire acinus
  - Biopsies of alcoholic hepatitis may show hepatocytes that are swollen with areas of necrosis, associated with inflammation (PMNs)
  - Hepatocytes may also contain **Mallory hyaline:** (also found in other causes of liver injury, as noted above)
    - Irregular ropelike strings of eosinophilic material in cytoplasm representing aggregates of microfilament cytokeratin
  - Although fat and neutrophils can resolve relatively quickly after alcohol abstinence, hyaline can take up to 6 weeks to disappear
  - Progression: initial scarring around central veins with spider web-like fibrosis long sinusoids; eventually bridging fibrosis connects central veins and portal tracts and adjacent portal tracts; When cirrhosis fully develops, most of the native central veins are obliterated
  - Alcoholic cirrhosis is Micronodular because scarring is relatively uniform throughout liver
  - If you get a biopsy report that says: 'alcoholic hepatitis': Caution! Better term is steatohepatitis, over 20 conditions can show hyaline with fatty change:
    - Obesity, Diabetes, Drugs/Vit A toxicity, Wilson's, Prolonged cholestasis (PBC), Jejunal-ileal bypass/gastric stapling
    - Most common are obesity and DM; those <40 consider Wilson's; Isolated Periportal Zone (1) consider PBC, Drugs/Toxins
- **Non-Alcoholic fatty liver disease (NAFLD)** *See also Liver- NAFLD (Chapter 4.22)*
- **Microvesicular steatosis:** AFLP, Meds (valproic acid, tetracycline), Reye's syndrome, Jamaican vomiting sickness, Mitochondrial disorders

VIRAL HEPATITIS
- Those with viral hepatitis, a biopsy can help assess amount of inflammation (grade), degree of irreversible fibrosis/cirrhosis (stage) and chronicity
- HAV: rarely need biopsy 2° rarely causing chronic liver disease; may help distinguish severe cholestasis in HAV from large duct obstruction
  - Acute hepatitis has predominantly parenchymal inflammation
- HBV/HCV: can cause chronic liver disease ± acute/fulminant disease; the histological features can help determine both treatment and prognosis
  - Chronic hepatitis (of any cause): a necroinflammatory process in which hepatocytes are preferentially injured compared with bile ducts
    - Associated with varying degrees of portal and periportal inflammation, parenchymal hepatitis, and fibrosis
    - The inflammation is usually in the form of lymphocytes, plasma cells, and PMNs
      - Once these cells cross limiting plate, there is hepatocyte damage, piecemeal necrosis, and lobular inflammation
      - Lobular inflammation is associated with hepatocellular necrosis (Acidophilic or Councilman bodies)
    - With time, chronic hepatitis leads to progressive fibrosis, and without treatment, cirrhosis
      - Fibrosis begins in portal areas, extends to periportal areas and begins bridging to other portal tracts & central veins
  - Specifics HBV: **'ground-glass,'** reflects accumulation of HBsAg within the endoplasmic reticulum of hepatocytes
    HCV: 'lymphoid aggregates within portal tracts, occasionally bile duct damage', although not as severe as seen in PBC/PSC
    AIH: the inflammatory infiltrate shows typically a predominance of **plasma cells**
- Batts & Ludwig system for evaluating inflammation (grade) and fibrosis (stage)

Inflammation:	Grade 1	Minimal patchy, piecemeal necrosis and lobular inflammation/necrosis
	Grade 2	Mild portal inflammation with piecemeal necrosis involving some or all portal tracts with focal hepatocellular damage
	Grade 3	Moderate piecemeal necrosis involving all portal tracts with increased hepatocellular damage
	Grade 4	Severe portal inflammation with piecemeal necrosis; bridging fibrosis and diffuse hepatocellular damage may be present

SECTION IV LIVER

Fibrosis:	Stage 1	Portal fibrosis (fibrous portal expansion)
	Stage 2	Periportal fibrosis (periportal fibrosis with rare portal-portal septa)
	Stage 3	Septal fibrosis (fibrous septa with architectural distortion)
	Stage 4	Cirrhosis

CHOLESTASIS
- Clinical/Lab findings (hemolysis) can help, Radiographic findings (extrahepatic obstruction) diagnose the easy cases; Cases for a liver biopsy are very difficult to diagnose based upon histology
- Question for pathologist: Inflammation or noninflammation (Bland Cholestasis)
  - Are there clues from large duct obstruction or interlobular duct inflammation (? missed ampula mass or stones)
  - Is there evidence of hepatitis; has viral injury been excluded
  - What are any potential toxic exposures at work, home, or play
  - Have granulomatous causes been excluded

DRUG INJURY
- Three conditions should make a pathologist to press the clinician to 'find the drug':
  - Significant fatty change, most often related to toxic ethanol injury
  - Features of hypersensitivity reaction: abundance of eosinophils (also present in nonspecific viral hepatitis, MCTD, Hodgkin's)
  - The look of recovering from a point-in-time injury, with numerous liver cell mitotic figures: suggest single/short episode of toxin exposure

BILE DUCT DISORDERS
- Neutrophils within edematous portal stroma are a feature of large duct obstruction (even when frank cholangitis is not present)
- PBC stages:
  1. Early, damage to septal and larger interlobular bile ducts, characterized by biliary epithelial damage with lymphocytes, plasma cells, PMNs
     The inflammation may include granulomas and lymphoid follicles (Florid Duct Lesion); This stage is confined within the portal tract
  2. Inflammation extends beyond the portal tract; piecemeal necrosis may be seen; bile ducts disappear
  3. Associated with increasing fibrosis and bridging fibrosis; decreased amounts of inflammation
  4. 'Biliary' (micronodular) cirrhosis
- PSC stages:
  1. Early, damage to bile duct and inflammation confined within portal tracts
  2. Periportal fibroinflammatory process
  3. Associated with increasing fibrosis and bridging fibrosis; bile ducts disappear
  4. End stage disease, cirrhosis
     - 'Onionskin' is rarely seen! Most common findings is nonspecific fibrosis with inflammation of portal tracts and paucity of normal bile ducts!
     - The major goal of biopsy is to consider PSC and then suggest ERCP/MRCP to confirm the diagnosis
     - Chronic cholestasis (PBC, PSC) may also have elevated liver copper levels (range 150-350 mcg/gm)

GRANULOMATOUS INFLAMMATION
- A granuloma is a sharply (or fairly sharply) defined aggregate of histiocytes; found in up to 10% of routine liver biopsies
- Most systemic granulomatous diseases involve the liver to some extent
- Liver granulomas: Most common are TB and sarcoid (I.e. think infection, drug, sarcoid); Other DDX:
  -Infectious: Viruses (CMV, EBV), Bacteria *(brucellosis, nocardiosis, tularemia)*, Spirochetes, Protozoa, Various fungi, *Rickettsia* (*Coxiella* – Q fever)
  -Noninfectious: Drugs, PBC, Extrahepatic inflammatory disease (IBD, Rheumatoid), Neoplasms (Hodgkin's), Foreign substance (talc, mineral oil)
- Patients with fever of unknown origin and negative fungi and acid-fast stains: must wait for cultures (more sensitive than staining);
  - Biopsy should be sterile and submitted without fixative to micro lab

CHAPTER 4.19 HISTOPATHOLOGY OF LIVER

INHERITED LIVER DISASE
- **Hemochromatosis:** Biopsy may be normal or show bridging fibrosis or even micronodular cirrhosis
  - The DDX of increased hepatic iron is long, the pattern of iron distribution may help:
    - Predominantly hepatocellular distribution: Genetic hemochromatosis, Alcoholic liver disease, Porphyria cutanea tarda
    - Predominantly in Kupffer cells: Multiple transfusions, Hemolytic anemias
    - Mixed hepatocellular and Kupffer cell distribution: Megaloblastic anemia, Anemia secondary to chronic infection
- **Wilson's Disease:** Biopsy shows a range of findings:
  - Children: Macrovesicular fatty change; Younger adults: chronic hepatitis with piecemeal necrosis; Adults: cirrhosis ± Mallory hyaline
  - Quantitative copper testing: levels typically >250 mcg/gm dry weight on liver biopsy (normal is 38 mcg/gm)
    - Chronic cholestasis (PBC, PSC) may also have elevated liver copper levels (range 150-350 mcg/gm)
  - Other helpful measurements include serum ceruloplasmin and 24 hr urinary copper levels
- **α-1 Antitrypsin Deficiency:** Biopsy show classic PAS-positive, diastase-resistant globules with periportal hepatocytes
  - Portal fibrosis and chronic hepatitis may also be present; Older patients, especially males, are at risk for developing HCC

NEOPLASMS
- **Metastatic neoplasms:** an adequate sample must be obtained for the diagnosis of metastasis
- **Primary liver tumors:** Vascular tumors generally are better diagnosed with radiologic methods; Three other types of tumors should be noted:
  - Hepatocellular Carcinoma:
    - Low-grade lesions can be difficult to distinguish from normal tissue or regenerative nodule in setting of cirrhosis
    - AFP and other tumor markers may help differentiate
  - Liver Cell Adenomas: women taking OCP may show characteristic features
    - Occasionally well-differentiated HCC can resemble adenomas
  - Focal Nodular Hyperplasia: localized lobulated nodule of hyperplastic liver cells surrounding a central scar
    - Can be confused with macronodular cirrhosis; Definitive classification may require excision of the nodule

TRANSPLANTATION
- **Acute rejection:**
  - Preferentially injure biliary epithelial cells of both interlobular and septal bile ducts; Hepatocytes & sinusoidal linings are not prime targets
  - Three main features: Predominantly mononuclear with mixed portal inflammation (lymphocytes, plasma cells, PMNs, eosinophils)
    Subendothelial inflammation (**endothelialitis**), which may involve both portal and central veins
    Bile duct infiltration by inflammatory cells with associated damage
- **Chronic rejection:** classically characterized by bile duct loss in more than 50% of portal tracts and is likely irreversible
  - Characterized histologically:
    - Ductopenic: loss of small bile ducts, seen on biopsy
    - Obliterative vasculopathy: affecting hilar structures, difficult to see on biopsy
  - May first manifest as prominent bile duct abnormalities
  - Unlike acute rejection, bile duct damage is typically out of proportion to the degree of inflammation
- **Distinguishing recurrent HCV from allograft rejection:** can be very difficult
  - HCV is characterized by mononuclear rather than mixed portal infiltrate, lobular hepatitis, and perhaps hepatocyte necrosis
- **Veno-Occlusive Disease (VOD):** usually a complication of bone marrow transplant (usually develops within 1-4 weeks after transplant)
  - Occlusion of central veins, sinusoidal fibrosis, and pericentral hepatocyte necrosis
- **Graft Vs. Host Disease (GVHD):** may be a complication of bone marrow transplant (usually develops within 6 weeks after transplant)
  - Degenerative bile duct lesions with some degree of mononuclear inflammation; Cholestasis may be present
  - Chronic GVHD develops 80-400 days after transplant, often preceded by acute GVHD; Bile ducts may be reduced in number or destroyed

4.20 LIVER FUNCTION TESTS

(Gastroenterology. 2002;123:1364-1384; Clin Chem 2000;12:1-60)
Adapted, in part, from Pocket Medicine 2nd ed. 2004. Lippincott Wilkins & Williams

TESTS OF HEPATIC FUNCTION:
- **Albumin:** general marker for liver protein synthesis, ↓ slowly in liver failure ($T^{1}/_{2}$ ~20d); A rapid ↓ can occur in the setting of sepsis
- **Prothrombin Time (PT):** depends on synthesis of coagulation factors that are Vitamin K dependant
  - An abnormal PT from liver dysfunction occurs in the setting of inadequate Vit K (Normally Vit K po/IV normalizes PT in ~48 hrs)
  - Because $T^{1}/_{2}$ of some factors (i.e., V, VII) is short, ↑ PT can occur within hours of liver dysfunction
  - **Factor 8** (only factor synthesized in vascular endothelium, not in liver): Therefore it is normal in FHF! Consumed/Low in DIC!
- **Bilirubin:** product of heme metabolism in liver via hepatocyte, not bile duct cells; unconjugated (indirect) or conjugated (direct - water soluble)

ABNORMAL LIVER TESTS:
- **Aminotransferases**
  (**ALT** [SGPT], **AST** [SGOT]): intracellular enzymes released 2° necrosis or inflammation (i.e. injury)
  - ALT relatively specific for liver
  - AST found in liver, heart, skeletal muscle, kidney, and brain
  - ALT > AST » viral hepatitis or fatty liver/nonalcoholic steatohepatitis (pericirrhotic)
  - AST:ALT >2:1 » alcoholic hepatitis (ALT production depends on B6, which is depleted with ETOH, therefore ↓ levels)
  - ↑↑↑ LDH » ischemic or toxic hepatitis
  - NOTE: ALT/AST lab assay tests don't indicate the quantity, rather how quickly it causes an enzymatic reaction:
    - Assumption is, the faster the reaction, the more enzyme is present

- **Alkaline phosphatase (Aϕ):** enzyme bound in hepatic canicular membrane
  - Aϕ also found in bone, intestines, placenta (these will have normal GGT)
  - Confirm liver origin: ↑ **5'-NT**, ↑ **GGT** (GGT very sensitive for hepatobiliary disease), or heat fractionation (liver: lives, bone: burns)
  - ↑ levels seen with biliary obstruction or intrahepatic cholestasis (ie. hepatic infiltration)

PATTERNS OF LIVER INJURY: OVERVIEW (See Detailed explanation of each below)
Hepatocellular: Damage or destruction of liver cells; ↑ aminotransferases, ± ↑ bilirubin or Aϕ
- Acute: less than 3 months (i.e. HAV, HBV, Meds, ETOH, Ischemia) or Chronic (HCV, HBV, NASH, ETOH, Hemochromatosis, AIH)
- ↑↑↑ aminotransferases (>3000): toxic hepatitis (i.e. acetaminophen), ischemia, or severe/abnormal viral hepatitis (i.e. herpes)

Cholestasis: Impaired bile transport; ↑↑ Aϕ & GGT and ± bilirubin (*don't* depend on bili to show cholestasis pattern); ± ↑ aminotransferases

Isolated hyperbilirubinemia: ↑↑ bilirubin, near normal Aϕ and aminotransferases
  Jaundice is a clinical sign seen when bilirubin >2.5 mg/dl (especially sclera); part of either cholestatic pattern or isolated hyperbilirubinemia

Infiltrative: ↑ Aϕ, ± ↑ bilirubin or aminotransferases

Hepatocellular Injury: predominantly ↑↑ AST & ALT, ± ↑ Bili & Aϕ
- Viral Markers » Viral hepatitis: HAV, HBV, HCV, HDV, HEV, CMV, EBV, HSV, VZV
- Auto Antibodies » Autoimmune (+ASMA)
- Toxic Screen » Drugs/Toxins: ETOH, Acetaminophen, Meds, Toxins
- Obesity, DM, Lipids » NASH
- Hypotension/CHF » Vascular: Ischemic, Congestive, Budd-Chiari, VOD
  Note with ischemia/shock liver typically AST & ALT rise within a day or so followed by normalization, then increase in bilirubin
- Systemic Disease » Inherited Liver Diseases: Hemochromatosis, α1-AT deficiency, Wilson's disease
  Others: Celiac sprue

Cholestasis: predominantly ↑↑ Aφ and GGT, ± Bili, ± ↑ AST & ALT
- **Ductal Dilation** » Biliary obstruction: Choledocholithiasis, Cholangiocarcinoma, Pancreatic cancer, Primary sclerosing cholangitis
  - Biliary stone often see AST/ALT >1000 with a rapid decrease within 24-48 hrs
- **NO Ductal Dilation** »
  - ↑↑ Aφ » Intrahepatic Cholestasis: Medication (sex hormones, erythromycin, PPIs, ETOH), Sepsis, CHF, Post-Op, PBC, TPN
  - ± ↑ Aφ » Biliary epithelial damage: Hepatitis (↑ ALT), Cirrhosis (↑ PT, ↓ Alb)

Isolated Hyperbilirubinemia: predominantly ↑ bili, near normal Aφ, AST & ALT
- **Conjugated** ("direct", water soluble, not bound to albumin, excreted in urine and bile) »
  - **Hepatocellular disease:** Hepatitis, Cirrhosis, ETOH, Toxic (acetaminophen, Jamaican bush tea, Arsenic), Sepsis/ischemia, HCC, Cystic fibrosis, Bacterial/parasitic/fungal, TPN
  - **Defective excretion:** Dubin-Johnson, Rotor's syndrome, Alagille syndrome
  - **Intrahepatic cholestasis:** Medication, PSC, PBC, NASH, Sarcoid/Amyloid, Lymphoma, Cholangiocarcinoma, Biliary atresia
  - **Extrahepatic cholestasis:** Stones, PSC, Cholangiocarcinoma, Pancreatic cancer, Acute/Chronic pancreatitis, Ampullary neoplasm/stenosis/sphincter of Oddi dysfunction (SOD), Parasite (Ascaris/Flukes), AIDS cholangiopathy, Stricture post procedure
- **Unconjugated** ("indirect", not water soluble, bound to albumin, excreted in bile) »
  - **Overproduction:** Hemolysis (total <4 mg/dl), Ineffective erythropoiesis, Hematoma reabsorption, PE
  - **Impaired uptake:** CHF, Portosystemic shunt placements (TIPS), Medications (rifampin, probenecid)
  - **Defective conjugation (Hepatocellular):** Gilbert's (total <5 mg/dl) & Crigler-Najjar I&II (cause of both: bilirubin UGT gene), Hyperthyroid, Prematurity/Newborn, Ethinyl estradiol, Liver diseases: Chronic persistent hepatitis, Advanced cirrhosis, Wilson's disease

Infiltrative Pattern: predominantly ↑ Aφ, can be near normal bili, AST & ALT (but if they ↑ don't be fooled)
- Malignancy » HCC, Metastatic, Lymphoma
- Granulomas » TB, Sarcoid, Histoplasmosis
- Abscess » Amebic, Bacterial
- Other » Medications, Idiopathic

LFT ALGORITHMS

General Questions to Ask Yourself with Abnormal Liver Tests:
Biggest questions: Medications, ETOH, Obesity (NAFLD)
Risk factor questions (for viral): History of blood transfusions, IVDA, Tattoos, Travel (HAV), Sexual behavior (HBV), IBD, Family history

Evaluation of Isolated Chronic Elevation of Serum Aminotransferases
These steps of workup can have a timeline of 3 months to 3 years, depending on physician's comfort level
Many practitioners may alter step order due to history or experience; These are general guidelines at best
Up to 25% of abnormal LFTs are unknown; May be due to 'normal' range of numbers; Tincture of time may be best

Step 1.
-Review possible link to medications, herbal therapies or recreational drugs; Ask about blood transfusions, tattoos, high-risk sexual behavior
-Screen for ETOH abuse (tox screens, AST:ALT >2:1)
-Evaluate for fatty liver/NASH: body habitus/metabolic with history of DM, cholesterol; (AST/ALT usually <1, obtain RUQ U/S)
-Obtain serology for Hepatitis B and C (HBsAg, HBsAb, HBcAb, HCV Ab); many will not do serologies until step 2
-Screen for hemochromatosis (FE/TIBC >45% i.e. Transferrin saturation) (Don't do Ferritin first, it is acute phase reactant)

Step 2.
-Exclude muscle disorders and confirm the source is hepatic (obtain creatinine kinase or aldolase)
-Obtain thyroid function tests (TSH if hypothyroid suspected, otherwise full thyroid function tests)
-Consider celiac disease (especially with history of diarrhea or iron deficiency anemia: serum anti-tissue transglutaminase IgA or small bowel biopsy)
-Consider adrenal insufficiency
-Many will consider Wilson's or AIH here depending on history and gender

Step 3. Consider less common causes of liver disease; Heightened suspicion for AIH or other inherited disorders (Wilson's, α1-AT, Hemochromatosis)
-Autoimmune hepatitis, particularly in women and those with a history of other autoimmune disorders; Check SPEP, If positive obtain ANA and ASMA
-Consider Wilson's disease in those <40, especially males (check ceruloplasmin, evaluate for Kayser-Fleischer rings)
-Consider α-1 Antitrypsin deficiency (especially with history of emphysema out of proportion to age and smoking history; Obtain α-1antitrypsin phenotype)

Step 4. Observe or obtain a liver biopsy
-Observe if ALT and AST are less than 2-fold elevated
-Otherwise consider liver biopsy and/or imaging if not done (i.e. U/S)

Evaluation of Elevated Serum Aφ
-Rule out physiologic causes (pregnancy, post prandial (up to 2 × ULN), repeat a fasting test)
-Determine the source (GGT) is from liver
- Normal: Aφ likely bone origin, test for bone disorders
- Increased: Aφ likely hepatobiliary origin
    - Check RUQ and AMA
        - AMA positive & RUQ normal -OR- AMA negative & RUQ abnormal: Liver biopsy
        - Dilated bile ducts: ERCP
        - AMA negative and RUQ normal: Assess degree of elevation of the Aφ:
            - >50% elevated: Liver biopsy, ERCP or MRCP
            - <50% elevated: observe

Evaluation of Conjugated Hyperbilirubinemia
-Normal liver enzymes:
- Sepsis, Dubin-Johnson syndrome, Rotor's syndrome
-Abnormal liver enzymes:
- Persistently high ALT
    - Pursue causes of hepatitis
- Elevated Aφ ± transient increase in ALT
    - U/S or CT
        - Dilated ducts: ERCP
        - Normal ducts: MRCP or consider biopsy

LIVER BIOPSY:
Methods: Percutaneous, Transjugular, Intraoperative
- Indications:
  - Intraoperative findings suggested of cirrhosis
  - Staging/Grading of HCV, HBV, NASH
  - Focal liver lesions
  - High LFTs in normal patient or history of OLT (serologic workup negative)
- Absolute contraindications:
  - Coagulopathy (PT >3 sec of control, Plts <50 K), Lack of transfusion support, Documented hemangioma, Uncooperative
- Relative contraindications:
  - Ascites, Infection in right pleural space or right subdiaphragmatic space, Morbid obesity
- Complications: 60% occur within 2 hours and 96% within 24 hours
  - Pain at site in 10-25% (2% need hospitalization), Intraperitoneal hemorrhage in 0.3%, Pneumothorax (rare); Mortality 1 in 10,000

NOTES

4.21 MASS (FOCAL LIVER) EVALUATION

DEFINITION:
- Benign or Malignant, Primary (originating in the liver) or Secondary (metastases), lesions of the liver

EPIDEMIOLOGY:
- See Etiologies below for specific conditions

ETIOLOGIES:
- Differential Diagnosis

	Benign	Malignant		Benign
Epithelial	Hepatic adenoma	Hepatocellular carcinoma	Other:	Focal nodular hyperplasia (FNH)
	Bile duct adenoma	Cholangiocarcinoma		Liver abscess
	Biliary cystadenoma	Biliary cystadenocarcinoma		Regenerative nodule(s) of cirrhosis
	—	Squamous carcinoma		Focal fatty infiltration
Mesenchymal	Cavernous Hemangioma	Angiosarcoma		Simple hepatic cysts
	Fibroma, Lipoma	Fibrosarcoma, Liposarcoma		
	Leiomyoma	Leiomyosarcoma		**Malignant**
	—	Primary hepatic lymphoma	Other:	Metastatic tumors

Modified from Kew MC: Tumors of the liver. In Zakim D, Boyer TD (eds): Hepatology: A Textbook of Liver Disease, 3rd ed. Philadelphia, W.B. Saunders, 1996, pp 1513.

- Cavernous hemangiomas: **most common benign cause,** more common in ♀ as solitary (60%) or multiple asymptomatic masses
  - Most <3 cm, right lobe; Microscopically consist of blood-filled vascular sinusoids separated by connective tissue septae
  - Seldom estrogen sensitive, rarely cause symptoms and do not pose a threat for rupture or malignant degeneration; No therapy

- Focal nodular hyperplasia (FNH): **second most common benign lesion,** over 90% occur in ♀, between 20-60 years
  - Round, nonencapsulated mass, usually with vascular *central scar* with fibrous septae radiating out, including Kupffer cells
  - Theorized to result from hyperplastic tissue response to a congenital arterial malformation
  - CT/MRI show "spoke wheel" in arterial phase, T2 demonstrates hyperintense (opposite of Fibrolamellar hepatocellular cancer)
    - Confirm with *technetium-sulfur (nuclear medicine)* scan: exploits the Kupffer cells as they uptake sulfur
  - Often associated with hemangiomas (22%) or very rarely Fibrolamellar HCC
  - Does not pose a threat for rupture or malignant degeneration; Difficult question is distinguishing from Adenoma
    - FNH: central scar on CT/MRI, ↑ uptake on Tc 99 m sulfur colloid scintigraphy, biopsy shows bile ducts in fibrous septa
  - Resection usually not necessary

CHAPTER 4.21 MASS (FOCAL LIVER) EVALUATION

- Hepatic Adenomas: Women and related to OCP use, benign tumor but often symptomatic, 4 per 100,000 ♀ (anabolic steroids in males is a risk factor)
  - Microscopically they are monotonous sheets of normal or small hepatocytes with no bile ducts, portal tracts, or central veins
  - CT demonstrates enhancement without central scar during arterial phase
  - Surgical resection recommended (even with stopping OCP): spontaneous rupture/hemorrhage up to 30%, ? HCC risk
  - Hepatic Adenomatosis (>10 adenomas) is extremely rare and considered a distinct entity from Hepatic Adenoma

- Liver Cysts: prevalence in general population 3–4% and increase with age; more common in ♀
  - Usually asymptomatic and frequency occur with other liver lesions/masses
  - Characterized by thin-walled structures lined with cuboidal bile duct epithelium and filled with isotonic fluid (lucent on U/S)

- Fatty infiltration: occurs with obesity, diabetes, ETOH intake, chemotherapy (especially with altered nutrition status)
  - Can be focal in nature producing appearance of a mass on imaging

- Metastatic liver disease more common than primary hepatic tumors; Cancers: colon, stomach, pancreas, breast, lung, esophageal, renal
  - Multiple liver defects suggest metastases, only 2% are single lesions; Involvement of both lobes is common, but 20% right lobe only

- Hepatocellular carcinoma (HCC) is by far most common malignancy originating in liver; accounts for 80% of primary liver cancers
  - Most are age >55, ♂ > ♀, Approximately 80% of patients with HCC have cirrhosis; *See also Liver- Hepatocellular Carcinoma (Chapter 4.17)*
  - Types of cirrhosis associated: Chronic HCV, Chronic HBV, Hemochromatosis, α1-AT, Alcoholic cirrhosis

- Cholangiocarcinoma: ~10% of primary liver cancers; jaundice is most frequent clinical presentation; *See also Pancreas/Biliary- Cholangiocarcinoma (Chapter 5.01)*
  - Risk factors: PSC, Ulcerative Colitis, Liver fluke ingestion, Congenital cystic liver disease, Choledochal cysts
  - Delayed tumor enhancement with IV contrast is noted in approximately 75% of intrahepatic cholangiocarcinomas
  - Klatskin tumors: cholangiocarcinomas at hilar bifurcation of hepatic ducts
  - Desmoplastic reaction accompanying these tumors make them poorly visible on imaging studies and difficult to diagnose on biopsy
  - Only 25% occur in setting of cirrhosis; most are unresectable at diagnosis and require palliative drainage of obstructive jaundice

- Hepatic lymphomas: Primary hepatic lymphoma is much less common than secondary liver involvement from Hodgkin's and non-Hodgkin's
  - Primary is typically large, solitary mass; Secondary spread is characterized by multiple nodules or hepatomegaly
    - Secondary lymphoma can be so diffuse, imaging can be normal; OLT and AIDS increase the risk of primary lymphoma

- Liver Abscess: *See also Liver- Abscess of Liver (Chapter 4.02)*
  - Two general types: Pyogenic (intraabdominal infections) & Amebic (colonic infections with invasive Entamoeba histolytica)

CLINICAL MANIFESTATIONS/PHYSICAL EXAM:

- Abdominal pain (RUQ pain) is most common but not specific; Fever is very common with abscess
- Common with malignant disease: night sweats, low-grade fever, involuntary weight loss, anorexia, diarrhea
- Common with intra-adenoma or intrahepatic hemorrhage: acute and severe abdominal pain

SECTION IV   LIVER

LABORATORY STUDIES:
- LFTs are usually normal in benign liver tumors (except GGT); Aϕ is often elevated with hepatic metastases, but not in all cases
- Hepatitis serology and Iron studies (for Hemochromatosis and IDA/Colon cancer)
- Tumor markers:
    Alpha-Fetoprotein (AFP) & CA19-9: markers of 1° hepatic malignancy; used when radiographic studies indicate originating focal liver lesion *See also Liver- Hepatocellular Carcinoma (Chapter 4.17)*
    - AFP best diagnostic marker of hepatocellular carcinoma (HCC), and used for screening test for high-risk patients
    - AFP >500 ng/ml is virtually diagnostic

    CA19-9: best diagnostic marker for cholangiocarcinoma and bile duct tumors; more sensitive in those with PSC (a risk factor for Cholangiocarcinoma)
    - CA19-9 >100 U/ml found in >50% of patients and values >1000 suggest unresectability
    - Also serves as a tumor marker for pancreatic carcinoma

    CEA (gastrointestinal metastatic adenocarcinoma) may be elevated

DIAGNOSTIC STUDIES:
- First step is accurate history and physical: age, sex, birthplace are important clues to etiology; i.e. viral hepatitis/cirrhosis ↑ risk of 1° malignancy

- Overall goal is to distinguish benign from malignant:
    - Is it simple cysts, hemangioma, focal fatty change, FNH all of which can be reassured and don't require intervention/monitoring
    - On the other hand is it abscess, adenoma, cholangiocarcinoma, HCC or metastases that need further investigation/treatment

- CT: Allows contrast injection to be viewed in both arterial (early) and portal/venous phases of perfusion
    - Arterial phase: HCC & hypervascular lesions appear
    - Venous phase: maximal enhancement of normal liver or hypovascular lesions
    - Cavernous hemangioma: Nodular peripheral enhancement in arterial phase with delayed venous filling
    - Intrahepatic Cholangiocarcinoma: no arterial enhancement but displays venous phase enhancement, high tumor markers
    - Fatty infiltration: hypodense because the fatty infiltration density is not as low as adipose tissue (hyperechoic on U/S)

- MRI: Contrast allows use in manner analogous to CT; Gadolinium-enhanced MRI used for those with contraindication to iodine or ARF/CRF
    - On horizon: Ferumoxide scans; dextran-coated iron oxide particles given by IV and taken up by Kupffer cells in normal liver & FNH
    - Focal Nodular Hyperplasia: Isointense on T1 & T2, after gadolinium injection: prominent arterial phase enhancement (hyperdense) with rapid washout during venous phase (isodense), Central scar usually present (but only 20% with small lesions)

- U/S: many liver masses found incidentally on U/S; however cannot fully characterize lesions; does have role in verifying simple cysts

- Fine needle aspiration (FNA): literature reveals a wide range of sensitivity for diagnosis of primary hepatic lesions (60-90%)
    - Hemangiomas: if need to know is absolute, can be done by experienced radiologist; acellular biopsy ("dry aspirate") is normal
    - Other controversies are needle-tract seeding and tumor spread (problematic if OLT and risk of metastasis)
    - FNA plays dominant role in setting of suspected metastatic disease to the liver and inoperable cancers

<u>Screening Strategies for HCC:</u>
- All patients with cirrhosis: especially with those with HBV, HCV and cirrhosis-related metabolic liver disease
- Strategy: Serial AFP and hepatic U/S every 6 months is common

CHAPTER 4.21 MASS (FOCAL LIVER) EVALUATION

Logical Approach to Evaluation of Focal Hepatic Mass:
Incidental lesions:
- Simple cysts » verify with U/S
- Hemangiomas » CT with and without contrast » MRI (gadolinium-enhanced)
- Focal nodular hyperplasia (FNH) » CT w/wo contrast » MRI (ferumoxide-enhanced)
- Hepatic Adenoma » History of OCP? » Rule out hemangioma and FNH » ? Biopsy/resection

Symptomatic lesions:
- Hepatic Adenoma » History of OCP? » Rule out hemangioma and FNH » Resection
- Liver Abscess » Sepsis » U/S » CT w/wo contrast (rim enhancement); *See also Liver- Abscess of Liver (Chapter 4.02)*

Cirrhosis and Risk Factors for Cholangiocarcinoma:
- HCC » AFP level » CT or MRI w/wo contrast
- Cholangiocarcinoma » CA19–9 » CT w/wo contrast (delayed phase)

History of Malignancy:
- Metastases » CT w/wo contrast » If resection is considered, MRI (ferumoxide-enhanced) may be best to rule out multiple metastasis

TREATMENTS:
- Hemangiomas: no intervention other than observation; Rarely a symptomatic giant cavernous hemangioma requires surgical enucleation/resection
- Adenoma: most recommend resection or ablation because of the risk of rupture or associated malignancy
- Cysts: those that are large and cause pain may be treated with surgical fenestration or percutaneous aspiration ± ethanol ablation
- For HCC, *See also Liver- Hepatocellular Carcinoma (Chapter 4.17)*

4.22 NON-ALCOHOLIC FATTY LIVER DISEASE (NAFLD)/NON-ALCOHOLIC STEATOHEPATITIS (NASH)/NON-ALCOHOLIC FATTY LIVER (NAFL)

(Dig Dis Sci 2005:50;171–80. Clin Gastroenterol Hepatol. 2004;2:1048–58. Gastroenterology. 2002:123: 1702–04 & 1705–25)

DEFINITION:
- The presence of **macrovesicular** fatty changes without inflammation **(steatosis)** and lobular inflammation in the absence of alcohol
- NAFLD can be divided into NASH or NAFL
  - NASH: 10–20%, biopsy proven, is macrovesicular steatosis *with inflammation* and **can progress to cirrhosis**
  - NAFL/Steatosis: 80%, comprising the majority of NAFLD, typically does not progress to NASH or cirrhosis
- Classifications of NASH:
  - Primary NASH: Obesity, Diabetes, Hyperlipidemia
  - Secondary NASH: Drug therapy: See Associated Meds, under Etiologies
    Surgical procedures: Jejunal bypass, Gastric bypass, Extensive small bowel resection
    Other Metabolic: TPN, Acute starvation, Rapid weight loss
    Miscellaneous: Bacterial overgrowth, Abetalipoproteinemia, Weber-Christian disease

EPIDEMIOLOGY:
- Prevalence of NAFLD: 7–9%; Most are Women (60–95%) but the gap is closing so that men = women
- Mean age at diagnosis: 50 years (range 16–80)
- Most common adolescent liver disease and increasing due to obesity epidemic (adolescents with abnormal LFTs, 60% are obese/overweight)
- A substantial portion of cases of cryptogenic cirrhosis may be 'burnt-out' NASH, as many are associated with obesity, DM, Lipids

ETIOLOGIES:
- Accumulation of fat in the liver can occur because of:
  - Increased delivery of free fatty acids (FFAs) to the liver
  - Increased synthesis of fatty acids in the liver
  - Decreased oxidation of FFA (oxidative stress on hepatocytes results in activated stellate cells production of collagen/inflammation)
  - Decreased synthesis or secretion of very-low-density lipoprotein (VLDL)
- Associated conditions: Metabolic syndrome-like: Obesity (50–95% of patients), DM (20–75% of patients), Hyperlipidemia (20–80% of patients)
- Associated Meds: Diltiazem/Nifedipine, Amiodarone, HAART, Glucocorticoids, Tamoxifen, Estrogens
  - Classic causes of *microvesicular* steatohepatitis: valproic acid and tetracycline

PATHOPHYSIOLOGY:
- Biopsy findings in fatty liver disease: (definitive diagnosis of steatohepatitis can only be made with a liver biopsy)
  In general: Macrovesicular steatosis, Mallory bodies, Lobular neutrophilic inflammation, Ballooning degeneration, Perisinusoidal fibrosis
  - Type 1: fatty liver alone (37%); Macrovesicular steatosis; Benign
  - Type 2: fat accumulation and lobar inflammation (7.5%)
  - Type 3: fat accumulation and ballooning degeneration (14%)
  - Type 4: fat accumulation, ballooning degeneration and either Mallory hyaline or fibrosis (41%); Highest proportion of cirrhosis
  Note: Type 3 and 4: NASH by definition

- Grading of Necroinflammatory activity of NASH; 1: mild, 2: moderate, 3: severe
  - Grade 1: Steatosis (predominantly macrovesicular); no or mild portal chronic inflammation
  - Grade 2: Steatosis of any degree; ballooning of hepatocytes; portal and intra-acinar chronic inflammation (mild-moderate)
  - Grade 3: Panacinar steatosis; ballooning and disarray; scattered PMNs

CHAPTER 4.22 NAFLD/NASH/NAFL

- Staging of Fibrosis
  - Stage 1: Portal fibrosis (fibrous portal expansion)
  - Stage 2: Periportal fibrosis (periportal fibrosis with rare portal-portal septa)
  - Stage 3: Septal fibrosis (fibrous septa with architectural distortion)
  - Stage 4: Cirrhosis

CLINICAL MANIFESTATIONS/PHYSICAL EXAM:
- Associated conditions- Metabolic syndrome-like: Obesity (50-95% of patients), DM (20-75% of patients), Hyperlipidemia (20-80% of patients)
- Usually asymptomatic (48-100%)
- Most diagnosed when LFTs done as part of management of other conditions associated with NASH (i.e. diabetes)
- ± RUQ pain is most common symptom
- Caution: 3-40% may not have DM and have normal lipid levels and lean body weight
- Caution: FHF and/or rapid progression to cirrhosis suggest drug-induced steatosis or Wilson's disease

LABORATORY STUDIES: (lack of specificity, makes it difficult to distinguish NASH from NAFL)
- Transaminitis of 2-3 × ULN; AST/ALT <1 (Total values <300); A ratio of >2 is strongly suggestive of ETOH liver disease
- Bilirubin: normal (rarely exceeds 3.0 mg/dl); INR: normal; Albumin: normal (i.e. most are normal values, unless decompensated cirrhosis)
- Aφ: modest increase in 40-60% of patients up to 3 × ULN
- ANA may be positive in low titers (1:40 to 1:320) in 40% of patients
- Hyperlipidemia in 20% of patients; Lipoprotein abnormalities
- Iron studies (elevated ferritin and transferring saturation) in 58% of patients

DIAGNOSTIC STUDIES:
- Exclusion of other causes of hepatitis or cirrhosis, including:
  - Negligible (<20 g/day) ETOH consumption; Negative HBV, HCV; Normal α1-AT phenotype and Ceruloplasmin level
  - No evidence of Hemochromatosis; Autoimmune serology (AMA, ANA, ASMA, ALKMA) negative
- MRI = CT = U/S (All equal in detecting fatty liver infiltration, however ? if NASH vs. NAFL)
  - U/S » hyperchoic = fatty change (30% of hepatocytes must be infiltrated, so negative U/S doesn't exclude NAFLD)
- Biopsy (See Pathophysiology above)
  - Rationale for biopsy: rule out other diagnoses, prove NASH or NAFL and provide prognostic information
- Usually if all serologic tests for other liver diseases are negative, and risk factors present (obesity, DM, etc), diagnosis of fatty liver or NASH as cause of elevated LFTs is made with some degree of certainty (but in the strictest sense, the diagnosis requires a biopsy)

TREATMENTS:
- **Weight loss** (diet/exercise), glycemic and lipid control; Use statins even with elevated ALT!
  - For significant obesity (75% overweight) gastric bypass may significantly reduce steatosis
- Stop any alcohol or hepatotoxic drugs
- Possible roles for Vitamin E, thiazolidinediones, fish oils, flax seed oils
- Ursodeoxycholic acid (UDCA) may have membrane-stabilizing effect and cytoprotective effect; Not promising
- Metformin: some evidence suggest improved LFTs
- Transplant is warranted for decompensated cirrhotics; It is possible for NASH to reoccur in the graft

PROGNOSIS:
- No prospective studies on natural history, retrospective studies suggest:
  - No change in patient status (54%), Progress to fibrosis (23%), Progress to cirrhosis (15%), Improvement (12%)
- Significant inflammation on biopsy are more likely to progress to cirrhosis
- ? if any progress to HCC or have increased risk

4.23 PRIMARY BILIARY CIRRHOSIS (PBC)

(NEJM 2005;353:1261-73. Hepatology. 2000;31:1005-13)

DEFINITION:
- PBC: Autoimmune destruction of *intrahepatic* bile ducts (small bile ducts)
- Autoimmune Cholangitis or AMA-Negative PBC: (may see positive ANA and/or ASMA)
  - Patients with PBC and non-detectable serum AMA; Response to therapy is the same as PBC
- Overlap or Variant Syndrome: presence of features of both Autoimmune Hepatitis (AIH) and PBC
  - Positive ANA and AMA; Piecemeal necrosis and coexistent periductal/portal inflammation with bile duct destruction

EPIDEMIOLOGY:
- Middle-aged *women* (age 40-60) occurring in 150-300 per million persons
- Concomitant autoimmune disease (See also Pathophysiology section below)
- Can see familial clustering

ETIOLOGIES:
- A chronic cholestatic liver disease of unknown etiology

PATHOPHYSIOLOGY:
- Autoimmune destruction of interlobular and septal *(intrahepatic)* bile ducts
- Frequent association with other autoimmune diseases:
  - Sicca syndrome, RA, Hypothyroidism, Sjogren's, Scleroderma, CREST, Dermatomyositis, MCTD, SLE, Lichen planus, Pemphigoid
- DDX: Other causes of chronic cholestasis:
  - Biliary stones, Iatrogenic strictures (i.e. biliary surgery), Tumors; Drug-induced: phenothiazines, estrogens, etc.

CLINICAL MANIFESTATIONS/PHYSICAL EXAM:
- **Fatigue and Pruritus** (both often intractable); RUQ pain and Anorexia; Liver can be enlarged and firm to palpation
- Jaundice as primary manifestation is uncommon, yet often heralds the presence of advanced histological disease
- Hypercholesterolemia: Xanthomas (extensor surface cholesterol deposition), Xanthelasma (eyelid cholesterol deposition)
- Fat malabsorption: 8% have concomitant celiac sprue
- Late symptoms: those of end-stage liver disease: GIB, ascites, PSE
- Look for other autoimmune diseases: RA, Sjogrens, Hypothyroid, GN, and CREST occurs in up to 8% of PBC patients

LABORATORY STUDIES:
- ↑ Aφ and ↑ bilirubin, some ↑ in ALT/AST
- Liver synthetic function, PT, Albumin, remain normal unless the disease is advanced
- Auto-antibodies: + **AMA (anti-mitochondrial ab) in 95%;** 9 subtypes M1-9 (M2 most common), titer doesn't correlate with disease severity
  Others: ANA, ASMA, RA, Thyroid-specific antibodies; **Increased IgM in 90%**
- ↑ **cholesterol,** interestingly however, the associated hyperlipidemia does not appear to place patients at increased risk of CAD (No treatment needed!)

DIAGNOSTIC STUDIES:
- RUQ U/S: usually adequate to exclude the presence of extrahepatic biliary obstruction
- ERCP/MRCP: used to distinguish from PSC in atypical patients: male gender, AMA negative, associated IBD
- Liver bx: (diagnostic) bile duct destruction and granulomatous cholangitis **("Florid Duct Lesion");** also seen with allograft rejection
  Staging: 1. inflammation confined to portal areas   3. bridging fibrosis
            2. inflammation confined to portal & periportal areas   4. cirrhosis

CHAPTER 4.23 PRIMARY BILIARY CIRRHOSIS (PBC)

TREATMENTS:
- **Ursodeoxycholic acid (UDCA)** (13–15 mg/kg/day): prolongs the time to treatment failure, improves overall survival, cost-effective, life-long
  - Hydrophilic nonhepatotoxic compound that acts by attenuating the effect of hepatotoxic hydrophobic bile acids; In other words, reduces the overall toxicity of bile salt pool since cholic and ursodeoxycholic acid are least toxic of bile salts
- Fat soluble vitamins:
  - Vit A: 25–50K U 2–3/wk (monitor for hepatic toxicity); Vit D: 50K U 3/wk; Vit E: 400 U/day; Vit K: If PT corrects, should be on indefinitely
- Pruritus: Cholestyramine: ↓ serum bile levels via binding, ↑ intestinal excretion by preventing absorption; 4 gm doses TID/QID
  - Given 1½ hours before/after other medication to avoid binding; Once itching decreased, reduced dose to lowest effective dose
  - Antihistamines: diphenhydramine 25 mg qhs
  - Rifampin (150–300 mg BID) may also be effective: p450 induction or inhibition of bile uptake; Liver toxicity in 15% of patients
- Lipid-lowering agents; Patients not at higher risk of CAD, and therefore not generally recommended
- Colchicine, MTX in selected case
- TIPS: in general the same indications for any other type of cirrhosis: GIB, refractory ascites, etc.
- Liver transplant: treatment of choice in end-stage disease; *See also Liver- Transplantation (Chapter 4.28)*
  - Among the highest in survival rate (85% at 5 yr, 70% at 10 yr); 7–12% post-transplant get histologic recurrence; ? role of UDCA

COMPLICATIONS:
- Hepatocellular carcinoma: higher risk than previously appreciated; Screen (cirrhotics only) q12–24 months: U/S, AFP level
- Bacterial cholangitis: very rare in PBC (small duct disease)
- Fatigue: (no treatment); Sjogren's/Sicca Syndrome: 60% (artificial tears); Thyroiditis/Hashimoto's (Endocrine Consult); Steatorrhea: (pancreatic enzymes, antibiotics)
- Fat-soluble vitamin deficiency: Vit A: night blindness, Vit D: bone disease, Vit K: prolonged prothrombin time, Vit E: neurologic abnormalities
  - Consider screening for Celiac Sprue (occurs in 8%)
- Metabolic bone disease:
  - Hepatic osteodystrophy/arthritis: occurs 10%, polyarticular, symmetrical, rarely erosive, occasional RF +
  - Avascular Necrosis (AVN): Therapy with Ca/VitD/Bisphosphonates; HRT; CREST can occasionally occur

PROGNOSIS:
- Both PBC and PSC eventually progress to end-stage liver disease, requiring consideration for liver transplant (can reoccur after transplant)
  - Overall median survival without liver transplant: 10–12 years from time of diagnosis
  - If total Bili >10 mg/dl, median survival 2 years without transplant
- Follow-up: Visit (q 6 mon), LFTs (q 3–6 mon), TSH (q 12 mon), Abdomen U/S & AFP (q 12 mon)

4.24 PRIMARY SCLEROSING CHOLANGITIS (PSC)

DEFINITION:
- Idiopathic cholestasis with fibrosis, stricturing and dilation of ***intra- and extrahepatic*** bile ducts (small and large bile ducts)

EPIDEMIOLOGY:
- Young *men* (age 20-50)
- May be autoimmune-linked: **Associated IBD (U/C more common than CD) in 70% of cases** usually appears before PSC; If not get colonoscopy at PSC diagnosis
- Some believe there may be a viral connection with CMV, REO (respiratory enteric orphan virus)

ETIOLOGIES:
- A chronic cholestatic liver disease of unknown etiology
- **Secondary sclerosing causes:** choledocholithiasis, biliary tract surgery, AIDS cholangiopathy, chemotherapy, OLT (ischemia, CMV)

PATHOPHYSIOLOGY:
- Idiopathic diffuse inflammation and fibrosis of the entire *(intra- and extrahepatic)* biliary tree
- Frequent association with other diseases:
  - Ulcerative colitis >> Crohn's disease; Rarely scleroderma, MCTD
- DDX: Other causes of chronic cholestasis:
  - Biliary stones, Iatrogenic strictures, Tumors; Drug-induced: phenothiazines, estrogens, etc.

CLINICAL MANIFESTATIONS/PHYSICAL EXAM:
- Pruritus and Fatigue
- RUQ pain and Anorexia
- Cholangitis (recurrent fever, RUQ pain, and jaundice) may occur
- Cholangiocarcinoma superimposed
- Liver is enlarged and firm to palpation
- Late symptoms: those of end-stage liver disease: GIB, ascites, PSE

LABORATORY STUDIES:
- ↑ Aφ and ↑ bilirubin, some ↑ in ALT/AST
- Liver synthetic function, PT, Albumin, remain normal unless the disease is advanced
- Auto-antibodies: **+p-ANCA in 70-80%,** low but detectable levels of ANA, ASMA may be found in <2% of patients

DIAGNOSTIC STUDIES:
- **ERCP/MRCP or Transhepatic Cholangiography:** multifocal beaded bile duct strictures **(diagnostic)**
  - Diffuse stricturing of both intra/extra hepatic ducts with subsequent saccular dilation of intervening areas: beads-on-string
  - 20% of patients may only have intrahepatic or hilar involvement with extrahepatic sparing
  - Presence of a dominant stricture should raise the question of **cholangiocarcinoma** as a complication of PSC!
- **Liver bx:** portal tract edema, ↑ connective tissue, proliferation of interlobular bile ducts: **Fibrous obliterative cholangitis** or **'onion-skin'**
  - As opposed to PBC a biopsy with PSC is not necessarily diagnostic
- Staging:
  1. Edema & scarring of portal triads & some piecemeal necrosis
  2. Expansion of portal triads & fibrosis extending into parenchyma
  3. Bridging fibrosis
  4. Cirrhosis (end stage of disease, much like PBC)
- **CT Scan:** suggestive if intra & extrahepatic dilations, however not detailed enough to confirm as with ERCP/MRCP

CHAPTER 4.24 PRIMARY SCLEROSING CHOLANGITIS (PSC)

TREATMENTS:
- High dose **Ursodeoxycholic acid (UDCA)** (20-30 mg/kg/day)
  - Not yet proven; No good medical therapy for PSC
- Fat-soluble vitamins:
  - A: 25-50K U 2-3/wk (monitor for hepatic toxicity); D: 50K U 3/wk; E: 400U/day; K: If PT corrects, should be on indefinitely
- Pruritus: Cholestyramine: ↓ serum bile levels via binding, ↑ intestinal excretion by preventing absorption; 4 gm doses TID/QID
  - Given $1\frac{1}{2}$ hours before/after other medication to avoid binding; Once itching decreased, reduce dose to lowest effective dose
  - Antihistamines: diphenhydramine 25 mg qhs
  - Rifampin (150-300 mg BID) may also be effective: p450 induction or inhibition of bile uptake; Liver toxicity in 15% of patients
- Cholangitis: may need prophylactic therapy (i.e. Cipro) with history of recurrent bacterial cholangitis
- Endoscopic or transhepatic dilation and short term stenting of dominant bile duct strictures if symptomatic, otherwise stay out of the biliary tree!
- TIPS: in general the same indications for any other type of cirrhosis: GIB, refractory ascites, etc
- Surgery: choledochoduodenostomy, palliative measure to alleviate symptoms of biliary obstruction; Rarely done due to complications
  - Colectomy does not favor a beneficial outcome with PSC in those with UC; No indication to remove colon to benefit liver disease
- Liver transplant (↑ risk of post-transplant duct strictures): treatment of choice in end-stage disease; *See also Liver- Transplantation (Chapter 4.28)*
  - Among the highest in survival rate (85% at 5 yr, 70% at 10 yr); 20% post-transplant get histologic recurrence

COMPLICATIONS:
- Cholangiocarcinoma: occurs in 10-15% of patients; Highest incidence in patients with long-standing UC *or* cirrhotic-stage PSC
  - Difficult to diagnose due to insensitivity of current techniques: brush cytology or mucosal biopsy; High CA19-9 may be a clue
- Hepatocellular carcinoma: higher risk than previously appreciated; Screen (cirrhotics only) q12-24 months: U/S, AFP level
- Recurrent bacterial cholangitis: frequent in those with prior biliary surgery
- Dominant stricturing of extrahepatic ducts: occurs in 15-20% of patients
- Fatigue: (no treatment); Sicca Syndrome: (artificial tears); Steatorrhea: (pancreatic enzymes, antibiotics)
- Fat-soluble vitamin deficiency: Vit A: night blindness, Vit D: bone disease, Vit K: prolonged prothrombin time, Vit E: neurologic abnormalities
- Metabolic bone disease (Hepatic osteodystrophy) or Avascular Necrosis (AVN); Treatment: Ca/VitD/ Bisphosphonates, HRT
- Colon cancer: 50% risk of colon cancer – even without UC! Probably should get yearly screening colonoscopy

PROGNOSIS:
- Both PSC and PBC eventually progress to end-stage liver disease, requiring consideration for liver transplant (can reoccur after transplant)
  - Overall median survival without liver transplant: 9-12 years from time of diagnosis
- Follow Up: Visit (q 6-12 mon), LFTs (q 3-6 mon), Abd U/S & AFP (q 12 mon), Colonoscopy with biopsy (q 12 mon), BMD (at diagnosis and q 24 mon)

4.25 PREGNANCY PEARLS

(Am J Gastroenterol. 2004;99:2479-88 & 1999;94:1728-32)

GENERAL
- Liver histology and function do not change during pregnancy
- Maternal blood volume and cardiac output increase, without corresponding increase in hepatic blood flow = net decrease in blood flow to liver
- Labs remain normal: AST, ALT, GGT, Bili, PT/INR
  - Aϕ can ↑ 2-4x (due to placenta source), return to normal within 20 days; Also ↑ α1-AT, Ceruloplasmin, Fibrinogen, Cholesterol
  - Albumin can decrease slightly, due to dilution, contributing to ~20% decline in total serum protein concentration; Also ↓ ferritin
- Can see small esophageal varices in 50% of pregnant women
  - Maternal blood volume and cardiac output ↑ significantly, without a corresponding ↑ in hepatic blood flow = net decrease in fractional blood flow to liver
  - Enlargement of the uterus makes venous return via the IVC progressively more difficult
  - Hence, blood is shunted via the azygous system and the development of esophageal varices
- Avoid estrogen-based contraceptives if history of acute liver disease: After 5 years of OCP use, risk of hepatic adenoma ↑ 116-fold
  - Hepatic adenomas often regress with stopping estrogen, but can recur during pregnancy; surgical resection recommended
  - Peliosis hepatic: small venular cavities or lakes within the liver arising from injury to sinusoids: OCP & Anabolic steroid use

ACUTE FATTY LIVER OF PREGNANCY (AFLP)
- Sudden catastrophic illness occurring late in pregnancy with microvesicular fatty infiltration resulting in liver failure with PSE
- Rare disorder–rapid progression of liver failure in **3rd** trimester (can develop post-partum); Most are nulliparous (unlike HELLP)
  - Recessive disorder, recurrence rate of 15-25%; Women with AFLP should undergo genetic counseling
- Etiology: Fetal-maternal interaction; Fetus has deficiency in long-chain hydroxyacyl co-A dehydrogenase (LCHAD),
  - Leads to abnormal mitochondrial B-oxidation of FFA that accumulate in the mother and are highly toxic to maternal liver
- Histology: Microvesicular steatohepatitis with mild-modest necrosis *See also Liver- Histopathology of Liver (Chapter 4.19)*
- Clinical:
  - Largely non-specific; jaundice in most patients, N/V, malaise, thirst, altered mentation, RUQ pain
  - Severe: FHF, DIC, ARF, Coma, Death
  - Can occur with coexistent preeclampsia (50-100%): hypertension, proteinuria and edema
- Labs: ↑ PT, AST/ALT (<1000), Bili (<5), Ammonia, Uric acid, WBC; ↓ Platelets, Glucose; Viral serologies negative; ± DIC
  - *More severe synthetic dysfunction of AFLP helps distinguish from HELLP (the two are often difficult to distinguish)*
- Treatment: Immediate delivery of baby, Supportive ICU care, Recovery is usually complete and transplant rarely necessary
- Maternal mortality can range from 10-33%; AFLP may reoccur with subsequent pregnancies but its reoccurrence is very rare
- Child outcome: Previous mortality high as 90%
  - Child presents about 8 months with acute hepatic dysfunction: HSM, PSE, Fatty liver
    - Avoid this child's morbidity by testing for long-chain 3-hydroxyacyl-CoA dehydrogenase deficiency
  - Prompt dietary intervention by treating with medium-chain fatty acids equates to a much longer survival

AUTOIMMUNE HEPATITIS
- Usually not a problem, but may worsen
- Continue immunosuppressive drugs; Azathioprine/Imuran usually safe, but try to lower prednisone dose

CHAPTER 4.25 PREGNANCY PEARLS

BUDD-CHIARI SYNDROME: *See also Liver- Clots (Chapter 4.09)*
- Presents in **3rd** trimester to 3 months after delivery
- Pathology: centrilobular hemorrhage and necrosis, sinusoidal dilation, RBCs in space of Disse
- Clinical triad: *sudden onset* of abdominal pain, hepatomegaly, and ascites
- Labs show ascites with high protein in ~50% of patients; Hypercoagulable state is common
- Imaging: CT: compensatory hypertrophy of the caudate lobe due to its separate drainage into the IVC
  Doppler of portal and hepatic vessels and MRI establish hepatic vein occlusion

GALLSTONES
- Higher cholesterol saturation in bile; 30% have biliary sludge
- Increased progesterone leads to increased fasting gallbladder volume and reduced gallbladder emptying
- ERCP is generally safe as radiation exposure for fluoroscopy is below the fetal safety level
- Biliary colic tends to continue once it starts (30% recurrence) and if complicated by pancreatitis is an indication for ERCP/cholecystectomy
  - Pancreatitis has high maternal (10%) and fetal (13%) mortality in pregnancy
  - Impacted common bile duct stone with pancreatitis is an indication for ERCP with antibiotics
  - Cholecystectomy is best done in 2nd trimester either laparoscopically or by open method

INTRAHEPATIC CHOLESTASIS OF PREGNANCY (IHCP):
*Most common liver disorder **unique to pregnancy**, can occur anytime during pregnancy*
- Benign for mother, Higher fetal distress/prematurity (50%) requiring C-section in 30-60% and fetal loss (9%, higher if untreated)
  - Elective Delivery at 36-37 weeks
  - Recurrence rate of about 40-70% of subsequent pregnancies
- Etiology: **3rd** trimester or OCP use (Cholestasis effects of estrogen)
  - Defect in multi drug resistance 3 (MDR3) gene: a canalicular phospholipids/bile acid transporter
- Pathology: Bland cholestasis without necrosis or inflammation
- Clinical: **Severe pruritus** (worse at night) in 2nd or more commonly 3rd trimester, Visible jaundice (rare: 10-15%, but 2nd most common cause after viral)
  - Indicating Probably NOT IHCP: Fever, HSM, Pain, Jaundice without or preceding the severe pruritus
- Labs: AΦ ↑ 3-7 times (usually with normal GGT), Modest ↑ AST/ALT (up to 1000), Bili usually <5 mg/dl (again, jaundice is rare)
  - Labs may persist for months after delivery
- Treatment of pruritus: UDCA (8-15 mg/kg/day); Cholestyramine 4 gm 4/day (falling out of favor to use); Atarax/Vistaril minimal relief
  - Vit K before delivery to minimize bleeding or prn if bleeding (may be malabsorption via UDCA)
  - Pruritus should improve promptly after delivery (within 24 hours)
- Prognosis: Usually there is resolution immediately after delivery
  Recur with subsequent pregnancies and/or estrogen replacement in 40-70%; ? increased risk of other liver/biliary diseases

PRE-ECLAMPSIA/ECLAMPSIA/HELLP
- Pre-Eclampsia (triad): hypertension, proteinuria and edema
  - Risk factors: nulliparity (75%), multiple gestation (30%), maternal age >40, positive family history, chronic HTN, diabetes
  - Clinical also includes: nausea/vomiting, abdominal pain, blurry vision, sudden increase body weight, shock, renal failure
  - Presents in **3rd** trimester, but may occur up to 7 days postpartum (watch for it after delivery)
  - Wide spectrum of hepatic disease from mild elevations in LFTs to liver failure (20-30%)
    - ↑ AST/ALT (usually <10 × ULN), ↑ bili (usually <5 mg/dl)
  - Most feared complications: Eclampsia, HELLP syndrome, AFLP, Hepatic infarction, Subcapsular hematoma/Hepatic rupture
- Eclampsia: severe hypertension (>160/100 mmHg), Proteinuria (>5 g/24 hrs), Organ damage
  - Seizures: 25% before labor, 50% during labor, 25% within 72 hours postpartum
- HELLP (hemolysis (hence unconjugated bili), elevated liver enzymes, low platelets)
  - Incidence of HELLP occurs in: 0.5% of all pregnancies, 4-12% of preeclamptic patients; Recurrence: 3-25%
  - Occurs 70% prepartum (between 27-36 weeks), 30% post partum (up to 48 hrs after delivery)
  - Can occur in absence of hypertension (20%) and may precede other features of pre-eclampsia
  - Risk factors: Multiparty (unlike AFLP), Caucasian race, Age >35
  - Clinical: RUQ pain (60-90%), malaise/flu-like symptoms (90%), weight gain (60%), nausea/vomiting (35-50%), headache (30%)

- Labs: ↑ AST/ALT 2-50 × ULN, Other liver *function* remains normal (Bili, PT, Albumin); Jaundice is rare occurring in only 5%
  - Diagnosis: 1. Hemolysis on smear, ↑ LDH, ↑ Indirect bili; 2. AST >70 U/L; 3. Plts <100 × 10^9
- CT indicated to detect any liver rupture, subcapsular hematomas and intraparenchymal hemorrhage or infarction
- Biopsy (high risk & generally not needed) findings can be patchy: periportal hemorrhage, fibrin deposition, necrosis, ± steatosis

■ Treatment:
  - Stabilize mother, IVF, correct coagulopathy, Mg for seizure prophylaxis, HTN treatment
  - Early imaging to rule out infarcts/bleeds
  - Fetal monitoring; Beyond 34 weeks and evidence of lung maturity, delivery; If premature lungs, deliver after 48 hrs of steroids
  - Termination of pregnancy if evidence of fetal or maternal distress

■ Complications:
  - Spontaneous Intrahepatic hemorrhage: 1-2% of pre-eclamptic patients
  - Hepatic infarction (fever, leukocytosis, abdominal pain, AST/ALT >3,000); CT or MRI to rule out
  - Other maternal complications: DIC, abruptio placentae, ARF, pulmonary edema/ARDS, ascites, liver failure
  - Maternal mortality 3-40%, Fetal mortality 60%; Once delivered most babies with mature lungs do well
    - Improved mortality with awareness, imaging studies, aggressive surgical management with massive transfusions

VIRAL HEPATITIS:
*Most common cause of **jaundice in pregnancy**, can occur any time during pregnancy*

■ Hep A, B, C run a similar course, including the frequency, in pregnant and non-pregnant women
  - No need for early delivery or cesarean section; Breast-feeding should not be discouraged
■ Hepatitis E (India/Asia): Higher risk of fulminant hepatic failure 20% (<1% in non-pregnant)
  - Mortality: 1st trimester: 1.5%, 2nd: 8.5%, 3rd: 21% (2% of non-pregnant women)
■ Vertical Transmission of Viral Hepatitis; See also corresponding chapters
  - Hep A: Rare;
    - HAV vaccine and/or HAIG (passive immunization) is safe and recommended during pregnancy
    - Newborn of mother with HAV should be given HAIG within 48 hours of birth
  - Hep B: Transmission 1st Trimester (10%), 3rd Trimester (90%); All women tested in 3rd trimester
    - Test mom for HBsAg, if +, Protect baby after delivery with HBIG (0.5 ml) and Vaccine (0.5 ml at birth and 1 & 6 months)
    - Test mom for HBsAg, If -, Baby should only get full dose of Hep B Vaccine (not HBIG) at delivery
    - Hep B Vaccine is safe in pregnant patients
  - Hep C: Transmission is 5% (RNA levels >1 million can be associated with 50% transmission rate); No prophylaxis available
    - According to CDC, breastfeeding is not contraindicated; No documentation via breastfeeding has been reported
■ Herpes (HSV): can be fulminant in pregnant women, with high mortality
  - Present in 3rd trimester: fever, systemic symptoms, vesicular cutaneous rash may or may not be present
  - Can be association with encephalitis, pneumonitis
  - Liver enzymes may be as high as 25-40 × ULN; Bilirubin levels usually low, <3 mg/dl (*Anicteric liver failure*)
  - Biopsy: necrosis with viral inclusion bodies in viable hepatocytes
  - Treatment should be immediate with acyclovir (without there is 50% maternal mortality)
    - No need for termination of pregnancy unless no response to antiviral therapy

WILSON'S DISEASE
■ Ceruloplasmin gradually increase during pregnancy, reaching a maximum at term
  - Therefore will not be low with suspected diagnosis, and cannot be used as a good diagnostic marker in pregnancy!
■ Must continue therapy throughout pregnancy; D-penicillamine, Zinc (reduced dose in 3rd trimester and nursing)

DIFFERENTIAL DIAGNOSIS: FIRST TRIMESTER
- Nausea/vomiting: Hyperemesis gravidarum
- Elevations in LFTs: Viral hepatitis (HAV, HBV, HEV)
- RUQ pain: Gallstones

DIFFERENTIAL DIAGNOSIS: SECOND TRIMESTER
- RUQ pain: Gallstones
- Elevations in LFTs: Viral hepatitis: HAV, HBV, HEV, HSV (low bili); Pre-eclampsia, IHCP

DIFFERENTIAL DIAGNOSIS: THIRD TRIMESTER
- RUQ pain: Gallstones, Pre-eclampsia (hematoma, rupture)
- Elevations in LFTs:
  - Aφ: IHCP
  - AST/ALT: Viral hepatitis (A-E), HSV (low bili), Pre-eclampsia, HELLP, AFLP

4.26 PULMONARY COMPLICATIONS

HEPATOPULMONARY SYNDROME (HPS)
Definition:
- HPS triad:
  - History of chronic liver disease; Arterial hypoxemia on room air; Presence of intrapulmonary vascular dilation
- Types of HPS:
  - Type 1: Diffuse pulmonary vascular dilation; Microscopic; Common
  - Type 2: Discrete arteriovenous communications; Macroscopic; Uncommon

Epidemiology:
- Reported incidence between 4–29%

Etiologies:
- Develops independent of the cause of liver disease

Pathophysiology:
- Primary problem with intrapulmonary **vascular dilation** (as apposed to Portopulmonary hypertension) leading to AV shunting and hypoxemia; Two types of dilation:
  - Type 1: diffusion-perfusion defect
  - Type 2: anatomic shunt
- Why intrapulmonary vascular dilation: Not definitively known; Nitric oxide (NO) likely plays a role:
  - Exhaled NO levels are increased in those with HPS and normalize after transplant
  - Methylene blue (NO inhibitor) transiently improves HPS

Clinical Manifestations/Physical Exam:
- Varied symptoms: may complain of symptoms of chronic liver disease and/or have several pulmonary complaints (dyspnea, platypnea)
- Signs: dyspnea, telangiectasias, cyanosis, clubbing, pulmonary dysfunction that improves with O^2 (hypoxia, orthodeoxia)
  - Heart and lung exam is generally normal

Laboratory Studies:
- ABG (PaO_2 < 80 mmHg)

Diagnostic Studies:
- Blood gas on room air is first diagnostic test (PaO_2 < 80 mmHg) – hypoxia
- CXR: usually normal, unless concomitant disease present; may show increased bibasilar interstitial markings
- Pulmonary function testing (PFTs): restriction is common in liver disease; may show low diffusion capacity for carbon monoxide
- Contrast-enhanced echocardiography ("bubble-echo"): preferred modality for demonstrating intrapulmonary vascular dilation
  - Can also evaluate cardiac function and pulmonary artery pressures; Transesophageal more specific than transthoracic
  - Positive in up to 40% of cirrhotic patients with a normal ABG (Qualitative)
  - Concept: contrast (indocyanine green dye or agitated saline) injected with one of three scenarios:
    - Normal: contrast seen in right heart, but not in left heart (filtered by pulmonary capillaries)
    - Intracardiac shunt: contrast seen almost immediately in left heart
    - HPS: **contrast seen in left heart after 3–6 heart cycles** (dilation of pulmonary vasculature doesn't allow for filtering)
- Technetium-labeled macroaggregated albumin scan (Tc-MAA): less sensitive than contrast echo for detecting intrapulmonary vascular dilation
  - Can't evaluate cardiac function or pulmonary artery pressures; Positive scan is specific for HPS even with concomitant lung disease
  - Concept: ^{99m}Technetium-labeled albumin is injected and then a body perfusion scan is done with one of two scenarios:
    - Normal: technetium detected almost exclusively in lungs
    - HPS: technetium is detected in other organs as well (brain, spleen) due to limited lung filtering
      - Use Tc-MAA to calculate shunt index (% of uptake in brain compared to lungs): >6% is abnormal (Quantitative)

CHAPTER 4.26 PULMONARY COMPLICATIONS

- Pulmonary angiography: most invasive; not a standard diagnostic tool in HPS
  - May help to exclude other causes of hypoxia or identify focal AV malformations amenable to embolization (Type 2 shunt)
- Algorithm: Hypoxia confirmed » Contrast Echo:
  (−): Not HPS
  (+) » PFT's: (−): HPS
              (+): Tc-MAA scan » (<6%): HPS is minor contributor to hypoxia
                                 (>6%): HPS is a substantial contributor to hypoxia

Treatments:
- Supportive care with **oxygen**
- Medical therapy has been disappointing: beta blockers and nitrates have no benefit, NO inhibitors have no practical role
- Interventional radiology: TIPS may help, but is controversial and generally not recommended; Embolization of type 2 shunts may be an option
- Liver transplant: Treatment of choice; Complete resolution after OLT is possible; Improved oxygenation may take months or years
  - HPS is a strong risk factor for increased peri- and postoperative mortality and morbidity

Prognosis:
- Carries a moderate-poor prognosis (but better than PPHTN); median survival ~11 months
  - PaO_2 levels correlate with survival (i.e. lower PaO_2 = lower survival time)

PORTOPULMONARY HYPERTENSION (PPHTN)

Definition:
- Presence of Portal HTN inferred by cirrhosis on liver biopsy or clinical/radiographic evidence (absence of other causes of pulmonary HTN)
- Altered hemodynamics on right heart: - Elevated PAP (>25 mmHg mean at rest, >30 mmHg mean with exercise)
                                          - Elevated PVR (>240 dynes/sec/cm^5)
                                            - Normal PCWP

Epidemiology:
- Reported incidence between 0.7-16%

Etiologies:
- Develops independent of the cause of liver disease

Pathophysiology:
- Primary problem with intrapulmonary **vascular constriction** (as apposed to Hepatopulmonary Syndrome) leading to obliteration of arterioles
- Lung pathology: Plexiform lesion; Intimal and medial thickening
- What causes this series of events: Not definitively known; Humoral substances produced by splanchnic bed, bypass liver reaching the pulmonary endothelium and through portosystemic collaterals, cause:
  - Endothelial proliferation, Vasoconstriction, In situ thrombosis, Obliteration of blood vessels
  - Substances responsible: serotonin, interleukin-1, endothelin-1, glucagons, secretin, thromboxane B2, VIP

Clinical Manifestations/Physical Exam:
- Varied symptoms: may complain of symptoms of chronic liver disease and/or have several cardiac complaints (dyspnea, chest pain, syncope)
- Signs: Elevated JVP, edema and ascites can be signs of either cirrhosis or RHF
  - Heart exam abnormal: right ventricular heave, accentuated second heart sound, TR murmur
  - Lung exam is generally normal

Laboratory Studies:
- ABG (Respiratory alkalosis)

SECTION IV LIVER

Diagnostic Studies:
- Blood gas on room air may show respiratory alkalosis, but less hypoxia than HPS
- CXR: RV enlargement, prominent hilar pulmonary arteries, peripheral hypovascularity (pruning)
- EKG: right axis deviation, right atrial enlargement, right ventricular hypertrophy, right ventricular strain
- Echocardiography: may be diagnostic demonstrating elevated pulmonary pressures
- **Right heart catheterization:** if uncertainty with echo, cath can conclusively rule-in or rule-out the diagnosis
  - ↑ PAP, PVR; Normal PCWP
  - Gold standard; Determines severity with improved accuracy, measures degree of portal hypertension
- Must rule out other causes of pulmonary hypertension!
  - PFTs, Sleep study, VQ scan, Autoantibody testing, HIV testing, Left heart catheterization with ventriculogram

Treatments:
- Mild (mPAP <35 mmHg): Annual to biannual echocardiography
- Moderate (mPAP 35-50 mmHg): Supplemental oxygen, anticoagulation, pharmacotherapy, liver transplant
- Severe (mPAP >50 mmHg): Contraindication to liver transplant

- Anticoagulation of PPHTN (goal INR 1.5-2.0)
  - Proven survival benefit in patients with primary pulmonary hypertension; However, no studies specifically in patients with PPHTN
  - May be difficult to monitor therapy in PPHTN: ↑ risk of hemorrhagic complications and inherent coagulopathy with liver disease

- Prostanoids (Prostacyclin, Flolan): potent vasodilator with anti-platelet properties requiring continual IV infusion; Best studied drug in PPHTN
  - Improves hemodynamics and exercise tolerance, but may not improve long term survival
  - Side effects/Complications: line infections, flu-like symptoms, hypotension, hypersplenism

- Endothelin receptor antagonists (Bosentan/Tracleer): oral administered
  - Improves hemodynamics and exercise tolerance, but initial trials excluded patients with liver disease
  - Limited approval by FDA for patients *without* severe liver impairment

- Phosphodiesterase inhibitors (Sildenafil/Viagra): novel and promising medication for treatment of pulmonary hypertension

Prognosis:
- Carries a poor prognosis; median survival for severe PPHTN: 6 months; overall 5-year survival: <10%
  - Main cause of death is right-sided heart failure and infection
- Liver transplantation:
  - Pulmonary pressures often improve or normalize; 3 yr survival is not significantly different when compared to those *without* PPHTN
  - Severe PPHTN (mPAP >50 mmHg): nearly 100% mortality with that high of PAP
    - Vasodilator therapy followed by OLT may improve outcomes; combined liver/lung might be considered

NOTES

4.27 TRANSPLANT IMMUNOSUPPRESSION

- Steroids: broad immunosuppressive antibodies
  - Suppress antibody production and ability to recognize antigen, inhibit IL-2 release from macrophages
  - Used for both acute rejection and maintenance
  - Dose varies widely; As usual, minimal dosing or avoidance is best
  - S/E: hypertension, osteopenia, diabetes, dyslipidemia

- Tacrolimus (FK506/Prograf) Broadly referred to as "calcineurin inhibitor"
  - Prevents T-cell activation though inhibition of several critical transcription factors, including IL-2
  - Used for maintenance therapy and/or rejection (unlike Cyclosporine)
  - Dose 0.1 mg/kg daily in BID doses is a starting dose
  - S/E: Neurotoxicity (seizures, paresthesias, delirium, tremor; usually subsides with dosage reduction), DM, HTN, **Nephrotoxicity**
    Metabolized by P450, therefore meds that inhibit P450 will raise drug levels, meds that induce P450 will lower levels and ↑ rejection
    - Increased drug levels: erythro/clarithromycin, keto/fluconazole, metoclopramide, verapamil, diltiazem, amiodarone
    - Reduced drug Levels: phenytoin, carbamazepine, phenobarbital, rifampin, isoniazid, warfarin
  - Tacrolimus levels after transplant: During 0-6 months: 10-15; After 6 months: 5-10

- Cyclosporine (Neoral): Broadly referred to as "calcineurin inhibitor"
  - Prevents T-cell activation though inhibition of several critical transcription factors, including IL-2
  - Used for maintenance therapy, not rejection (unlike Tacrolimus)
  - Dose for maintenance generally: 8 mg/kg daily in BID doses
  - S/E: Neurotoxicity (seizures, paresthesias, delirium, tremor; usually subsides with dosage reduction), DM, HTN, **Nephrotoxicity**
    Metabolized by P450, therefore meds that inhibit P450 will raise drug levels, meds that induce P450 will lower levels and ↑ rejection
    - Increased drug levels: erythro/clarithromycin, keto/fluconazole, metoclopramide, verapamil, diltiazem, amiodarone
    - Reduced drug Levels: phenytoin, carbamazepine, phenobarbital, rifampin, isoniazid, warfarin
  - Cyclosporin levels after transplant: During 0-6 months: 200-225; During 6-12 months: 180-200; After 12 months: 150-180

- Azathioprine (Imuran): Broadly referred to as "antiproliferative agent"
  - Metabolized to 6MP in liver; Interferes with DNA synthesis: Inhibits purine biosynthesis & inhibits T-lymphocytes
  - Used for maintenance therapy, not rejection
  - Dose for maintenance generally: 2 mg/kg daily (po or IV)
  - S/E: bone marrow suppression; *See also IBD- Treatment: Crohn's and U/C (Chapter 3.03)*

- Mycophenolate (Cellcept): Broadly referred to as "antiproliferative agent"
  - Impairs lymphocyte function by blocking purine biosynthesis via inosine monophosphate dehydrogenase; Inhibits B & T lymphocytes
  - Used for maintenance therapy, not rejection
  - Dose for maintenance generally: 1 gm BID
  - S/E: diarrhea, leucopenia, opportunistic infections (does not cause CRF)

- Sirolimus (Rapamune): A macrolide antibiotic
  - Structurally related to Tacrolimus and shares same binding site, inhibits both B & T cells
  - Useful alternative to calcineurin inhibitors
  - Dose for maintenance: 2-10 g/day
  - S/E: Less renal toxicity; Many don't use 2° to ↑ risk of **hepatic artery thrombosis** post-op and hypertriglyceridemia
  - Sirolimus levels after transplant: During 0-6 months: 10-12; After 6 months: 5-10 with goal being less than 5 mg/day after 6 months

CHAPTER 4.27   TRANSPLANT IMMUNOSUPPRESSION

- Muromonab-CD3 (OKT3)
  - Mouse antibody against human T3 cells
  - Generally used for steroid resistant rejection with a 10 day course
  - Dose is 5 mg/day IV for 10 days
  - S/E: anaphylaxis, long term risk of lymphoproliferative disease after transplant

- **Typical regimes:** Calcineurin inhibitor (Tacrolimus or Cyclosporine) plus Antiproliferative agent (Azathioprine or Mycophenolate) plus Steroids
  - Example: Prednisone, Cyclosporine and Azathioprine
  - Some only use two agents, such as: Prednisone and Tacrolimus

4.28 TRANSPLANTATION

(Hepatology. 2005;41:1-26)

REFERRAL:
- Decision ultimately rests with the transplant center
  - Transplant when the natural history of liver disease suggest a better survival with transplant
- United Network for Organ Sharing (www.UNOS.org): develops minimum criteria for listing
- Evaluate for listing when Child-Pugh ≥7 (B) or MELD ≥10, or evidence of decompensation (i.e. GI bleed, PSE, Ascites)

INDICATIONS:
- Acute liver failure/Fulminant hepatic failure (7%): These patients are assigned the highest priority (called Status 1)
  - Cryptogenic, HAV, HBV, Drug induced (acetaminophen), Metabolic (Wilson's), Vascular (ischemia), Toxin (Amanita)

- ESLD: Cirrhosis with liver failure (80%); **Those with Child-Pugh ≥7 (B) or MELD ≥10–15 should be considered for transplant**
  - **HCV** (50% of the 80%), ETOH, HBV, Autoimmune, PBC, PSC, NASH, Budd-Chiari, Sarcoid, Polycystic liver disease, Cryptogenic

- Congenital:
  - Hemochromatosis, Wilson's, α1-AT, Cystic fibrosis, Congenital hepatic fibrosis, Oxylosis, Hereditary/Familial amyloidosis

- Hepatic Tumor (10%):
  - Hepatocellular carcinoma (HCC): can be associated with: HBV, HCV, Heriditary Hemochromatosis, NASH with Cirrhosis
    - Milian Criteria (represent those acceptable to transplant): 1 tumor <5 cm, 2 or 3 tumors <3 cm; No metastasis
  - Hepatic adenoma, Carcinoid tumor

- Other: Recurrent or severe encephalopathy, Refractory ascites, SBP, Recurrent variceal bleeding
  Hepatorenal syndrome
  Bilirubin >10 mg/dl, Albumin <3 g/dl, PT >3 sec above control

CONTRAINDICATIONS:
- Absolute:
  - Uncontrolled sepsis/infection, Active ETOH/Substance abuse, Extrahepatic malignancy, Inadequate social support
  - Hepatocellular carcinoma (see Milian criteria, above); Extensive portal and/or mesenteric vein thrombosis
  - Severe comorbidities: advanced cardiac disease (CAD, CHF, Cor pulmonale), Advanced HIV/AIDS
- Relative (depends on severity of conditions and experience of center)
  - Cholangiocarcinoma, Pulmonary hypertension (uncontrolled), Previous extensive abdominal surgery, Advance age (?)
  - Thrombosis: Portal vein, Hepatic artery; HIV/AIDS infection

EVALUATION/SCORING: The sickest first . . .
- **Child-Turcotte-Pugh class** (A: 5-6, B: 7-9, C: 10-15); *See also Liver- Cirrhosis & Encephalopathy (Chapter 4.08)*
  Generally those B or C are considered for transplant
- **MELD: Model for End Stage Liver Disease** (originally used for pre-mortality risk with TIPS)
  - Used to stratify patients on liver transplant list; Removes subjectivity of physician bias
  - Continuous measurement of disease activity; Independent of complications of PHTN such as varices, SBP
  - Based on Cr, INR & total bilirubin to predict 3 month survival in patients with a variety of underlying forms of liver disease
    - Will probably incorporate the use of sodium (and hence indirectly, ascites) in the future (Gastroenterology. 2006;130:1652-1660)

CHAPTER 4.28 TRANSPLANTATION

- Calculate: Yahoo/Google search 'MELD score' for free online calculators
  Mayo MELD Score = 11.2 ln (INR) + 3.78 ln (Bilirubin) + 9.57 ln (Cr) + 6.43 (rounded to nearest integer)
- **PELD:** Pediatric model for end stage liver disease; Based on bili, INR, albumin, age, growth failure (no creatinine used)
- Blood Type
- Kings College Criteria/Acute Liver Failure; *See also Liver- Acute Liver Failure (Chapter 4.03)*

WORK UP/LABORATORY STUDIES:

- Studies: CT brain (rule out bleed and for ICP monitoring in Acute Fulminant patients)
  Liver Vascular/Doppler ultrasound, CT or MRI abdomen, DEXA scan
  TTE, EKG, CXR, Spirometry

- Labs: PT/PTT, CMP/LFT, CBC/Diff, Type/Screen, ABG, CMV IgG, Vitamin: A,E,D25, TSH, HIV, RPR, VZV titer, AFP, CA19-9
  Hepatitis Panel (Acute and Remote), HCV Quant (viral load) & genotype, HBV DNA, Amylase/Lipase, Lactate, Ammonia
  Urine/Blood toxicology (acetaminophen levels q 1–2 hr until peak determined), Random cortisol, Blood/Urine cultures
  Possibly needed: Iron studies, ANA, AMA, ASMA, Ceruloplasmin/serum copper, α1-AT, HCG (♀), CK/Troponin

- Consults: Cardiology/Anesthesia
  Psychiatry if appropriate
  Social Service, Chemical dependency if appropriate

POST-OP (1–4 WEEKS): *See also Liver- Transplant Immunosuppression (Chapter 4.27)*
Rejection
- 30–60% experience acute cellular rejection within first 3 months (histological diagnosis); Occurs most common with FHF transplants
- Elevated liver enzymes within first 7–10 days post-op, may be first indication of problem with graft and warrants a biopsy
- Liver biopsy is gold standard for diagnosis of cellular rejection
  - DDX of rejection: Hepatic artery or portal vein thrombus, biliary leak, cholangitis, drug toxicity, recurrent viral hepatitis, infection
  - Workup: drug levels, ultrasound, cholangiogram, cultures, liver biopsy is only way to prove rejection
- Early recognition key; Treat with **steroid pulse** (85% response rate) or alternatively **Muromonab-CD3 (OKT3)** (90% response rate)

Other Acute Complications
- Central Pontine Myelinosis:
  - Chronic ↓ Na » brain secretes osmoles/help ↓ swelling » rapid correction » ↑ serum osmo » rapid H_2O egress » acute brain dehydration
  - Mostly seen as a complication of fulminant patients, after new liver, rapid overcorrection of low Na; Prior to OLT, Na should be >120

POST-OP (>4 WEEKS): *See also Liver- Transplant Immunosuppression (Chapter 4.27)*
Rejection
- Chronic rejection characterized by: insidious but progressive rise in Aφ and bilirubin, *i.e. rejection is typically a biliary phenomenon;* Synthetic function usually intact until late stages
- Liver biopsy is gold standard for diagnosis of cellular rejection
  - DDX: **CMV infections,** Incomplete treatment of rejection
    Post-op (hepatic artery or portal vein thrombus, biliary leak)
    Medications (Tacrolimus, Cyclosporine), other opportunistic infections: EBV, fungal
- Treatment of chronic rejection:
  - Steroid pulse and consider need for re-transplantation

SECTION IV LIVER

COMPLICATIONS:

- Medical complications:
  - Osteoporosis: Steroids ↓ bone formation, ↑ bone resorption; Tacrolimus/Cyclosporine promote rapid bone turnover
    - Treat with bisphosphonates and/or calcium with vitamin D
  - Diabetes: Steroid use promotes hyperglycemia, 33% of patients in first year; Insulin resistance ↑ with Tacrolimus/Cyclosporine
    - Treat with diet and exercise
  - Obesity: 20-40% of post OLT patients become obese (BMI >30)
    - No difference between OLT and Non-OLT patients: OLT patients have new lease on life and ↑ food consumption
    - Treat with diet and exercise
  - Hyperlipidemia: After 1 year, hyperlipidemia in 24% of patients taking Cyclosporine, 5% of patients taking Tacrolimus
    - Treat with diet and exercise; Statins
  - Hypertension: Tacrolimus/Cyclosporin thought to promote renal vasoconstriction, Steroids ↑ Na retention, weight gain
    - Treat 1st line: CCB (dihydropyridine preferred): decreases vasoconstriction which is thought to be the cause
    - Others: Thiazides with CCB, ACE-I (can ↑ K and ↓ GFR), BB (not as effective due to post OLT low rennin state)
- Need for retransplant (10%):
  - Early transplant:
    - For primary nonfunctioning graft and/or **hepatic artery thrombosis** (common in children/size-mismatched grafts)
  - Late transplant:
    - Recurrence original disease: Hep B/C, Autoimmune, PBC/PSC, NASH, Hemochromatosis, Malignancy, Chronic rejection
  - Diseases that do NOT reoccur after transplant, and therefore not requiring retransplant:
    - Wilson's, α1-AT, Fulminant of unknown cause, Glycogen storage disease, Extrahepatic biliary atresia, Benign tumors
- CMV Infection:
  - Most occur 1-4 months after transplant; Greatest risk: D+/R−; Prophylaxis with ganciclovir or acyclovir
  - Symptoms: fever, malaise, leucopenia, thrombocytopenia, organ involvement (hepatitis, pancreatitis, retinitis, gastroenteritis)
  - Liver Biopsy: viral inclusions; Labs: CMV DNA assay correlates with viremia
  - Treatment: 2-4 week course of ganciclovir
- Pneumocystis Carinii Pneumonia (PCP) infection:
  - Symptoms: fever, shortness of breath, nonproductive cough
  - Diagnosis: bronchoscopy with bronchoalveolar lavage
  - Prophylaxis: Bactrim; If noncompliant, should have high index of suspicion
- Hepatitis C:
  - Almost all patients with HCV, have recurrent disease (nearly 100%); Treatment may be necessary; **See also Liver- Hepatitis C (Chapter 4.15)**
- Posttransplant Lymphoproliferative Disorder (PTLD) occurs in 10%: most are B cell type related to EBV and Immunosuppression (OKT3 use)
  - Symptoms: fever, LAN
  - Diagnosis: biopsy
  - Treatment: reduce immunosuppression; Referral to oncology is necessary for consideration of chemo or radiation
- Malignancy (due to immunosuppression): 40% get skin cancers (squamous cell) & should avoid UV light; Cervical cancer common too!

PROGNOSIS:

- Survival: 1-yr survival up to 90%, 5-yr survival up to 80%
  - Best to worst survival based on reason for transplant: Familial amyloid > PBC/PSC > ETOH > HCV > FHF
  - <2% of grafts lost to rejection

NOTES

4.29 WILSON'S DISEASE

(Hepatology. 2003;37:1475-92)

DEFINITION:
- Autosomal recessive inherited disorder of **copper overload** secondary to deficiency of an enzyme derived from liver cells (↓ secretion)
- Other inheritable forms of liver disease: α1-AT, Hemochromatosis

EPIDEMIOLOGY:
- 1 in 30,000 is homozygous and 1 in 100 is a heterozygous carrier
- Usually manifests before age 30; almost always before 40

ETIOLOGIES:
- Autosomal recessive; Gene located on chromosome 13, codes for P-type adenosine triphosphatase, a copper-transport protein
  - Most likely causes a defect in transfer of hepatocellular lysosomal copper into bile, thereby resulting in copper retention
  - i.e. impaired copper secretion into the bile, thereby resulting in copper retention

PATHOPHYSIOLOGY:
- Impaired copper transport and *secretion* (Hereditary Hemochromatosis is increased iron *absorption*)
  - Copper homeostasis is achieved via biliary secretion; Intestinal absorption is normal but biliary secretion is decreased
  - ↓ ceruloplasmin is not the cause of Wilson's rather it is an effect of the abnormal cellular trafficking of copper
- ATP-7B gene involved, located on chromosome 13
  - The number of clinically important mutations makes genetic testing less useful (as opposed to genetic testing for HH)

CLINICAL MANIFESTATIONS/PHYSICAL EXAM:
- May be completely asymptomatic or have devastating neurological symptoms
- Copper retention in liver:
  - Chronic hepatitis and cirrhosis, rarely fulminant hepatic failure (♀ > ♂) which is uniformly fatal without transplant
  - Always get a ceruloplasmin in young people with hepatitis or steatosis
- Copper retention in CNS/Neuro:
  - Neuro psych disorders: psychosis/depression
  - Tremor, ataxia
  - Kayser-Fleischer rings in eyes (copper deposition in periphery of cornea) or sunflower cataracts (do not interfere with vision)
  - Dementia
- Hemolytic anemia (coombs negative)
- Other systems involved: Joints (arthropathy), Kidneys (nephrolithiasis), blue discoloration of base of fingernails (Azure lunulae) is rare

Always have high index of suspicion in patient with unexplained hepatic, neurological or psychiatric disease

LABORATORY STUDIES:
- If ↓ **ceruloplasmin or ↑ 24 hr urine copper = liver biopsy for histology and quantitative copper determination**
- ↓ serum ceruloplasmin (copper binding protein); therefore ↑ serum & urinary copper
  Diagnostic criteria (any one of below):
  - Ceruloplasmin <200 mg/L (normal is 230-500 mg/L or 21-45 mcg/dL) and KF rings
  - Ceruloplasmin <200 mg/L and Hepatic copper content >250 mcg/gm dry weight on liver biopsy (normal is 38 mcg/gm)
  - Ceruloplasmin <200 mg/L and Urinary excretion > than 100 mcg copper in 24 hrs w/o administering penicillamine (normal is <30 mcg/dl)
  - Normal Ceruloplasmin and abnormally low incorporation of ^{64}CU into ceruloplasmin despite the normal level (rarely, if ever, used)

CHAPTER 4.29 WILSON'S DISEASE

- **Biopsy changes:** hepatic steatosis, chronic hepatitis, cirrhosis, hepatic concentration >250 mcg/gm and can be as high as 3,000 mcg/gm
- **Aφ often low** in Wilson's, especially fulminant disease (i.e. a liver problem that causes a low Aφ); Low uric acid
- AST/ALT >1 because of hemolysis
- Can see elevated copper in other cholestatic liver disease (PBC, extrahepatic biliary obstruction): usually clinical presentation can differentiate
- Often have hemolysis with fulminate Wilson's: ? plasmapheresis as a treatment

DIAGNOSTIC STUDIES:
Algorithm of suspected Wilson's with unexplained liver disease ± Neurological/psychiatric symptoms
- Check: AST, ALT, Bilirubin, Albumin, INR, CBC, Serum ceruloplasmin, 24 hr urinary copper, slit lamp exam for KF rings:
  - Low serum ceruloplasmin and KF rings present » Diagnosis established: treat patient and screen family
  - Normal ceruloplasmin, 24 hr urinary copper, LFTs, KF rings absent » Continue evaluation for alternative diagnosis
  - Any of these three scenarios:
    -Normal ceruloplasmin, KF rings present, LFTs abnormal OR
    -Low serum ceruloplasmin, KF rings absent, Normal LFTs, Persistent symptoms (hemolysis, splenomegaly, etc) OR
    -Low serum ceruloplasmin, KF rings absent, LFTs abnormal or elevated urinary copper
      » Liver biopsy with histology, histochemistry and copper quantification:
        -Copper content >250 mcg/gm and consistent histology » Diagnosis established: treat patient and screen family
        -Copper content <250 mcg/gm or histology not consistent » Continue evaluation for alternative diagnosis

TREATMENTS:
- D-penicillamine + Pyridoxine (Vit B6): Chelation therapy that induces cupriuria, also has some immunosuppressant actions
  - Side effects: fever, rash, neutropenia/thrombocytopenia (aplastic anemia), nephrotoxicity (proteinuria), Lupus-like syndrome
    - Occasionally up to 20% of patients may have irreversible worsening of their neurological symptoms
  - Dosage: start with divided doses: 250-500 mg/day, increased by 250 mg increments every 4-7 days to max: 1000-2000 mg/day
    - Maintenance is usually 750-1000 mg/day divided into BID doses
    - Food inhibits absorption, so give 1 hour prior or 2 hours after meals
    - Best monitor of therapy: Urine copper (should be in vicinity of 200-500 mcg per day on treatment)
    - CBC should be checked weekly for 1 month then every 1-2 months for 6 months
  - Pyridoxine (Vit B6) should be given 25-50 mg/day (to blunt side effects and prevent B6 depletion)
- Trientine (if intolerant of penicillamine, **most use as 1st line therapy**): Chelation therapy that induces cupriuria
  - Side effects (fewer): gastritis, sideroblastic anemia, aplastic anemia (rare); Pregnancy: risk unknown and it shouldn't be used
  - Dosage: start with divided doses: 750-1000 mg/day
    - Maintenance is usually 750-1000 mg/day divided into BID doses
    - Food inhibits absorption, so give 1 hour prior or 2 hours after meals
    - Also chelates iron, and their coadministration should be avoided since the complex with iron is toxic
    - Best monitor of therapy: Urine copper (should be in vicinity of 200-500 mcg per day on treatment)
- Oral zinc acetate, normally used for maintenance/asymptomatic; dosage: 50 mg po TID
  - Does not help in chelation, rather ↓ gut copper absorption and prevents more uptake
  - Side effects (very few): gastric irritation, not to be given with chelators as rendered ineffective
  - Good alternative to maintaining copper load in females that are pregnant
- With hemolysis (subfulminate or fulminate cases): ? plasmapheresis
- Fulminant Wilson's disease should be treated promptly with transplant as recovery is unusual without a transplant
  - Can often occur in young persons who are non-compliant with their meds because they feel well

SECTION IV LIVER

- Genetic counseling/screening for family members; 25% of siblings and treatment before cirrhosis is essentially curative
  - Screening after age 5 with LFTs, ceruloplasmin, and slit-lamp exam: if normal repeat every 5 years until age 20

COMPLICATIONS:
- This is an inheritable disease; Once patient is diagnosed, all first-degree relatives should be screened!
  - If low ceruloplasmin, 24 hr urinary copper followed by liver biopsy for histology and quantitative copper
- Patients presenting with complications of chronic liver disease or fulminant hepatic failure should be quickly considered for OLT
- Reports of HCC are rare, even though they may have liver fibrosis at a young age

PROGNOSIS:
- Neurological symptoms usually improve with therapy
- If liver transplant, it is considered a cure like α1-AT (and unlike Hemochromatosis which needs to periodically be followed)

V

PANCREAS/BILIARY

5.01 CHOLANGIOCARCINOMA

DEFINITION:
- Bile duct cancers that arise from the epithelial cells of the bile ducts (does not include gallbladder or ampullary cancer)
- Classification:
  - Intrahepatic: originate from small or large intrahepatic ducts proximal to right and left hepatic duct bifurcation
  - Perihilar Extrahepatic (65%): includes the confluence of the right and left hepatic duct bifurcation
    - Further classified according to involvement of the hepatic ducts: Bismuth Classification (Figure)
    - Type I: tumors below the confluence
    - Type II: tumors reaching the confluence
    - Type IIIA & IIIB: tumors occluding the common hepatic and Right or Left hepatic duct
    - Type IV: tumors that are multicentric or involving confluence and both hepatic ducts
    - Klatskin tumors: term used to define involvement of the common hepatic duct bifurcation
  - Distal Extrahepatic: from common bile duct to the point where the bile duct lies posterior to the duodenum

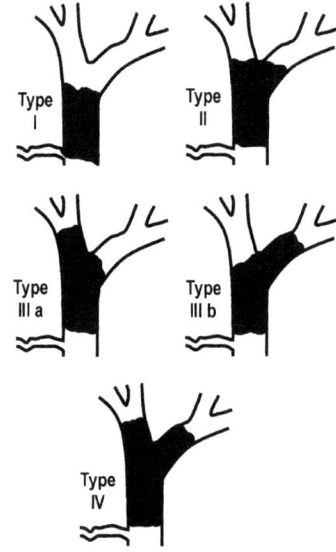

EPIDEMIOLOGY:
- Rare; Represent 3% of GI malignancies with an incidence of 1-2 per 100,000; ♂ > ♀
- Nearly all (>90%) are adenocarcinomas, further divided into:
  - Sclerosing: invade bile duct early, associated with low respectability and cure rates
  - Nodular: constricting annular lesion of the bile duct and highly invasive
  - Papillary: rare, present as bulky masses in the common bile duct and early presenting symptoms

ETIOLOGIES:
- Several risk factors identified:
  - PSC/UC patients represents 30% of all diagnosed cholangiocarcinoma (lifetime risk is 10-15% for PSC/UC patient)
    - Difficult to diagnose since biliary tree is abnormal to begin with; >30% diagnosed within 2 years of PSC diagnosis
    - Screening suggested by some clinicians: US and CA19-9 annually or semi-annually if cirrhotic
    - A CA19-9 >100 U/ml and a malignant appearing stricture has been used in lieu of tissue diagnosis to begin treatment

CHAPTER 5.01 CHOLANGIOCARCINOMA

- Choledochal cysts, Caroli's syndrome, Congenital hepatic fibrosis: 15% risk of malignant change (average age at diagnosis is 34)
  - Unclear why; could possibly be related to biliary stasis or chronic inflammation via pancreatic juice reflux
- Parasitic infection:
  - Infection with liver flukes (Clonorchis and Opisthorchis) is associated with intrahepatic bile duct cancer, especially in Asia
  - Consuming undercooked fish leads to adult worms laying eggs in the biliary system leading to chronic inflammation
- Hepatolithiasis and Cholelithiasis:
  - Unclear if gallstones really predispose to cholangiocarcinoma
  - There is a clear association with intrahepatic stones (much higher prevalence in Asia) and cholangiocarcinoma
- Toxic exposures:
  - Thorotrast, an old radiologic contrast agent banded in the 1960's showed a clear association
  - Association of smoking and alcohol are conflicting as is occupational exposures (auto, rubber, wood)
- Lynch syndrome II and Multiple biliary papillomatosis
  - Have an associated increased risk
- Chronic liver disease:
  - HBV, HCV, and Cirrhosis regardless of etiology are believed to be risk factors
- Other possible risks:
  - Diabetes, HIV infection

PATHOPHYSIOLOGY:

- Conversion from normal to malignant bile epithelium is probably a stepwise accumulation of genetic mishaps similar to colon cancer
  - Evidence of such genetic abnormalities is poorly understood
  - Evidence of oncogenes (K-ras) and tumor suppressor genes (p53) have been described

CLINICAL MANIFESTATIONS/PHYSICAL EXAM:

- Usually symptomatic when there is obstruction of the biliary system causing **painless jaundice** and:
  - Pruritus-intermittent (66%), abdominal pain (30-50%), weight loss (30-50%), fever (10-20%), clay-colored stools and dark urine
- Signs include jaundice (90%), hepatomegaly (25-40%), and rarely a RUQ mass (10%) or Courvoisier's sign (palpable gallbladder)
- The **triad of cholestasis, abdominal pain, and weight loss** is suggestive of hepatobiliary or pancreatic malignancy
  - The differential also includes choledocholithiasis, secondary biliary strictures (postoperative), PSC, pancreatic (chronic/cancer)
- Those affecting only the intrahepatic ducts (<10%) are less likely to present with jaundice, rather they have RUQ pain, weight loss and ↑ Aφ

LABORATORY STUDIES:

- Suggest biliary obstruction: total bili frequently >10 mg/dl with ↑ direct bili, Aφ (2-10 × ULN), GGT
  - ALT/AST may be normal; Chronic biliary obstruction often leads to liver dysfunction with ↑ ALT/AST and PT

Tumor markers: most have been studied/used with PSC patients who have an increased incidence of cholangiocarcinoma

- CEA: a level >5.2 ng/ml has been suggested to be 68% sensitive and 82% specific (not very good)
- CA19-9: a level >180 U/ml has been suggested to be 67% sensitive and 98% specific; Some use a value >400 U/ml
  - May also be useful for following the effect of treatment and to detect recurrent disease
- The use of combined CEA and CA 19-9 formula for PSC patients has been suggested; Formula = CA19-9 + (CEA × 40)
  - Value >400 (specificity 100%, sensitivity 66%); Gastro 1995;108:865-9

DIAGNOSTIC STUDIES:

- U/S: demonstrates duct obstruction (89% of the time) and localization of obstruction (94% sensitivity)
  - Obstructing mass is suggested by duct dilation (>6 mm) in the absence of stones/GB Surgery
  - Intrahepatic appear as mass lesion; perihilar and extrahepatic may not be detected
  - Color doppler has added an adjunct: invasion of portal vein or hepatic artery indicates unresectability

SECTION V PANCREAS/BILIARY

- CT: Useful for detecting intrahepatic tumors and level of biliary obstruction:
  - Delayed tumor enhancement with IV contrast is noted in approximately 75% of intrahepatic cholangiocarcinomas
  - Klatskin: intrahepatic ductal dilation (without extrahepatic dilation) with a contracted gallbladder
  - Cystic duct stone/tumor: Intrahepatic and extrahepatic duct not dilated with a distended gallbladder
  - Common bile duct/ampulla/pancreatic mass: dilated intrahepatic and extrahepatic ducts and a distended gallbladder
  - Invasion of portal vein: dilated intrahepatic and extrahepatic ducts with a atrophied hepatic lobe and hypertrophic contralateral lobe
  - Note: abdominal LAN does not always mean malignancy
- MRCP: Noninvasive means for evaluating intrahepatic, extrahepatic and pancreatic ducts; ERCP should be reserved for therapeutic options
  - Hypointense lesion on T1, Hyperintense on T2
  - While the role of MRCP for preoperative evaluation is evolving, it likely will be the primary test
- Cholangiography via ERCP (Endoscopic retrograde cholangiopancreatography) or PTC (percutaneous transhepatic cholangiogram)
  - Preoperative cholangiography may be indicated either diagnostically or therapeutically for any patients with biliary obstruction
  - Which to do depends largely on level of each expertise available; However, in PSC patients percutaneous approach is difficult
  - Both can provide bile samples, cytology (sensitivity 35-69%) and biopsy (only raises sensitivity to 43-88%) and stenting
    - In other words, a negative test does not rule out malignant disease
    - Combining brush cytology and an abnormal CA19-9 has a sensitivity of 88% and specificity of 97%
- EUS: best for distal bile duct lesions with visualizing the local extent of the primary tumor and status of lymph nodes
  - Also allows for FNA of tumor or lymph nodes which provides better sensitivity for detecting malignancy compared to ERCP brushing
  - The role for imaging and staging proximal bile duct lesions is uncertain and based upon clinical experience
- PET scan: permits visualization due to high glucose uptake in bile duct epithelium
  - Better for staging rather than diagnosing
  - False positives may occur with acute cholangitis (especially with PSC patients who are prone to repeat cholangitis)
- Angiography: can accurately document vascular encasement or thrombosis of the portal vein and hepatic artery
  - Rarely needed due to CT and MRCP non invasive studies
- Bottom-line with diagnostic modalities
  - Unless evidence of metastases, true respectability can only be determined by operative evaluation (laparoscopy or laparotomy)
- Is tissue the issue?
  - Biopsies obtained by a variety of means can be difficult
    - May not be necessary in those with characteristic findings or those who are planning palliative therapy
  - A tissue diagnosis is important in:
    - Strictures with indeterminate origin (those with a history of bile duct surgery, bile duct stones or PSC)
    - Patient or Surgeon are reluctant to proceed with surgery without a firm diagnosis
    - Prior to chemotherapy or radiation therapy, especially if taking place in research protocol

TREATMENTS:
- Surgery provides the only possibility for cure
  - Distal Extrahepatic have highest respectability rates, while Perihilar have lowest
  - Traditional guidelines for respectability:
    - Absence of nodal, distant liver, or disseminated metastases, no invasion into portal vein or hepatic artery
  - Preoperative biliary stenting/decompression is debated: some surgeons feel it is a hindrance to determining tumor extent
    - In general, it is preferable to avoid stents if possible; However, cholestasis and liver dysfunction can develop rapidly
    - Some surgeons proceed directly to surgery without preoperative biliary drainage
    - Some perform nonoperative biliary drainage in those with a bilirubin >10mg/dl and stage Laparoscopically

- Surgery:
  - Whipple's for distal lesions: Five-year survival 15–25%, but high as 50%
  - Hepatic resection for intrahepatic lesions: Three-year survival 22–66% depending on lymph node status
  - Bismuth classification serves as a guide for perihilar:
    - Type I & II: en block resection of extrahepatic bile ducts and gallbladder with Roux-en-Y hepaticojejunostomy
    - Type III: similar to above but may require hepatic lobectomy
    - Type III & IV are potentially curative within highly specialized centers with expertise
  - Liver transplant is not considered a standard form of therapy due to high recurrence rates (virtually 100%)
- Adjuvant treatment: after surgical resection, most recurrence is local
  - Radiation therapy: retrospective series suggest a benefit for incomplete resection
  - Chemotherapy: most studies fail to show a benefit
  - Chemoradiotherapy: remains unproven
  - Several possibilities exist however, depending on resection margins following surgery
- Neoadjuvant treatment
  - Usually not an option as most are jaundice with poor performance status; Currently not a standard approach

■ Palliative Treatment: 50–90% of patients present with unresectable disease and life expectancy is only months
- Goal: improve symptoms of pain, pruritus, jaundice, and improve quality of life
- Endoscopic stenting is possible in 70–95% of patients
  - Unilateral stenting (either right or left hepatic duct) appears to be sufficient (only 25% of liver needs drainage for relief)
  - MRCP often helps guide decision making on which side to stent to give maximal drainage potential
  - Metal (as opposed to plastic) stents are associated with longer patency rates (they can not be removed once deployed)
- Biliary-enteric bypass rather than endoscopic stenting is an option for some, particularly those with unresectable hilar cancer
- Photodynamic therapy is emerging and may be an important palliative option in those with unresectable cancer

PROGNOSIS:
■ Highly lethal because most are locally advanced at presentation; Average 5 year survival: 5–10%

5.02 CHOLECYSTITIS & CHOLANGITIS

CHOLECYSTITIS

Definition:
- Inflammation of the gallbladder

Etiologies:
- *E. coli*, Klebsiella, Enterococcus, and Enterobacter are the usual pathogens
- DDX: hepatitis, liver mets, pancreatitis, pseudocyst, PUD, pyelonephritis, renal stones, pneumonia, pulmonary embolism, myocardial infarction, pre-eruptive zoster
- Rheumatalogic disease association: Polyarteritis nodosa results in vasculitis of cystic duct artery and causes cholecystitis

Pathophysiology:
- Obstruction of the cystic duct by a gallstone
- Acalculous with sludge (? Ischemic)
- Erythromycin hepatotoxicity can present with symptoms mimicking acute cholecystitis; Important to elicit antibiotic history during evaluation
  - A consistent history and associated eosinophilia may assist in identifying the syndrome

Clinical Manifestations/Physical Exam:
- History: nausea/vomiting (>50% patients), fever, steady sever epigastric and **RUQ pain** usually lasting longer than 4-6 hours
- Jaundice may be present
- **Murphy's sign:** ↑ RUQ pain on inspiration, ± palpable gallbladder

Laboratory Studies:
- ↑ WBC, ± ↑ bilirubin and Aφ, and ± ↑ amylase (even in absence of pancreatitis)
- Transaminases (ALT/AST) >500 or Bilirubin >4 mg/dl » choledocholithiasis

Diagnostic Studies:
- **RUQ U/S:** high sensitivity and specificity for gallstones
  - Specific signs of cholecystitis include pericholecystic fluid, edema of the gallbladder wall, and sonographic Murphy's sign
- **HIDA** (hepatobiliary iminodiacetic acid scan): most sensitive test for acute cholecystitis
  - Procedure involves IV injection of radio-labeled HIDA, which is selectively secreted into biliary tree
  - In acute cholecystitis, HIDA enters the common bile duct (CBD) but not the gallbladder

Treatments:
- NPO, IV fluids, antibiotics targeting Enterobacteriaceae (68%), Enterococci, Bacteroides, Clostridium:
  - Piperacillin/tazobactam (Zosyn), Ampicillin/sulbactam (Unasyn), 3rd gen cephalosporin + clindamycin, Imipenem (life threatening)
- ERCP or CBD exploration to rule out choledocholithiasis in patients with jaundice, cholangitis or stone in CBD on U/S
- Semiurgent Cholecystectomy (usually within 72 hours) may be needed
- Cholecystostomy tube and percutaneous drainage in patients too sick for surgery

Complications:
- Perforation
- Empyema
- Emphysematous gallbladder due to infection by gas-forming organisms
- Cholecystenteric fistula (to duodenum, colon, or stomach): can see air in biliary tree
- Gallstone ileus: bowel obstruction (usually at terminal ileum) due to stone in intestine that passed through a fistula

CHOLANGITIS

Definition:
- CBD obstruction with infection proximal to the obstruction; I.e. "pus under pressure"

Etiologies:
- CBD stone (most common)
- Occurs infrequently with Stricture, Neoplasm (biliary or pancreatic), Infiltration with flukes *(Clonorchis sinensis, Opisthorchis viverrini)*

CHAPTER 5.02 CHOLECYSTITIS & CHOLANGITIS

Pathophysiology:
- *E. coli* and Klebsiella (70%), Enterococcus and Anaerobes (15%)
- Weil's Syndrome: caused by Leptospirosis, characterized by fever, jaundice, azotemia, RUQ pain-may mimic acute cholangitis
  - Clues to diagnosis: history of exposure risk, myalgias, ocular pain, photophobia, azotemia, and abnormal urinalysis

Clinical Manifestations/Physical Exam:
- **Charcot's triad:** RUQ pain, jaundice, fever/chills (present in 60% of patients)
- Reynold's pentad: Charcot's triad with shock + mental status changes
- Medical emergency if: fever >40°C or associated with sepsis, hypotension, peritoneal signs, or bilirubin >10 mg/dL

Laboratory Studies:
- CBC (WBC), LFTs

Diagnostic Studies:
- RUQ U/S or MRCP initially, but all will require decompression, typically with ERCP

Treatments:
- Antibiotics: same as Cholecystitis above (85% respond to initial antibiotics and supportive therapy before biliary intervention)
- Mandatory: decompression of biliary tree via ERCP, percutaneous transhepatic biliary drainage, or surgery

5.03 CHOLELITHIASIS & CHOLEDOCHOLITHIASIS

CHOLELITHIASIS

Definition:
- "Gallstones"
- "Sludge" (microlithiasis): super-concentrated mixture of bile acids, bilirubin, cholesterol, mucus, and proteins
  - Discharge into cystic duct & CBD can cause **Acalculous Cholecystitis** or **'Idiopathic Pancreatitis'**; Often after feeding from being NPO

Epidemiology:
- >10% adults in U.S. have gallstones, however only 20% of these persons develop symptoms (1-2% chance per year)
- ↑ prevalence in women, Native Americans, and with increasing age, obesity and pregnancy
- 500,000 cholecystectomies are performed each year in the United States

Etiologies:
- Drug/Medical therapies associated:
  - Ceftriaxone, OCPs, Octreotide impairs emptying, TPN & fasting promote gallbladder atony and sludge formation

Pathophysiology:
- Bile Physiology: Liver synthesizes 0.2-0.6 g/day; Pool of bile in body is about 3 grams
  - Biliary secretion = pool × cycles (pool is 3 g, cycles occur 4-12 times/day, slowing during fasting, accelerating with meals)
    - Hence, there are 12-36 grams of bile secreted and absorbed per day
  - Bile composed of bile salts, phospholipids, cholesterol; ↑ cholesterol saturation in bile promotes gallstones
- Enterohepatic circulation: Biliary secretion occurs, Ileal absorption returns 97% of intraluminal bile acid back into circulation via portal vein
  - (90% are extracted from portal circulation on their first pass through the liver)
  - Fecal excretion (0.2-0.6 g/day), Urinary excretion via systemic circulation (<0.5 mg/day)
  - In health, hepatic synthesis of bile acids is equivalent to enteric losses (0.2-0.6 g/day)
- Gallbladder:
  - In health, the gallbladder concentrates bile 10-fold for efficient storage during fasting
  - Intraduodenal fat and protein release cholecystokinin (CCK) which stimulates gallbladder contraction, sphincter-of-Oddi relaxation
- Principle factors involved in gallstone formation: cholesterol supersaturation, crystal nucleation, gallbladder hypomotility
  - Cholesterol supersaturation: result from deficient bile secretion or hypersecretion of cholesterol
    - Bile secretion reduced with age or liver disease, reduced enterohepatic circulation (TI disease)
    - Cholesterol secretion increased with hormones (female, sex, pregnancy, exogenous estrogens), obesity, liver disease
  - Nucleation: formation of insoluble deposits from supersaturated bile within biliary system
  - Gallbladder hypomotility: pregnancy, prolonged TPN, somatostatin therapy
  - Other influencing factors: bile transit time, gallbladder contraction, presence of bacteria, mucin, glycoproteins such as IgA
- Types of gallstones; including color of stone
  - Mixed (80%): multiple stones, composed of 80% cholesterol and 20% unconjugated bilirubin, may calcify (15-20%); Yellow
  - Cholesterol (10%): usually single stone, large, uncalcified; Yellow
  - Pigment (10%): unconjugated bilirubin (hence seen in chronic hemolysis) and cirrhosis; Calcium too; Black & Radiopaque
  - Infectious: colonization of bile with enteric bacteria and/or parasites; Soft clay-like in ducts, not gallbladder; Asian population; Brown

Clinical Manifestations/Physical Exam:
- Asymptomatic:
  - Most are found incidentally and remain asymptomatic in 80% of patients: require no treatment Prophylactic cholecystectomy: travel to remote areas (i.e. outer space!) or American Indians (stone associated cancer 20-fold ↑)
  - When symptoms do develop, only 2%/year present with acute cholecystitis or other complications

CHAPTER 5.03 CHOLELITHIASIS & CHOLEDOCHOLITHIASIS

- Biliary Colic: episodic RUQ or epigastric abdominal pain that begins abruptly, continuous, resolves slowly, lasts 30 min–6 hrs
  - Most patients with recurrent biliary colic have histology compatible with chronic cholecystitis

Laboratory Studies:
- Predominantly ↑↑ AΦ and GGT, ± Bili, ± ↑ AST & ALT; *See also Liver- LFTs (Chapter 4.20)*
- If transient passage of gallstone (i.e. ↑ amylase/lipase) then ↑ AST/ALT with normal bilirubin; AΦ with quick normalization in a day or two

Diagnostic Studies:
- Plain X-ray: detects only 10-15% of gallstones, which are calcified sufficiently to appear radiopaque
- RUQ U/S: sensitivity and specificity >90-95%, can also show complications (cholecystitis and cholangitis)
  - Most sensitive (90-98%) for detecting gallbladder stones; Widely variable (20-80%) for detection of common duct stones
- EUS: highly sensitive for detecting intraductal stones and slightly less for gallbladder stones depending on anatomy
  - Optimal screening tool when suspicion for duct stones is low-moderate, examination of gut also needed, risk of ERCP unacceptable
  - Can also detect sludge & microlithiasis with symptoms and negative RUQ: Acalculous Cholecystitis or 'Idiopathic Pancreatitis'
- HIDA (hepatobiliary iminodiacetic acid scan): scanning of gamma emissions after IV administration, hepatic uptake, and biliary excretion
  - Failure to visualize gallbladder is 97% sensitive and 96% specific for acute calculous cholecystitis
    - False negative: acalculous cholecystitis
    - False positive: chronic cholecystitis, chronic liver disease and during TPN or fasting states
  - Can also be used to confirm an intra-abdominal bile leak
- CT: best imaging method for evaluation of possible complications of biliary stone disease if U/S is compromised or suboptimal
- Cholangiography: invasive or non-invasive
  - ERCP favored in patients with suspected periampullary or pancreatic neoplasia, non-dilated ducts, anticipated need for therapeutic maneuvers (stone removal, stenting), hypersensitivity to contrast agents or failed percutaneous routes
    - Purely diagnostic use is rapidly diminishing because of MRCP and EUS
  - MRCP favored in frail patients who are not candidates for conscious sedation and in those with coagulopathy or need for concurrent evaluation of the hepatic parenchyma, especially when there is little likelihood for therapeutic intervention
- Percutaneous transhepatic cholangiography
  - Favored in patients with more proximal obstruction (hilar or above), surgically distorted gastro-duodenal anatomy (Roux limbs, Billroth II), and if ERCP fails

Treatments:
- Surgical:
  - Cholecystectomy (usually laparoscopic) if symptomatic
- Non-Surgical: requires patency of the cystic duct, as determined by HIDA scan; Recurrence of stones: 15% per year, 50% of all patients
  -ERCP ± papillotomy and basket/balloon extraction is procedure of choice
  -Stone destruction:
  - Mechanical lithotripter, laser, acoustic; Currently in U.S. only approved for duct stone applications, not gallbladder stones
  -Dissolution therapy: in patients who refuse or who are not surgical candidates
  - Oral: limited to small stones (<1 cm) which are comprised of cholesterol, non-calcified
    - Ursodiol (Actigall) for life: 7-8 mg/kg per day; Dissolves 30-80% of radiolucent stones over 6-24 months
  - Contact: uses solvents (methyl-tert-butyl ether) to solubilize pigment/cholesterol
    - Administered via radiologist with transhepatic catheter; Need oral therapy after or they return

Complications:
- Acute Cholecystitis (30% of symptomatic biliary colic » cholecystitis within 2 years)
- Cholangitis, Pancreatitis, Gallbladder carcinoma (~1%)
- If patient is on strict calorie restriction: ↑ hepatic cholesterol, ↓ gallbladder motility; Treatment: aspirin and UDCA can help prevent stones
- **Gallstone Ileus:** usual escape via cholocystoduodenal fistula (duodenum and gallbladder) and obstruct the terminal ileum
- **Bouveret's syndrome:** enter stomach via fistula and obstruct the pylorus

SECTION V PANCREAS/BILIARY

- **Mirizzi's syndrome:** stone impacting the neck of the GB or cystic duct with inflammation causing extrinsic compression of the CBD
  - Consider when cholecystitis is associated with higher than normal bilirubin (>5 mg/dl) or when CBD not dilated
- **Porcelain Gallbladder:** intramural calcifications or GB wall; Diagnosis via plain abdominal radiographs or abdominal CT
  - Prophylactic cholecystectomy is recommended to prevent development of carcinoma, which occurs in 20% of cases

CHOLEDOCHOLITHIASIS

Definition:
- Gallstone lodged in the common bile duct

Epidemiology:
- Occurs in 15% of patients with gallstones and 5-15% of those undergoing cholecystectomy

Pathophysiology:
- Types of gallstones: Cholesterol (70%) and Pigment (30%)

Clinical Manifestations:
- Asymptomatic (50%)
- Wide range of symptoms: Biliary colic with jaundice to overt cholangitis and pancreatitis
- Stone-related obstruction is typically recurrent with incomplete obstruction

Laboratory Studies:
- Aϕ and Bili are less marked than those for fixed obstructions (i.e. malignancy)

Diagnostic Studies:
- RUQ U/S: dilated ducts (but sensitivity only 33% for detecting CBD stones), i.e. sensitivity drops dramatically from cholelithiasis in gallbladder
- EUS detects over 90% of stones but cannot be treated with EUS
- Cholangiogram (ERCP, percutaneous, or operative), endoscopic lithotripsy can be clinically helpful
- CT has difficult time visualizing distal stones near the ampulla

Treatments:
- ERCP and sphincterotomy with stone extraction
- Dissolution therapy for Choledocholithiasis stones does not exist

Complications:
- Cholecystitis, Cholangitis, Pancreatitis, Biliary stricture

NOTES

5.04 CYSTIC DISEASE OF THE PANCREAS

(Surgical Oncology 2005;14:155-78. Pancreas 2002;25:217-21)

DEFINITION:
- **True pancreatic cyst** has epithelia cell lining (account for only 10-15% of all cystic lesions of the pancreas)
- **Pancreatic pseudocyst** is lined only by inflammatory tissue, it has no epithelium; Communicates with pancreatic duct (PD), so has high Amylase levels in fluid
  - Spontaneous resolution: 30%; Less likely with chronic pancreatitis or if developed as a consequence of trauma
- **Acute fluid collections** occur within 4 wks of pancreatitis, no well-defined wall and irregular, no communication to PD, low amylase content in fluid
  - Spontaneous resolution: 65%
- **Hemosuccus Pancreaticus** is major bleeding into the main PD from a pseudoaneurysm
  - Angiography is diagnostic/therapeutic; Rarely surgery

EPIDEMIOLOGY:
- Pancreatic cysts occur in up to 25% of patients undergoing abdominal imaging
  - Increasing resolution of CT and MRI allows detection of cysts less than 2 cm in size
- The prevalence increases with age

ETIOLOGIES: Differential of lesions of the pancreas:
- **Pancreatic pseudocyst (70-90%):**
  - Def: See Definition above; Often occur after episodes of acute or chronic pancreatitis
    Often contain inflammatory cells (PMN, leukocytes) with no evidence of mucin or epithelial cells
  - Clinical: Frequently (not invariably) associated with pain; Large cyst can compress adjacent structures (early satiety, jaundice)
  - Labs: $\downarrow > \uparrow$ CEA, $\downarrow > \uparrow$ CA 72-4, $\uparrow$ CA19-9, $\downarrow$ CA125, $\downarrow$ CA15-3, $\uparrow$ Amylase
    Fluid characteristics: thin, dark/muddy, nonmucinous, opaque
  - Dx: See Diagnostic Studies below; EUS: anechoic (black), thick walled, rare septations
  - Tx: See Treatments below

- **Cystic Neoplasms (10-15%): Benign or Malignant terminology**

  Serous cystic neoplasms (SCN) (32-39%): Serous Cystadenoma or Serous Cystadenocarcinoma
  - Def: Numerous small cyst filled with glycogen-rich (+PAS), low viscosity serous fluid, cuboidal epithelium lined
    Equal distribution throughout pancreas
  - Clinical: **Benign tumors,** ♀ > ♂, Average age at diagnosis is 50-60; May be associated with gene for von Hippel-Lindau disease
  - Labs: $\downarrow$ CEA (<5 ng/ml), $\downarrow$ CA 72-4, $\downarrow\uparrow$ CA19-9, $\downarrow$ CA125, $\downarrow$ CA15-3, $\downarrow$ Amylase
    Fluid characteristics: thin, clear, nonmucinous, bloody
  - Dx: CT/MRI/EUS: "Honeycomb with sunburst calcification in a central fibrotic or calcified scar"
  - Tx: Surgical if symptomatic, otherwise conservative observation (especially for elderly/high risk patients)

  Mucinous cystic neoplasm (MCN) (10-45%): Mucinous Cystadenoma or Mucinous Cystadenocarcinoma
  - Def: Most are single large mucin-filled; Columnar epithelium lined (dense ovarian-like stroma); Most in **body/tail;** No PD communication
    Subclassified: Benign/Adenomatous (44%), Borderline (8%), Malignant (48%): May contain both benign and malignant features
  - Clinical: Most considered potentially malignant; ♀ >> ♂, Age range at diagnosis is 40-60 years old
  - Labs: $\uparrow$ CEA (>800 ng/ml), $\uparrow$ CA 72-4, $\uparrow\downarrow$ CA19-9, $\uparrow\downarrow$ CA125, $\uparrow$ CA15-3, $\downarrow$ Amylase
    Fluid characteristics: viscous, stringy, clear, mucin
  - Dx: CT/MRI/EUS: most are incidentally found; May have thick walls/septations; Peripheral 'eggshell' calcification predictive of cancer
  - Tx: Surgical resection due to high risk of malignancy

CHAPTER 5.04 CYSTIC DISEASE OF THE PANCREAS

Intraductal Papillary Mucinous Neoplasm (IPMN) (21-33%): **Adenoma or Moderate dysplasia or Carcinoma (noninvasive/invasive)**

- Def: Appear cystic due to dilations of the ducts with mucus; Most arise in **head of pancreas with PD communication** (unlike MCN)
  Intraductal papillary growth of mucin-producing columnar epithelium; occurs in main PD or side ducts
- Clinical: Mucin extruding from ampulla of vater; ♀ = ♂; Mean age of Non-invasive: 63 yrs, Mean age of Invasive: 68 yrs
  75% have symptoms: abdominal pain (similar to chronic or relapsing pancreatitis), weight loss ± steatorrhea, DM, jaundice
  Obstructive pancreatitis often develops with atrophy of the gland
- Labs: ↑ CEA (>800 ng/ml), ↑ CA 72-4, ↑↓ CA19-9, ↓ CA125, ↓ CA15-3, ↑ Amylase
  Fluid characteristics: viscous, stringy, clear, mucin
- Dx: CT/MRI: suspected when dilated pancreatic duct or side ducts are seen, main differential is chronic pancreatitis
  EGD/ERCP: mucin extrusion from the ampulla (pathognomonic), dilation of main pancreatic duct or its major branches
  EUS: may be helpful in making diagnosis
- Tx: Surgical: hopes of preventing invasive carcinoma or curative for invasive IPMNs
  Operations: Overall Mortality 0-4% & Morbidity 35%
  Whipple's (pancreaticoduodenectomy): 50-70%; Distal pancreatectomy: 12-28%; Total pancreatectomy: 16-23%

- **True Cysts (rare)**
  - Associated von Hippel-Landau disease:
    Retinal angiomatosis, CNS hemangioblastomas, Multiple pancreatic serous cystadenomas
- **Miscellaneous cystic lesions (exceedingly rare)**
  - **Retention cyst:** dilated areas of the PD resulting from obstruction of the duct; Usually small (<1 cm)
    Associated with chronic pancreatitis, advanced cystic fibrosis, or duct obstructing carcinoma
  - Endometrial cysts, Parasitic cysts (*Echinococcus, Taenia solium*), Macrocysts associated with cystic fibrosis

PATHOPHYSIOLOGY:

- Pancreatic pseudocyst develops from necrosis of pancreatic tissue due to leakage of pancreatic enzymes from disrupted PD
  - Most ETOH related to pancreatitis
- Cystic neoplasms: unclear pathogenesis
  - Serous cystadenomas are strongly associated with mutations of the von Hippel Lindau (VHL) gene
  - MCN and IPMN may be associated with mutations of K-ras and p16 genes

CLINICAL MANIFESTATIONS/PHYSICAL EXAM:

- Most pancreatic-cystic lesions do not cause symptoms
  - When symptoms present most common: recurrent abdominal pain, nausea, vomiting, pancreatitis if invasion of main pancreatic duct
- See also Etiologies above

LABORATORY STUDIES:

- See Etiologies above

DIAGNOSTIC STUDIES:

- CT or MRCP (initial test if suspected diagnosis): anatomy landmarks, rule out pseudoaneurysm, look for gas in cyst (infection)
  - If no lesion seen in pancreas, it is very unlikely that a clinically significant neoplasm is present
  - If diagnosis made with certainty via characteristic findings, surgical resection without further testing is warranted in many cases
  - Indeterminate lesions should undergo further testing with EUS
- EUS ± FNA is an excellent tool for morphologic evaluation (most important part is the ability for FNA)
- ERCP for IMPN may be useful
  - May show characteristic findings of mucinous filling defects within the duct, diffuse dilation, and cystic dilation of side branches
- Note that transabdominal ultrasound is generally not helpful

TREATMENTS:
- **When to drain pseudocyst?** Three methods: surgical, percutaneous, endoscopic
  - When it causes significant symptoms, evidence of infection, critical compression of adjacent structures, internal hemorrhage
  - Asymptomatic pseudocyst can be observed carefully, regardless of size
- Surgical: best when cannot rule out cystic neoplasm (↑ suspicion when cyst not related to pancreatitis or enlarging), multiple or recurrent pseudocysts, concurrent PD stricture
  - Whipple's may be procedure of choice; Need experienced surgeon; No surgery if infection present (percutaneous drainage better)
  - Caveat with IPMN: most grow longitudinally along ducts (not radially into parenchyma), so frozen section during surgery is a must
  - Mortality 3%, Recurrence 8%
- Percutaneous: best for high risk patients, thin walled cyst (i.e. No sutures needed), **infected;** Mortality 2%, Recurrence 7%
- Endoscopic: dependent on skill of endoscopist; Mortality 1%, Recurrence 16%

COMPLICATIONS:
- Complications of untreated pancreatic pseudocyst:
  - Secondary Infection (10%)
  - Rupture (<3%)
  - Pancreatic ascites (leak from pseudocyst 70%, or PD 15%):
      Ascites with amylase >1000 u/dl & protein >2.5 gm/dl (i.e. low SAAG)
      Treat with TPN/Octreotide (100 mcg sq q 4 hr) or ERCP (stent site of leak)
  - Pancreatic fistulas: complication of drainage; Treat with octreotide or surgery
  - Obstruction of GI tract, urinary system, vena cava, portal vein; Necessitates drainage
  - Jaundice (10%): hepatic dysfunction, extrahepatic biliary obstruction, stenosis of distal CBD
  - Pseudoaneurysm: enzymes erodes into adjacent vessel (7%); Pain, hypotension, falling hematocrit (hemosuccus pancreaticus)

PROGNOSIS:
- Cystic neoplasms are slow growing and the risk of malignant change is probably small
  - Highest rate of malignancy, nearly 50%, is seen with main-duct IPMN lesions

NOTES

5.05 PANCREATIC CARCINOMA

(Gastroenterology 1999;117:1463-84)

DEFINITION:
- Adenocarcinoma, well-differentiated, arising from pancreatic ductal epithelium (90% of cases)
  - Most arise in the head of pancreas (80%)
- *See also Pancreas/Biliary- Cystic Disease of the Pancreas (Chapter 5.04)*

EPIDEMIOLOGY:
- 30,000 new cases a year
- 85% have distant metastases at diagnosis

ETIOLOGIES:
- Risk factors: smoking & working in chemical industry (aromatic amines), chronic pancreatitis, diets large in fats and meat products
  - Risks may also include Diabetes Mellitus, pernicious anemia, partial gastrectomy; ETOH has not been shown to be a proven risk
  - Hereditary pancreatitis is a risk, but is probably more related to chronic pancreatitis
  - Intraductal Papillary Mucinous Neoplasm (IPMN) are a risk factor, *See also Pancreas/Biliary- Cystic Disease of Pancreas (Chapter 5.04)*
  - Inheritance: 6-8% of patients have a family history in a first-degree relative, representing a 13-fold increase
    - Syndromes associated with increased risk: Peutz-Jeghers syndrome, BRCA2 mutations (most common inheritance risk)
    - No screening guidelines; Some recommend CT/EUS at regular intervals; CA19-9 are too insensitive and nonspecific
  - Protective: high intake of dietary fiber

PATHOPHYSIOLOGY:
- About 80% of pancreatic ductal adenocarcinomas occur in the head of the pancreas
- Histology varies from: well-differentiated with glandular structures to poorly differentiated that exhibit little or no glandular structure or stroma
- Metastases to liver and lungs; can also spread to adrenals, kidneys, bone, brain, and skin

CLINICAL MANIFESTATIONS/PHYSICAL EXAM:
- Abdominal pain (80% of patients), jaundice (50% of patients)
- Weight loss (with or without anorexia and usually without steatorrhea) and early satiety
- If pancreatic head cancer, then obstruction of distal CBD with development of **obstructive jaundice**
- Courvoisier's sign: palpable, distended gallbladder in RUQ and jaundice
  Usually result of malignant bile duct obstruction: pancreatic, cholangiocarcinoma or ampullary mass (not specific for cancer)
- Abdominal pain with radiation to back, weight loss, nausea, anorexia

LABORATORY STUDIES:
- CA19-9: sensitive >90%, specificity 75%; Often normal in early stages and small tumors (<1 cm)
  - False elevations: chronic pancreatitis, biliary disease or obstruction of any sort, other GI cancers
  - Predictive: usually falls after resection and persistent elevation indicates inadequate resection or metastatic lesions
  - Also a marker for Cholangiocarcinoma
- ↑ bilirubin and AΦ (obstructive pattern)
- Amylase is elevated in only 5% of patients
- Genetic markers (not commonly used due to low sensitivity and specificity):
  - K-ras: most common, present in 90% of patients
  - p53: present in 50-70% of patients

CHAPTER 5.05   PANCREATIC CARCINOMA

DIAGNOSTIC STUDIES:
- Transabdominal U/S: Highly sensitive for biliary dilation and level of obstruction
- CT: more sensitive than U/S; **Should be first test if clinically suspected as can diagnose and stage the tumor**
  - Pancreatic cancer is hypoattenuating on CT
  - Sensitivity for tumors smaller than 15 mm is 67%
  - If highly suspicious and resectable per CT, go right to surgery (do not need to biopsy first!)
- EUS: most accurate to diagnose small tumors (<3 cm) and to evaluate local spread of tumor to surrounding organs, vessels and lymph nodes
  - FNA: 100% specific, 80% sensitive (i.e. negative FNA does not rule out pancreatic cancer)
  - However FNA should be limited as those who are resectable should go right to surgery
  - Biopsy indications: locally unresectable, known metastases (i.e. liver), possibility of autoimmune pancreatitis
- ERCP: also highly sensitive/specific, used to perform palliative drainage of biliary system
  - **Double-duct sign:** stenosis of the CBD and PD at pancreatic head; With obstructive jaundice or mass: 85% specific for cancer
- PET scan: limited value/use; false negatives with hyperglycemic states; best for distant and peritoneal metastases
- Laparoscopic staging: may be necessary depending on surgeon

Staging:

Primary Tumor	Regional LN	Distant Mets:	Stages:	
Tx: Tumor can't be assessed	Nx: LN can't be assessed	Mx: Mets can't be assessed	0:	Tis, N0, M0
T0: No evidence of tumor	N0: No LN metastases	M0: No distant metastases	1:	T1 *or* T2, N0, M0
Tis: Carcinoma in situ	N1: LN metastasis	M1: Distant metastases	2:	T3, N0, M0
T1: Limited to pancreas, ≤2 cm			3:	T1 *or* T2 *or* T3, N1, M0
T2: Limited to pancreas, >2 cm				
T3: Extends to duodenum, bile duct, mesenteric vessels			4A:	T4, Any N, M0
T4: Extends to stomach, spleen, colon			4B:	Any T, Any N, M1

TREATMENTS:
- Surgery: only chance for cure; Only 15-20% are candidates for surgery
  - Perioperative biopsy or FNA is not required in most instances because the findings do not alter the decision to resect
  - At time of diagnosis, 40-50% already have locally advanced disease which precludes surgery (other than palliation)
  - Whipple's (pancreaticoduodenectomy): most commonly done for pancreatic head cancer
    - Mortality from surgery <5%, but Morbidity ~50%
      Experienced surgeon and high volume center is key
  - Distal pancreatectomy and splenectomy: most commonly done for body and tail pancreatic cancer
- Chemo:
  - 5FU (old standard): response rate <10%; No effect on quality of life or survival
  - Gemcitabine (new standard): slight increase in clinical benefit and median survival, but still only 5 year survival of <2%
- Radiation: Used in two situations:
  - Use as adjuvant therapy after resection for cure
  - Unresectable locoregional pancreatic cancer, combined with 5FU is superior to radiation alone for mean survival
    - Combination chemoradiation therapy survival 42 weeks versus 23 weeks with radiation alone
- Pain control:
  - Intraoperative splanchnicectomy
  - Celiac block (chemical splanchnicectomy): 50% alcohol injection on each side of aorta at level of celiac axis via EUS
    - Either block probably provides better pain relief and less complications of narcotic use (constipation, nausea)

SECTION V   PANCREAS/BILIARY

- Palliation with unresectable cancer with symptoms: obstructive jaundice, pruritus, cholangitis, duodenal obstruction
    - ERCP stent placement (best with expandable metal which is less likely to occlude than plastic stents)
        - or Interventional Radiology for transhepatic/transcutaneous stents (higher 30-day mortality and not procedure of choice)
    - Only 20% develop duodenal obstruction before they die, hence palliative prophylactic gastrojejunostomy is not standard
        - Duodenal stent via endoscopy is another option
        - Some have slow gastric emptying from metastases nerve infiltration, so a drainage procedure will not help
- Nutrition:
    - Pancreatic enzymes from unresectable cancer with symptoms of malabsorption
        - Viokase 8 tabs with meals (two after a few bites, four during the meal, two at end of meal)

PROGNOSIS:
- Fifth leading cause of death in U.S.
- Median survival is 4–5 months (less than 20% live for 1 year); only 1–3% survive 5 years
    - The lowest 5-year survival of any cancer!
    - Poor prognosis due to increased metastasis at diagnosis and low respectability rate

NOTES

5.06 PANCREATITIS: ACUTE

(Am J Gastroenterol 2006;101:2379-2400 & 1997;92:377-86. N Engl J Med 2006;354:2142-50. J Hepatobil Pancreat Surg 2006;13:56-60)

DEFINITION:
- Acute pancreatitis: inflammatory condition of the pancreas that may extend to local and distant extra-pancreatic tissues
    - Interstitial pancreatitis: mild acute pancreatitis, based on radiographic appearance; Implies preservation of pancreatic blood supply
    - Necrotizing (Severe) pancreatitis: implies presence of organ failure, local complications or pancreatic necrosis
- Acute recurrent pancreatitis: acute pancreatitis occurring two or more occasions (evidenced by elevation of the serum pancreatic enzymes)

EPIDEMIOLOGY:
- Over 200,000 new cases a year (80% are interstitial or edematous variety and 20% are necrotizing or severe variety)
- See also Etiologies below

ETIOLOGIES:
- Common:
    - Gallstones (**40% of cases,** typically women): usually small (<5 mm) stones are culprit; Mortality 12% during first attack
    - Alcohol (**30% of cases,** typically men, lower socioeconomic): usually chronic with acute flares
    - Idiopathic (20-25% of cases), however, in 2/3 of these patients
        - Microlithiasis ("Biliary sludge") is identified 70% with repeat U/S
- Rare:
    - Obstructive: ampullary or pancreatic tumors, pancreas divisum (controversial)
    - Metabolic: TG >750 for type I & V familial hypertriglyceridemia; TG usually ~ 4500; Hypercalcemia/Hyperparathyroidism
    - Meds (5% of case): furosemide, thiazides, azathioprine/6-MP, valproic acid, estrogens, didanosine, sulfa, protease inhibitors, ACE-I
    - Infection: *Echovirus, Coxsackievirus, Mumps, Rubella,* EBV, CMV, HIV, HAV, HBV, *Ascaris, Mycoplasma, Salmonella,* TB
    - Ischemia from any cause
    - Trauma: blunt abdominal trauma, **Post ERCP;** *See also Endoscopy & Procedures- ERCP (Chapter 7.06)*
    - Pregnancy: most occur in 3rd trimester or postpartum; Coexisting stones in 90% of cases
    - Scorpion sting (in Trinidad)
    - Post-transplant: think secondary hyperparathyroidism, hyperlipidemia, viral infections, vasculitis, immunosuppressive (Treatment with steroids)
    - In HIV/AIDS: think infection (CMV, fungal, MAI, Toxo, Pneumocystis), drugs (Didanosine, Bactrim), other (Kaposi's, lymphoma)
- DDX:
    - Biliary disease, PUD, perforated viscus, small bowel obstruction, mesenteric ischemia, MI, AAA leak, distal aortic dissection

PATHOPHYSIOLOGY:
- Premature activation of trypsin within pancreatic acinar cells » activation of digestive enzymes leading to pancreatic inflammation
- Two forms defined by inflammatory changes in the pancreatic parenchyma are "interstitial" and "necrotizing"
    - Interstitial (85%): edema and inflammation of the pancreatic parenchyma occur without death of pancreatic acini
    - Necrotizing (15%): extensive parenchymal destruction, frequency with peripancreatic fat necrosis

CLINICAL MANIFESTATIONS/PHYSICAL EXAM:
- Ranges from mild nonspecific epigastric pain to catastrophic acute medical illness
- In general: epigastric abdominal tenderness/pain, radiating to the back, constant, little change with position; ± guarding

CHAPTER 5.06 PANCREATITIS: ACUTE

- N/V & Fever is common
- Other clinical signs:
  - ↓ bowel sounds (adynamic ileus), ± palpable abdominal mass; ± jaundice if biliary obstruction
  - Signs of retroperitoneal hemorrhage are uncommon: *Cullen's* » periumbilical; *Grey Turner's* » flank ("turn" patient to see flank)
  - ± Hypotension or shock (tachycardia, tachypnea, hypotension) from cytokine release

LABORATORY STUDIES:
(Amylase and Lipase both secreted in active form, not a proenzyme; Checking them daily adds little to assessing clinical progress/prognosis)
- ↑ **Amylase:** levels >3 × ULN very suggestive of pancreatitis: rises 2–12 hours after symptom onset, but level *does NOT* equal severity
Continued elevation (several weeks) should make one think of PD duct blockage, pseudocyst, persistent pancreatic inflammation
  - False Neg Amylase: acute or chronic (i.e. ETOH); Hypertriglyceridemia (↓ amylase activity); May check urine amylase (will be high)
  - False Pos Amylase: other abdominal process (small bowel/colon tumors/perforation, ovarian cysts), salivary gland disease, lungs, acidemia, renal failure
    - Macroamylasemia: amylase binds to IgA, cannot be renally filtered, therefore low urinary amylase
- ↑ **Lipase:** may be only slightly more specific than amylase, stays elevated longer than the 3–5 days amylase takes to decline
  - Macrolipasemia: lipase binds to IgA; Also reported in cirrhosis, non-Hodgkins
- ALT >3 × ULN » **gallstone (biliary) pancreatitis;** Aφ and Bili not helpful (takes time to rise); Backup causes hepatocyte compression = ↑ ALT
- CRP predicts severity: a value >150 mg/L is considered diagnostic of severe acute pancreatitis when drawn <48 hrs after symptom onset
- Other labs depending on severity: ↑ Hct due to hemoconcentration/dehydration (very poor prognostic sign), ↑ WBC, ↑ BUN, ↑ Glucose
  - Check calcium after attack: levels can be spuriously low during an attack and hypercalcemia as the cause can be missed
- See Ranson's Criteria and CT Severity Index under Prognosis

DIAGNOSTIC STUDIES:
- **Abd U/S:** This is the *first test* to be done (not CT); To evaluate for gallstones, CBD dilation, ascites, pseudocyst
  - Pancreas can often be obscured by bowel gas; If and when seen features are consistent with enlarged, hypoechoic gland
- **Abd CT (with IV contrast):** When to obtain: 1. failure to improve clinically, 2. presence of organ failure, 3. suspicion of necrosis (F, ↑ WBC)
  - Purpose is to determine if necrosis is present, and if so, to do aspiration
Also to exclude other abdominal processes, stage severity, and look for complications
  - CT with IV contrast is generally avoided for 1st few days because theoretical concern of ↑ necrosis (and necrosis may not be radiographically apparent for 48–72 hrs) and until volume status is repleted and renal function is assessed
  - If you made decision to CT, then Radiology should be prepared to do aspirate at that time and general surgery should be onboard
- **Abd Plain Films:** may show "sentinel loop" which is a focally dilated small-bowel loop or Calcification 2^0 to chronic pancreatitis
  - **CXR:** pleural effusion in 1st 24 hours correlates with greater severity of necrosis, organ failure, and mortality
- **MRCP:** Reliable method for staging severity; Can also detect pancreatic duct disruption; Often done with secretin stimulation
- CT-guided abscess drainage and ERCP
  - See below, under Treatments
- Duodenal bile aspiration and microscopy is gold standard for diagnosis of biliary sludge (microlithiasis)– rarely performed

SECTION V PANCREAS/BILIARY

TREATMENTS: "Pancreas": **p**ain control, **a**ntibiotics, **n**po, **c**a/mg, **r**est, **e**lectrolytes, **a**cid (PPIs), **s**uction (Ng)

Acute Interstitial Pancreatitis:
- Supportive:
  - **IV Fluid resuscitation (may need up to *10 L/day*** if hemodynamically severe pancreatitis such as necrotizing)
  - **NPO;** Ng suction if protracted vomiting only, not as a standard; Electrolyte repletion
    Consider feeding by day 3 if non-severe with no pain and near normal amylase
    - **Nutrition:** Enteral feeding beyond the ligament of Treitz is better than TPN (decreased infection complications)
  - **Analgesia** with meperidine; There is no evidence that morphine actually worsens the disease
  - **Thiamine** (if ETOH)
- Antibiotics:
  - Not to be used with acute interstitial pancreatitis as they do not alter outcome
- ERCP:
  - Generally NOT indicated except in gallstone pancreatitis with biliary obstruction (i.e. total bili >1.35 mg/dl on hospital day 2)
  - Little effect on local or systemic pancreatitis, rather stone removal probably ↓ biliary sepsis in gallstone pancreatitis
  - Reserved for those with biliary obstruction suspected on the basis of hyperbilirubinemia and clinical cholangitis
- Cholecystectomy
  - Should be performed before discharge to prevent recurrent attacks
  - ERCP with sphincterotomy may be a good alternative if U/S shows stones and patient is poor surgical candidate

Acute Necrotizing Pancreatitis:
- Same as Acute Interstitial Pancreatitis, along with Intensive Care Unit monitoring and the following:
- Antibiotics:
  - Prevention of infection is critical
  - Gut decontamination with oral non-absorbable antibiotics may be efficacious
  - Systemic Antibiotics: **Imipenem (or meropenem)** with severe necrotizing pancreatitis (>30% necroses by CT) may ↓ morality
- CT-guided abscess drainage or FNA if pancreatic necrosis present on CT to rule out infection (96% sensitive, 99% specific)
  - Perform in those patients with persistent fevers, high WBC, organ failure–not responding to therapy
- Surgical
  - Sterile Necrosis: see Complications below
  - Infected Necrosis: see Complications below

COMPLICATIONS: *See also: Pancreas/Biliary- Cystic Disease of the Pancreas (Chapter 5.04)*
- Systemic: shock, ARDS, Renal failure, GI hemorrhage
- Metabolic: hypocalcemia, hyperglycemia (i.e. DM), hypertriglyceridemia
- **Acute Fluid Collection** (30–50%): seen early, low attenuation, non-encapsulated, treatment not generally required
- **Pseudocyst** (10–20%): fluid collection that persists for 4–6 wks & becomes encapsulated
  - Suggested by persistent pain or persistent elevation of amylase or lipase; Most resolve spontaneously
  - If >6 cm *or* persists >6 wks with pain » internal/percutaneous drainage; However **most only drained if persistent symptoms**
- **Sterile Necrosis** (20%): area of non-viable pancreatic tissue; 30–50% *will become infected necrosis*; Mortality 9%
  - Treat conservatively with prophylactic antibiotics (i.e. Imipenem) and supportive measures for as long as possible
    - Surgery if patient not responding to conservative therapy or unstable
- **Infected Necrosis** (5% of all cases, 30–70% of acute necrotizing cases, most common cause of death): fever & high WBC
  - Pancreatic abscess: circumscribed collection of pus: Treat with antibiotics & drainage (CT-guided if possible)
  - Infected Necrosis (aspiration » +bacterial culture): Antibiotics & surgical debridement (100% mortality without debridement)
  - Organisms: usually $2°$ enteric GNR; Translocation of bowel wall, local lymph, hematogenous, biliary spread
    - *E. coli* (51%), Enterococcus (19%), Staph (18%), Pseudomonas spp. (16%)

CHAPTER 5.06   PANCREATITIS: ACUTE

- **Pancreatic ascites** or pleural effusion: indicates disrupted pancreatic duct; may need ERCP with stent placement across duct
- Scarring of pancreatic duct » stricture » **Chronic Pancreatitis;** *See also Pancreas/Billiary- Pancreatitis Chronic (Chapter 5.07)*
- **Coexisting ETOH and Cholelithiasis:** No cholecystectomy should be performed as does not prevent further attack; Attacks generally follow ETOH pattern
- **Massive UGIB:**
  Isolated gastric varices from splenic vein thrombosis: may need splenectomy
  Hemosuccus pancreaticus: bleed through the PD into duodenum due to erosion of a pseudocyst into adjacent vasculature

PROGNOSIS:
- Mortality (5% overall of all acute pancreatitis cases) occurs in two phases:
  - Early deaths (1-2 weeks after onset, 50% of all deaths): due to multisystem organ failure from release of inflammatory mediators (i.e. cytokines)
  - Late deaths resulting from local or systemic infections
- **Ranson's Criteria:** (originally described for ETOH pancreatitis, recent studies suggest poor positive predictive value)

  At Dx: Age >55; WBC >16K; Gluc >200; AST >250; LDH >350
  At 48 hrs: HCT ↓ >10%; Bun ↑ >5 mg/dl; Base deficient >4 mEq/L; Ca <8; Pa02 <60 mmHg; Fluid deficit >6 L

  Mortality: ≤2 findings: <5% mortality. 3-4: 15-20%. 5-6: 40%. ≥7: >99%
  Any score >3 should make you worry and think about ICU level care

- **APACHE-II** (Acute Physiology and Chronic Health Evaluation): based on 12 physiological variables
  - Cumbersome and clinically impractical

- **CT Severity Index** = pancreatitis grade (0-4) + necrosis degree (0-6) (Radiology 1990;174:331-6)

Grade of Pancreatitis:		Degree of Necrosis	
A: Normal pancreas (mild pancreatitis):	0	No necrosis:	0
B: Focal or diffuse enlargement:	1	Necrosis 1/3 pancreas:	2
C: Pancreatic or peripancreatic inflammation:	2	Necrosis 1/2 pancreas:	4
D: *Single* fluid collection:	3	Necrosis ≥1/2 pancreas:	6
E: *Multiple* fluid collections:	4		

Pancreatic necrosis: 30-50% infection rate; Total scores of 7-10 are associated with 92% Morbidity and 17% Mortality

5.07 PANCREATITIS: CHRONIC

DEFINITION:
- Chronic Pancreatic (CP) implies the presence of parenchymal fibrosis, and loss of glandular function

Marseilles-Rome/Sarles classification:
  Lithogenic (Calcifying) CP: Largest group, *ETOH is leading cause and is responsible for >70% of cases of chronic pancreatitis*
  - Chronic calcifying pancreatitis; Irregular fibrosis of the pancreas with pancreatic duct stones & protein plugs, ductal injury

  Obstructive CP: Intraductal tumor or benign ductal stricture in distal (tail end) of the gland; Obstruction is not from stones
  - Glandular changes: uniform fibrosis, ductal changes with dilation, acinar atrophy; Often improves when obstruction is relieved

  Inflammatory CP: Associated with autoimmune diseases such as Sjogren's, PSC, autoimmune pancreatitis
  - Characterized histologically by mononuclear cell infiltration, associated exocrine parenchyma destruction, diffuse fibrosis, atrophy

  Pancreatic Fibrosis: Also called **Idiopathic Senile CP**
  - Characterized by silent, diffuse perilobular fibrosis
  - Must rule out: nutritional/hereditary pancreatitis, hypercalcemia, trauma with duct injury, hyperlipidemia, autoimmunity, pancreatic divisum, obstruction, cancer

ETIOLOGIES: Other causes than those above:
- Hereditary CP (High risk for pancreatic cancer):
  - Three genes have been associated with chronic hereditary pancreatitis:
    - Cationic Trypsinogen gene: cause *autosomal dominant* form of chronic pancreatitis (i.e. many family members)
    - Cystic fibrosis transmembrane conductance regulator (CFTR) and Pancreatic secretory trypsin inhibitor (SPINK1) genes
      - Mostly found in apparent *sporadic* forms of pancreatitis because they have low penetrance
    - Mesotrypsinogen gene is NOT implicated
  - Affects both ♂ & ♀ equally; Can present as acute pancreatitis in childhood by age 10–12
- Cystic fibrosis: exocrine pancreatic insufficiency afflicts approximately 85% of CF patients
  - Reduced pancreatic duct secretions, leading to protein-rich acinar secretions becoming inspissated: proximal obstruction & fibrosis

PATHOPHYSIOLOGY:
- Trypsin (inhibit) and Food (stimulate): CCK releasing peptide » pancreatic enzyme secretion » pain

CLINICAL MANIFESTATIONS/PHYSICAL EXAM:
- Abdominal pain, Steatorrhea, Diabetes mellitus
- Weight loss: decreased intake due to fear of pain, malabsorption, uncontrolled diabetes
- Osseous abnormalities (5%): medullary infarcts or aseptic necrosis of femoral/humeral heads; From medullary fat necrosis during acute attacks
- Nephrolithiasis: with steatorrhea, long-chain fatty acids bind to intraluminal calcium; Less calcium available to bind oxalate = more oxalate in urine

LABORATORY STUDIES:
- Amylase and lipase not helpful: may be normal, elevated, or low
- ↓ Trypsin is suggestive of CP (although no serologic test is sensitive or specific for chronic pancreatitis)
- Steatorrhea: must lose 90% of exocrine function before steatorrhea develops (takes 5–12 years); Pancreas has great reserve!
- Fat soluble vitamin deficiency: although diminished, marked deficiency is UNcommon in chronic pancreatitis
  - Clinically easy bruising, bone pain, decreased night vision, is more suggestive of small bowel malabsorption, such as Celiac sprue
- B12 malabsorption: cobalamin-binding proteins, usually destroyed by pancreatic enzymes, are binding more B12
  - Treat with pancreatic enzymes

CHAPTER 5.07 PANCREATITIS: CHRONIC

DIAGNOSTIC STUDIES:
- In later stages of the disease when calcifications and steatorrhea are present, the diagnosis is relatively straightforward
  - Difficulty arises if pancreatic structure and function are not unequivocally abnormal; Histology is standard, but often not available
- KUB: focal or diffuse pancreatic calcification (30–40% of cases) makes the diagnosis of advanced CP, however not found in early CP
- U/S: PD dilation, calcifications, cavities and decreased parenchymal echogenicity; Sensitive: 70%, Specific: 90%
- CT: PD dilation, calcifications, cystic lesions, heterogeneous density of gland with atrophy or enlargement; Sensitive: 80%, Specific: 90%
  - Good starting point: can identify most complications such as peripancreatic fluid collections, bile duct obstructions, etc
- MRCP: close correlation with ERCP; Benefits: concomitantly evaluate both parenchyma and ducts; Often done with secretin stimulation
- EUS: features include ductal and parenchymal changes: echotexture of gland, calcifications, lobulations, bands of fibrosis
  - Problems can occur distinguishing senile changes, alcoholics who may have fibrosis without pancreatitis, recent acute attack
- ERCP: 'chain of lakes' in main PD; Sensitive: 90%, Specific: 100% (gold standard to test other imaging against)

Cambridge grading: based on PD and side branches normality or abnormalities:

Grade	Main Pancreatic Duct	Side Branches	Other
Normal	Normal	Normal	None
Mild	Normal	≥3 abnormal	None
Moderate	Abnormal-dilated, strictures	≥3 abnormal	None
Severe	Abnormal-dilated, strictures	≥3 abnormal	large cavity (>10 mm) or intraductal filling defects or duct obstruction/irregularities

- Pancreatic Function Test (Secretin Stimulation Test with or without CCK):
  - Measures volume of secretion and concentration of bicarbonate via direct endoscopic collection
    - Dreiling tube (old method): cumbersome, time insufficient, need fluoro to place tube
  - Usually positive with 60% exocrine function lost
  - False positive can happen with primary DM, Billroth II gastrectomy, celiac sprue, cirrhosis
  Bicarb: ≤50 mEq/L: Chronic pancreatitis, >50 and <70 mEq/L: indeterminate, ≥75 mEq/L: normal

TREATMENTS:
- Diet therapy: Increase carbohydrates/protein in meals
  - Low fat historically recommended–however, some argue the calories are worth the risk
  - Small frequent meals
  - Avoid any foods that are known to exacerbate symptoms
- Pancreatic enzyme replacement (replacing lipase): generics not FDA regulated; Avoid if possible
  - Non-enteric coated **(Viokase):** Better for pain via enzyme readily available in duodenum; however can cause stomach upset
    - Readily available protease » Inhibit CCK » Pancreatic function decreased
  - Enteric coated **(Creon):** do not dissolve in stomach, less susceptible to acid pepsin inactivation
  - Usual dose is 30,000 units *delivered and available to the duodenum* with each meal (i.e. TID with meals)
    - Reasons for pancreatic enzyme replacement failures:
      -Compliance, inadequate dose, delayed gastric emptying, increased gastric/duodenal acid, bacterial overgrowth
    - Solutions:
      -Alternative dose (up to 80,000 units/dose); Take 20,000 units: 1 before meals, 2 during meals, 1 after meals
      -Use enteric coating (Creon), Add PPI, Test/treat for bacterial overgrowth, Replace dietary fat with medium-chain TG
  - Loss of response to previously effective enzyme replacement with a normal CT (i.e. no pancreatic cancer)?
    - Suggests small bowel problem interfering with digestion/absorption such as bacteria overgrowth, ? trial of antibiotics

SECTION V PANCREAS/BILIARY

- Chronic pain control (in escalating order): (Gastro 1998:115:763-64 & 765-76)
  - **Stop ETOH and Smoking,** Non-narcotic analgesics, Celiac plexus block; Try to avoid narcotics
  - Correctable causes: presence of pseudocyst or duodenal/bile duct obstruction should be sought via CT scan
  - Pancreatic enzymes (replacing trypsin); For chronic pain, use of high-protease content preparations, preferably non-enteric coated
  - Celiac plexus block appears to have limited benefit in chronic pancreatitis
  - Endoscopic management (sphincterotomy, stenting PD, stone removal): good option before surgery, ? if predicts surgical response
    - 5 year follow-up pain relief: 65% continue to be pain free, 16% continue regular endoscopic therapy, 23% go to surgery
  - Puestow operation: preferred in patients with ductal obstruction in the head of the pancreas with distal duct dilation (>7 mm)
    - 5 year follow-up pain relief: 55% complete relief, 25% improved only, 20% failure of pain control
  - Future?: total pancreatectomy with auto-islet cell transplantation

COMPLICATIONS:
- Diabetes Mellitus: eventually develops in 85% of patients (Develops after Steatorrhea)
- Duodenal obstruction: potentially reversible gastric outlet obstruction can occur during an acute flare as a result of peripancreatic inflammation
- Pseudocysts (most common complication, 25%); *See also Pancreas/Biliary- Cystic Disease of the Pancreas (Chapter 5.04)*
- Pancreatic ascites; *See also Liver- Ascites & Portal Hypertension (Chapter 4.05)*
- Isolated gastric varices from splenic vein thrombosis occurs 5% of CP patients: may need splenectomy with gastric devascularization
- Chronic pancreatitis is a risk factor for pancreatic carcinoma; No good surveillance regimen for detecting cancer (i.e. CA19-9, U/S)
  - Highest risk factors: Hereditary pancreatitis, Smoking
  - Not proven to be risk factors: ETOH, Pancreatic calcifications

NOTES

5.08 SPHINCTER OF ODDI DYSFUNCTION

DEFINITION:
- The Sphincter of Oddi (SO) is a fibromuscular sheath that encircles the terminal portion of the common bile duct, pancreatic duct, and common channel in the second portion of the duodenum; It is made up of smooth muscle; Three interconnected sphincters exist: choledochus, pancreaticus, and ampulla
- SOD Dysfunction (SOD): a benign disorder characterized by functional or structural obstruction at the level of the sphincter; It is suspected in patients with RUQ pain suggestive of a biliary or pancreatic origin

EPIDEMIOLOGY:
- Risk for SOD: Females in 3rd to 5th decades of life (up to 90%)
- Symptoms often apparent after cholecystectomy; Incidence is approximately 1% in post cholecystectomy patients

ETIOLOGIES:
- Long-term opiate use can precipitate SOD due to increased pressures in the biliary ducts

PATHOPHYSIOLOGY:
- Function of SO: Regulates bile and pancreatic juice into the duodenum, reduces duodenal reflux into the pancreatic/biliary ducts, contracts tonically during the interdigestive portion to promote gallbladder filling, contracts phasically in the digestion period (cholinergic stimulation) to promote flow of bile
  - Endogenous substances effect on SO: Motilin ↑ intensity; Vasoactive intestinal peptide (VIP) and nitric oxide (NO) ↓ intensity
  - Cholecystokinin (CCK) is induced by food intake and stimulates contraction of the gallbladder and relaxation of SOD
- Two abnormalities that can lead to SOD:
  - Primary motor abnormality of the SOD, termed **Biliary dyskinesia** or spasm (elevated pressure)
  - Fibrosis or inflammation, most likely from recurrent passage of biliary stones/microlithiasis (may present post cholecystectomy)

CLINICAL MANIFESTATIONS/PHYSICAL EXAM:
- Symptoms can be biliary or pancreatic in nature: Pain in RUQ with radiation to back and may be meal related; episodic or continuous
- Symptoms of IBS often co-exist and it can often be difficult to distinguish SOD from Non-ulcer dyspepsia
- Another manifestation is "idiopathic" acute recurrent pancreatitis as a result of SOD
- Non-toxic physical exam during a flare with tenderness in epigastrium or RUQ
- Must rule out: costochondritis, PUD, GERD, malignancy, stones, chronic pancreatitis

LABORATORY STUDIES:
- LFTs, Amylase & Lipase should be obtained during or soon after any flare of pain (likely will see transient elevation)

DIAGNOSTIC STUDIES:
- Start with thorough H & P
- U/S or CT performed to excluded cholelithiasis, chronic pancreatitis, or other intra-abdominal pathology
  - With SOD typically dilation of pancreatic duct (PD) is seen
- Other tests as indicated: GES for predominate N/V, EGD or pH study (24 hr, BRAVO) for dyspeptic or reflux-type symptoms
- Optional tests based on institutions:
  -Secretin stimulated MRI: In general considered positive test if sustained dilation of more than 2 mm for more than 30 min
  -Timed HIDA scan (J Nucl Med 1992;33;1216–22)
  -SO manometry: mean basal pressure increase of >40 mmHg above the duodenal baseline for a 30 sec duration on two pull-throughs
  - Normal pressures does not rule out SOD (best done without an intact gallbladder so pressure can not be normalized by GB reservoir)
  - Narcotics and smooth muscle relaxants (i.e. glucagon) should be held prior to and during the procedure
  - ERCP has higher risk of pancreatitis with those who have SOD (15-30%); All other risks same: cholangitis, perforation, bleeding

CHAPTER 5.08 SPHINCTER OF ODDI DYSFUNCTION

- Milwaukee Classification (Labs during episodes of pain and normalize in absence of pain):

Biliary:		Pancreatic:
Type 1	Biliary type pain, ALT/AST/ Aφ >1.1 × ULN, bile duct >10 mm	Pancreatic type pain, ↑ amylase/lipase, dilated PD*
Type 2	Biliary type pain and *either* ALT/AST/Aφ >1.1 × ULN *or* bile duct >10 mm	Pancreatic type pain, *either* ↑ amylase/lipase or dilated PD*
Type 3	Biliary type pain only (typically more functional problem and ↓ pressures)	Pancreatic type pain only

*>6 mm in Head; >5 mm in Body

TREATMENTS:
- Because there often exists an overlap with IBS, antispasmodics, and low-dose antidepressants or SSRI should be tried initially
- Low fat diet may decrease pancreaticobiliary stimulation and improve symptoms; Nitrates, calcium channel blockers can be tried
- Narcotics can interfere with manometric studies (do these first before patient becomes narcotic dependant)
- Sphincterotomy for type 1 & 2 only with documented elevated pressures via manometry are expected to benefit from endoscopic therapy
  - If manometry is abnormal, pain relief with sphincterotomy:
    - Type 1: >90% relief; Type 2: ~85% relief; Type 3: ~55% relief
  - If manometry is normal, pain relief with sphincterotomy:
    - Type 1: >90% relief; Type 2: ~35% relief; Type 3: ~<10% relief
  - Failure?: incomplete sphincterotomy, restenosis, underlying chronic pancreatitis, disease unrelated to biliary/pancreatic system

PROGNOSIS:
- See Sphincterotomy for pain relief under Treatments above

5.09 POTPOURRI

PANCREAS ANATOMY AND PHYSIOLOGY
Anatomy
- Retroperitoneal, between L4-5 spine
- Arterial supply: gastroduodenal, SMA, splenic; Venous drainage: portal & splenic; Nerves: vagal (stimulatory), sympathetic (inhibitory)
- Note thrombosis of the splenic vein causes the splenic blood to drain through the short gastric veins which results in gastric varices

Overview
- Endocrine pancreas:
  - Islet cells produce insulin, glucagon, pancreatic polypeptide and somatostatin
    - Key molecule is Insulin and loss causes diabetes
- Exocrine pancreas:
  - Acinar cell produce digestive enzymes
    - Key molecule is Trypsinogen and premature activation of trypsinogen causes pancreatitis
  - Duct cells produce bicarbonate-rich fluid (~140 mMol bicarb)
    - Key molecule is CFTR and loss causes cystic fibrosis of pancreas

Pancreatic enzymes: lipase and amylase are synthesized in active form, all other are pro-enzymes
- Proteases (most): Trypsin (trypsinogen)
- Lipases: Pancreatic lipase
- Glycosidases: Pancreatic alpha-amylase (amylase is also produced in salivary glands)
- Nucleases: Ribonuclease and Deoxyribonuclease I

Activation Cascade:
Food » Enterokinase at brush boarder of intestine causes Trypsinogen conversation to Trypsin (master enzyme)
Trypsin then activates all Proenzymes to Enzymes (i.e. Chymotrypsinogen to Chymotrypsin)
Trypsin is regulated by Trypsinogen (inactive form), Serine Protease Inhibitor Kazal type 1 (SPINK1) (inhibitor), and Calcium ($\downarrow$ ca = $\downarrow$ trypsin)

GALLBLADDER POLYPS
- Prevalence 3-8% of population
- U/S: No shadowing on ultrasound with polyps (tissue only); Shadowing is present with gallstones due to calcium stone reflection
- Cholesterol polyps (63%), tubular adenoma (6%), adenocarcinoma (7%), metastasis (particularly melanoma)
Others: adenomyomatous lesions, hamartomas (esp. with Peutz-Jegher), carcinoid
- Malignant potential (risk factors): single polyp (sessile), larger (>1 cm), Age >50 yrs, Gallstones
Polyps >1.5 cm have about 95% chance of being malignant; CT or EUS may be helpful for differentiation
- Surgical Removal: all lesions >1 cm or Biliary dyskinetic symptoms (i.e. postprandial distress)
- Note: Gallbladder cancer 5 year survival: 5-10% if unresectable! 5 year survival: 60% if resectable
  - Polyps <1.0 cm = surveillance U/S q 3-6 months

VI

GI BLEED

6.01 ACUTE GI BLEED PEARLS

(Gastrointest Endosc 2004;60:497-504)

PRE-ENDOSCOPY

Questions to ask:
Nature and duration of bleed: When did it start? First time/Recurrent?
Symptoms: Fever, Pain, Dyspepsia, Hematemesis/Coffee grounds, Hematachezia/Melena/BRBPR, Clots
History: Past bleeds, Trauma, Surgery, Liver disease, Renal disease
Medications: NSAIDs, Coumadin, Antiplatelets
Physical Exam: Vital Signs! CV exam, Abdominal/Rectal exams
Labs: CBC/Chemistries, PT/INR, PTT, Type & Cross, EKG (if age >50 or CAD risk factors)
IV access: Fluids, Blood
NG tube needed?
Sclerosing agent needed at bedside? (i.e. liver patient)

Endoscopy Therapy Contraindications:
Risk > Benefit
Suspect perforation
Uncooperative
Irreversible coagulopathy
Lack of informed consent

See Each Corresponding Procedure for Indications, Contraindications and Risks
Endoscopy & Procedures Section 7: Balloon Tamponade, Capsule, Colonoscopy, EGD, ERCP, EUS

INTRA-ENDOSCOPY
Which bleeding stigmata require endoscopic therapy: See table below
-Active bleeding visible vessels (oozing or spurting)
-Non-bleeding visible vessels
-Adherent clot (depends on severity of bleed)
-Therapy: bipolar and heater probes: comparable efficacy

POST-ENDOSCOPY

Peptic Ulcer Disease

Description	Prevalence (%)	Re Bleed %	Mortality (%)	Triage	Endoscopic Therapy
-Clean base (white base)	42	3-5	2	Advance Diet Early Discharge	No
-Flat red spot or Black slough (pigmented spot)	20	7-10	3		
-Oozing (w/o stigmata)	–	10-27	–	Medical ward Observe 24-48 hr	Yes
-Adherent clot	17-25	10-36	7	ICU vs. Medical ward	
-Nonbleed visible vessel (pigmented protuberance)	17-50	40-50	7	Observe 48 hr	
-Active bleed (arterial)	18-20	55-90	11	ICU, Observe 72 hr	

NOTES

6.02 DIVERTICULAR BLEEDING

DEFINITION:
- Bleeding diverticulum; *See also Bowel- Diverticulosis & Diverticulitis (Chapter 2.14)*

EPIDEMIOLOGY:
- Those with diverticulosis will develop diverticular bleeding 3-5% of the time
- After angiodysplasia, diverticula hemorrhage is the second commonest cause of colonic bleeding representing 50% of acute lower GI bleeds
- Most are clinically insignificant bleeds, however 5% represent a massive bleed

PATHOPHYSIOLOGY:
- Erosion of blood vessels feeding diverticulum by a fecalith (i.e. not an inflammatory process)
- Diverticula more common in left colon; but bleeding diverticula are usually in **right colon**!

CLINICAL MANIFESTATIONS/PHYSICAL EXAM:
- Mostly **painless bleeding** (maroon-colored stools or hematochezia)
  - Can present with sudden onset of abdominal cramping followed by voluminous hematochezia
- Usually stops spontaneously (80%) but may follow a stuttering course for hours to days
- Physical exam is usually benign

LABORATORY STUDIES:
- Hb, Plts, PT/PTT

DIAGNOSTIC STUDIES:
- Colonoscopy: after acute bleeding has stopped and following oral prep
- For severe bleeding: mesenteric angiogram (± after bleeding scan)

TREATMENTS: *See also GI Bleed- UGIB & LGIB (Chapter 6.04)*
- Colonoscopy » epinephrine injection ± electrocautery, hemoclip placement, or banding
  - Signs of possible rebleed: active bleeding, nonbleeding visible vessel (pigmented or nonpigmented protuberances), adherent clots
  - Those with hemodynamic instability and severe LGIB and history of NSAID use should undergo EGD to rule out PUD
- Angiography (detects 0.5-1 cc blood/min) » also allows embolization or intraarterial vasopressin infusion
- Bleeding scan (tagged RBC scan) detects bleeding rates ≥0.1 cc blood/min
- Surgical resection may be necessary (generally subtotal colectomy)
  - Elective resection should be considered after two or more bleeding episodes requiring transfusion with an acceptable operative risk

COMPLICATIONS:
- Estimated rebleed risk: 20-30% after first episode; More than 50% after second episode

NOTES

6.03 OCCULT & OBSCURE BLEEDING

(Gastroenterol 2000;118:197-200 & 201-21)

DEFINITION:
- **Occult:** bleeding that is not visible or hidden and is manifested by positive fecal occult blood testing or iron deficiency anemia
- **Obscure:** clinically observable bleeding with a negative standard evaluation, including: EGD, Colonoscopy, SBS, etc.

ETIOLOGIES:
See Upper and Lower GI bleed etiologies in *GI Bleed- UGIB & LGIB (Chapter 6.04)*, also in the DDX:
- Gastrointestinal stromal tumors, leiomyomas, leiomyosarcomas cause >50% of bleeding neoplasms of small intestine
  - Those under 50 years often have small intestinal tumors as a cause of obscure bleeding
- Angiodysplasia (AVMs) or Osler-Weber-Rendu syndrome (OWR)
- Dieulafoy's lesions
- Cameron's erosions (associated with large hiatal hernias)
- GAVE (gastric antral vascular ectasia or "watermelon stomach")
- Nonesophageal varices
- Portal hypertensive gastropathy
- Crohn's disease
- Small bowel erosions, IBD or tumors (i.e. lymphoma, leiomyoma, carcinoid)
- Diverticula (Meckel's diverticulum in younger patients)
- Ulcers: small bowel, colonic
- Mesenteric ischemia
- Vasculitis
- Amyloidosis
- Hemorrhoids

PATHOPHYSIOLOGY:
- Depends on the particular etiology (above)

CLINICAL MANIFESTATIONS/PHYSICAL EXAM:
- Clues:
  - Facial/oral telangiectasias suggest hereditary telangiectasia (Osler-Weber-Rendu syndrome)
  - Perioral pigmented spots suggest hereditary hamartomatous polyposis (Peutz-Jeghers syndrome)
  - Acanthosis nigricans in axilla suggest possible malignancy
  - Purpura or ecchymoses implies possible bleeding disorder

LABORATORY STUDIES:
- Fecal occult blood testing (FOBT)
  Procedure: avoid false positive foods × 4 days; A stool sample is collected from 3 consecutive BMs; Cards developed with 6 days, no rehydration

  How much causes positive test? As little as 2 ml of blood in GI tract
  - False (+): foods with pseudoperoxidase: rare red meats, raw broccoli, turnips, cauliflower, radishes, cantaloupe; Card rehydration
  - False (−): vitamin C ingestion, delayed development of the card (>6 days), testing when lesion in bowel not bleeding!

  If one + finding, the test is positive and patient needs colonoscopy; If negative, consider EGD

- Iron deficiency anemia:
  Symptoms: fatigue, tachycardia (anemia), pica, pagophagia (ice eating)
  Physical signs rare: cheilitis, glossitis, koilonychias
  Labs: microcytosis, high TIBC, low ferritin, high platelets
  Work up if IDA and + FOBT » Colonoscopy; If negative FOBT » EGD (? Celiac Sprue) » consider Small bowel series
  Workup if only IDA: rule out Celiac Sprue, non-GI causes (menstrual, urinary), nutritional, infectious (hook worm, strongyloidosis); ? full GI workup

DIAGNOSTIC STUDIES:

Typical sequence:
- Repeat EGD/Colon: should be considered early in evaluation because yield is 35%
- Small Bowel Evaluation: Capsule Endoscopy, CT enterography, Enteroclysis/Small bowel series
  - Capsule is probably best method, yielding an abnormal finding 70% of the time
- EGD Push or Double Balloon Endoscopy
- Angiogram (look for abnormal 'vascular blush'); Positive if bleeding more than 0.5 cc/min
- Intraoperative endoscopy

More rarely used tests in clinical practice
- RBC bleeding scan (patient has to be actively bleeding); Positive if bleeding more than 0.1 cc/min
- Meckel's scan (Tc-pertechnetate scan), usefully only in young patients, rarely helps in middle-age or elderly

TREATMENTS:

- Angiodysplasia (AVMs): EGD with APC laser ***See also GI Bleed- Potpourri (Chapter 6.06),*** bipolar therapy, heater probe
  - ? estrogen/progesterone combinations, ? Octreotide therapy
  - Patients should avoid NSAIDs, Anticoagulants

6.04 UPPER & LOWER GI BLEEDING

(Gastrointest Endosc 2005;62:656-60 & 2004;60:497-504. Ann Intern Med 2003; 843-857.)

DEFINITION:
- Intraluminal blood loss anywhere from the oropharynx to the anus (i.e. mouth to butt)
- Classification: **Upper** » above the ligament of Treitz; **Small Bowel** » between lig of Treitz and IC valve; **Lower** » Colonic
- Signs: **Hematemesis:** blood in vomitus (UGIB); Can be bright red or coffee grounds (darkened due to acid exposure)
  Hematochezia: bloody reddish/maroon stools (usually LGIB, however 10-20% can be rapid UGIB or Small bowel bleed)
  Melena: black, tarry, stinky stools from digested blood (usually UGIB but can be anywhere above and including the right colon)
- Occult and Obscure, *See also GI Bleed- Occult & Obscure Bleeding (Chapter 6.03)*

EPIDEMIOLOGY:
- UGIB constitutes 75% of all acute GI bleeding; See also each etiology under UGIB and LGIB

UGIB ETIOLOGIES: (Am J Gastro 1998;93:1202-08)
- Always consider oropharyngeal bleeding or epistaxis leading to swallowed blood
- **PUD (40-50%):** Both Duodenal and Gastric!
  - Duodenal Ulcers (30%)
  - Gastritis/Gastrophathy: Gastric Erosions (27%) and Gastric Ulcers (22%) NSAIDs, *H. Pylori,* Stress-related mucosal disease
- **Erosive esophagitis** (11%)
  - Immunocompetent: GERD, BE, XRT; Immuno*compromised:* CMV, HSV, Candida
- **Duodenitis** (10%)
- **Varices** (5-30%); *See also GI Bleed- Variceal Bleeding (Chapter 6.05)*
- **Mallory-Weiss tear** (5-15%) GE junction tear due to retching against closed glottis
- **Vascular Malformations** (5%)
  - Dieulafoy's lesion (superficial submucosal artery, majority within 6 cm of GEJ (but can occur anywhere) » sudden, massive GIB)
  - AVMs (may be isolated or occur with Osler-Weber-Rendu syndrome)
  - Gastric antral vascular ectasia (GAVE), aka: Watermelon stomach; primarily involves antrum and crosses the pylorus
  - Portal hypertensive gastropathy (PHG); primarily involves proximal stomach (fundus)
  - Aorto-enteric Fistula (Abdominal aortic aneurysm or aortic graft erodes to 3rd portion of duodenum; presents with 'herald bleed': small, then massive bleed)
  - Hemobilia (liver or biliary trauma, including liver biopsy); EGD shows blood coming from ampulla
  - Hemosuccus Pancreaticus (bleeding from peripancreatic vessels into PD); Angiography is diagnostic/therapeutic; Rarely surgery
  - Neoplastic disease (esophageal or gastric)
- Other: Hiatal hernia ulcer (Cameron lesions), Vasculitis, Mixed connective tissue disease, Coagulopathy, Amyloid

LGIB ETIOLOGIES: (Am J Gastroenterol 1993;93:1202-08)
- **Hemorrhoids, Internal (most common cause in adults, 50-80%** of population): intermittent, sometimes massive, often with defecation
- **Angiodysplasia 41%** (age acquired, esp >50 years old; Most are in cecum and proximal ascending but can occur anywhere in GI tract)
  - Histologically: ecstatic, distorted thin-walled veins, venules, and capillaries in mucosa or submucosa
  - Most are subacute and recurrent bleeds, although 15% present with acute massive bleed, while 10% present with occult blood loss
  - Bleeding ceases spontaneously in >90% of cases

CHAPTER 6.04 UPPER & LOWER GI BLEEDING

- **Diverticular 23%** Right-side bleed more (occurs 3–5% of those with Diverticulosis; Bleeding reoccurs 25%, second recurrence is 50%)
  - Acute, massive, painless hematochezia; Stops spontaneously or with medical therapy in 75–95% of patients
  - Not a chronic process causing chronic occult blood loss; Surgical resection may be necessary; *See also GI Bleed- Diverticular Bleeding (Chapter 6.02)*
- **Neoplastic disease 15%** (most are occult blood loss and Iron deficient anemia rather than acute blood loss
  - Most have variable bowel habits, weight loss; Physical exam can show palpable mass or rectal mass
- **Colitis: 12%** infection, ischemic, radiation, IBD (UC much more common than CD)
- **UGIB accounts for 11% of "LGIBs"!**
- Rare: intussusception, colonic varices, solitary rectal ulcer syndrome, aortoenteric fistula, colonic endometriosis

CLINICAL MANIFESTATIONS/PHYSICAL EXAM:
- UGIB > LGIB: hematemesis, coffee-ground emesis (nausea, vomiting), melena, epigastric pain, syncope or vasovagal reactions
- LGIB > UGIB: diarrhea, tenesmus, BRBPR or maroon stools (melena can also be cecum/right colon)
- Acute blood loss: **Tachycardia** at 10% volume loss; **Orthostatic hypotension** at 20% loss; **Shock** at 30% loss
  - 500 cc: no detectable physiologic changes; 1000 cc: 10–20 mmHg ↓ in SBP & 20 bpm ↑ in pulse rate changes; ≥2000 cc: shock
- Pallor, telangectasias (alcoholic liver disease or Osler-Weber-Rendu syndrome/Peutz-Jeghers)
- Signs of chronic liver disease: jaundice, spider angiomata, gynecomastia, testicular atrophy, palmar erythema, caput medusae
- Localized abdominal tenderness or peritoneal signs, bowel sounds, masses, signs of prior surgery
- Rectal exam: appearance of stools, presence of hemorrhoids or anal fissures
  - BRBPR not associated with orthostatic BP changes or syncope is probably not from UGI tract

HISTORY:
- General:
  - Acute or chronic GIB, number of episodes, most recent episode
  - Use of anticoagulants, or known coagulopathy
  - Iron and Pepto-bismol can produce black stools
- UGI Bleed
  - As above under Clinical Manifestations/Physical Exam; *See also GI Bleed- Acute GI Bleed Pearls (Chapter 6.01)*
  - NSAIDs: prevalent use in up to 60% of PUD bleeding; E TOH and Cigarettes are NOT associated with PUD hemorrhage
    - Corticosteroids: no increased risk of PUD, however several fold increased risk *with concomitant* NSAID use
  - History of heartburn and abdominal pain before onset of bleeding strongly suggests peptic source
  - History of liver disease or heavy ETOH use raises the possibility of variceal bleeds
  - Vomiting and/or retching *prior* to hematemesis suggests a Mallory-Weiss tear
  - Prior GI or Aortic surgery
- LGI Bleed
  - As above under Clinical Manifestations/Physical Exam; *See also GI Bleed- Acute GI Bleed Pearls (Chapter 6.01)*

LABORATORY STUDIES:
- Hct (bleeding is whole blood, so Hct may be normal early in acute blood loss before equilibration, ↓ 2-3% with 500 cc blood loss)
  - 2 hrs: 25% of final fall/decrease is achieved; 8 hrs: 50%; 24–72 hrs: the final fall is achieved
  - Obviously time table is accelerated if IVFs given and dilution occurs earlier and quicker
- **Plt count, PT, PT T, Type/Cross**
- **BUN/Cr ratio:** ratio >36 in UGIB due to GI resorption of blood and/or prerenal azotemia
- Chronic blood loss: LFTs, Creatinine, Iron studies, RBC indices (MCV, RDW, Retic count)

DIAGNOSTIC STUDIES:
- Ng tube: useful for localization, can also clear GI contents prior to EGD and detect continual bleeding; No role for guaiac testing Ng aspirate (Non-bloody bile may exclude active bleeding proximal to the ligament of Treitz; False Negative if lower duodenal bleed or intermittent bleed)

SECTION VI GI BLEED

- UGIB
  - EGD (potentially also therapeutic); Get *H. Pylori* biopsies if ulcer disease!
- LGIB: In general, rule out UGIB before attempting to localize presumed LGIB
  - **Bleeding spontaneously stops:** Cscope (identifies cause in >70%, potentially therapeutic)
  - **Stable but continues to bleed:** Cscope after rapid purge; If source not found consider Bleeding scan ± repeat Cscope
    - Bleeding scan (tagged RBC scan) detects bleeding rates ≥0.1 cc/min, but actual localization difficult and often inaccurate
    - Follow with interventional radiology as bleeding scan is helpful to determine the best timing for angiography
  - **Unstable:** Angiography detects bleeding rates ≥0.5-1 cc/min and potentially therapeutic (embolization or intraarterial vasopressin)
    - Complications of angiography include: ARF, cholesterol plaque emboli, thrombosis of wrong vessel, bowel infarction
  - Exploratory laparotomy may be necessary; Get Colorectal surgery involved early

TREATMENTS:

- **Acute Treatment of GIB** is hemodynamic resuscitation with IVF/Crystalloids and blood
  - **Access** with 2 large-bore (18 g or larger) IV lines
  - **Volume resuscitation** with normal saline
  - **Transfusion** send blood for type & cross; O-neg if patient is exsanguinating
  - **Correct Couagulopathies** FFP to normalize PT, platelets to keep count >50K
  - Ng when? lavage for EGD if hematemesis; May be misleading; *Placing with suspected varices does not increase bleeding!*
  - Airway management as needed (i.e. intubation for ongoing hematemesis, decreased consciousness or loss of gag reflex)
  - Consult surgery early if needed
- **PUD:** *See also GI Bleed- Acute GI Bleed Pearls (Chapter 6.01)* for PUD classification/triage
  - Pharmacologic:
    - High dose PPI in IV form or until po; At gastric pH >6 there is functional coagulation and platelet aggregation; Evidence suggest PPI infusion before EGD therapy (NEJM 2007; 356: 1631-40)
    - May consider Octreotide 50 mcg IV bolus followed by » 50 mcg/hr infusion
  - Non-Pharmacologic:
    - EGD Therapy: injection with epi 1:10,000, endoclip, thermal: heater probe (30J) or bipolar electrocoagulation (14-16W)
      Removing an adherent clot is controversial, but more evidence favors clot removal and treatment
    - Angiography with embolization or infusion of vasopressin
    - Surgery if EGD, Angiography and Pharmacologic fails (clinical signs of bleeding persist)
- **Esophagitis/Gastritis/Duodenitis**
  - PPI better than H2-antagonist; Avoid NSAIDs!
  - ICU Acid suppression indications: coagulopathy, mechanical ventilation, extensive burn injuries
- **Varices:** *See also GI Bleed- Variceal Bleeding (Chapter 6.05)*
- **Mallory-Weiss Tear**
  - Usually stops spontaneously in 80-90%; EGD therapy if bleeding (injection/thermal); Rebleed: 2-5%
- **Angiodysplasia**
  - EGD with APC treatment, Angiography, Surgery, ? Estrogen (hormonal) therapy
- **Gastric antral vascular ectasia (GAVE):** Does not improve with TIPS; Treat with APC, rarely antrectomy/hormones
  Portal hypertensive gastropathy (PHG): Does improve with TIPS, BB, and Octreotide since related to high portal pressures
- **Diverticular Disease:** *See also GI Bleed- Diverticular Bleeding (Chapter 6.02)*
  - Usually stops spontaneously
    - Colonoscopy therapy (i.e. epinephrine injection), Angiography with embolization or infusion of vasopressin, surgery
- **Aortoenteric Fistula**
  - Etiology: thoracic aortic aneurysms/graft reconstructive procedure, esophageal foreign bodies, or neoplasms
  - 75% communicate with duodenum (3rd portion); 50% have herald bleed (bleeding that stops hours-months before massive bleed)
  - EGD first (positive <40%); Angiography rarely helpful and may delay therapy; CT may be helpful; Suspected patients need surgery

COMPLICATIONS:
- Poor prognostic signs:
  - Demographics: age >60 yrs, comorbidities, variceal bleed, neoplastic etiology
  - Severity: bright red blood in Ng not clearing, requiring ↑ transfusion requirements, hemodynamic instability
- Ulcer Appearances (best to worse): clean base » oozing without vessel » adherent clot » vessel » active arterial bleeding; *See also GI Bleed- Acute GI Bleed Pearls (Chapter 6.01)*

PROGNOSIS:
- Mortality from UGIB is low (5–10%) but hasn't changed much in the last several decades
- Re-bleeding: nearly 94% by 72 hours and 98% by 96 hours

6.05 VARICEAL BLEEDING

(Gastrointest Endosc 2005;62:651-5. NEJM 2001;345:669-81)

DEFINITION:
- Bleeding from varices
- For Portal Hypertensive Gastropathy (PHG) and Gastric antral vascular ectasia (GAVE), *See also GI Bleed- UGIB & LGIB (Chapter 6.04)*

EPIDEMIOLOGY:
- Varices:
  - Prevalence: 50% of all cirrhotics have varices (80% in Childs C, 20% in Childs A)
  - Incidence: 10% per year in cirrhotics
- Variceal Bleeding:
  - Incidence: 24% per 2 years with moderate to large varices
  - Mortality: >20% with first bleed; 70% 5-year mortality; 40-50% will re-bleed

ETIOLOGIES:
- In acute bleeds (causes): Varices 50%.
  - Nonvariceal source: Gastric erosions 50%, MWT 15%, Any PUD 14%, Erosive esophagitis 11%

PATHOPHYSIOLOGY:
- Hepatic Venous Wedge Pressure Gradient [HVWPG] = ~6 mmHg normally
  - >10 mmHg is required for variceal development; >12 mmHg is at high risk for bleeding
  - HVWPG represents the pressure difference between the wedged hepatic vein (which reflects the portal vein pressure) and the direct measurement of the abdominal IVC (or the free hepatic vein pressure)
  - Similar concept to a right heart catheterization (Swan-Ganz), in other words: HVWPG = Wedge Pressure (balloon up) − Free Hepatic Vein (balloon down)
- Types of **Gastric Varices** (Sarin classification):
  - GV-1: lesser curve (74%); GV-2: greater curve (16%)
  - Currently no data support use of prophylactic treatment of gastric varices
- **Isolated Gastric Varices (IGV):** usually complication of splenic vein thrombosis (especially IGV-1) or portal vein thrombosis
  - Cause: trauma, pancreatitis/pancreatic cancer, hypercoagulability/essential thrombocytosis, cirrhosis (schistosomiasis), idiopathic
  - Types: IGV-1: fundus (8%), IGV-2: antrum/pylorus (2%)
  - Therapy: splenectomy for isolated splenic vein thrombosis

CLINICAL MANIFESTATIONS/PHYSICAL EXAM:
- Upper GI Bleeding (may present as upper or lower GI bleed)

LABORATORY STUDIES:
- Hb, PT/PTT

DIAGNOSTIC STUDIES:
- All cirrhotics should be screened for varices at diagnosis of cirrhosis with **screening EGD:**
  - No varices: repeat EGD 2-3 yrs; No prophylaxis necessary
  - Small varices: repeat EGD 1-2 yrs (shorter interval if ETOH/severe liver disease or red-wale signs, etc)
    - Consider beta-blockers if Childs C
  - Medium-Large varices: 1° prevention: EBL, Beta blockers, etc (See Prognosis, below)

TREATMENTS: See also 1° prevention and 2° prevention below under Prognosis
- Beta-Blockers (non-selective): i.e. propranolol 10 mg TID or nadolol 40 QD
  - Goal is 20% reduction in HVWPG or 25% ↓ heart rate; This decreases bleeding risk 50-90%
    - However only 35% of patients achieve this goal!
  - A reduction in HVWPG to <12 mmHg equals nearly 100% no bleeding risk
    - However only 25% of patients achieve this goal!

- Beta-Blocker's, do NOT prevent the development of varices, but do prevent small varices to becoming large varices
- Problems: non-compliance, contraindications to beta blocker therapy
- Sclerotherapy
  - Not recommended for prophylaxis of initial variceal bleed (see Prognosis below)
- EGD and Esophageal Band Ligation (EBL)
  - 90% success, 26% rebleed; Has replaced Sclerotherapy which has 88% success, 44% rebleed
- TIPS (Transjugular Intrahepatic Portosystemic Shunt)
  - More effective than BB or EBL, however increased risk of encephalopathy, more expensive and NO improvement in survival
  - Indications: salvage in acute bleed and/or recurrent significant bleeding despite EBL and BB
- Cyanoacrylate Injection ("Glue")
  - Risks: systemic embolization (2%), bacteremia, needle fixation (need to flush continually), variability in polymerization time
  - Rebleed: 5-17% at 72 hrs, 17% at 1 yr; Not yet FDA approved
  - Contraindications: Hepatopulmonary syndrome, Cardiac septal defects (risks arterial embolization)

TREATMENTS CONTINUED:
- ACUTE bleeding:
  - Transfuse Hb to 8 gm/dl (more aggressive transfusion may precipitate further portal hypertension and bleeding)
    - Consider: Platelets, FFP, Lactulose, Endotracheal intubation
  - Pharmacologic (start immediately, do not wait for EGD to be performed):
    - **Octreotide:** 50 mcg IV bolus then 50 mcg/hr infusion (84% success); Continue for 4-7 days
    - **PPI:** IV drip until po can be taken (need to help cure the ulcer that banding will create)
    - **Antibiotics:** All variceal bleeds should get antibiotics against gut bacteria (3rd gen cephalosporin) during hospitalization for 4-7days
    - BB (non-selective i.e. propranolol or nadolol) ± nitrates once stable
    - Vasopressin & nitro less efficacious and more complications
    - ETOH/Cirrhotic more likely to have a coagulopathy needing correction (i.e. Vitamin K, FFP)
  - Non-Pharmacologic:
    - EGD with band ligation (>90% success, 26% rebleed) has replaced Sclerotherapy (88% success, 44% rebleed)
      - Repeat as outpatient every 2-4 weeks until varices obliterated
    - **EGD/band ligation with Octreotide** (>95% success)
    - Balloon tamponade (Sengstaken-Blakemore/Minnesota tube) if bleeding severe ***See also Endoscopy & Procedures- Balloon Tamponade (Chapter 7.02)***
    - Cyanoacrylate or Embolization or TIPS if EGD fails (Surgical shunts rarely done unless Childs-Pugh class A)

PROGNOSIS:
- **1° prevention of esophageal variceal UGIB**
Indicated in patients with moderate-large varices >5 mm in diameter
  - Non-selective BB, starting doses: Propranolol 10 mg TID or Nadolol 40 mg QD
    - Titrate to 25% ↓ heart rate (i.e. a resting pulse of 55-60 beats/min)
    - ~50% ↓ bleeding; addition of nitrates may further ↓ bleeding
  - Band Ligation: greater ↓ bleeding compared with BB, but no change in mortality, therefore reserve for those intolerant of BB
    - Second-line 1⁰ prevention
- **2° prevention of esophageal variceal UGIB**
Indicated in all patients who have previously bled; >80% of those who already bleed will bleed again within 2 years
  - Band Ligation ± BB & Nitrates; If continued to re-bleed » Tips or Transplant

6.06 POTPOURRI

ARGON PLASMA COAGULATION (APC) THERAPY
General recommendations for setting
(Do not use with pacemaker)

Condition	Probe (mm)	Wattage (W)	Gas Flow (L/min)
XRT Proctitis	3.2	65	1.5
GAVE	3.2	65–75	2
AVM: colon	3.2	20–30	1.5
AVM: small bowel	2.3	20–30	1–1.5
Polyp: colon	3.2	30–40	1–1.5
Polyp: small bowel	3.2	30	1.5
Polyp: papilla	3.2	30–40	1.5
Bleeding tumor	3.2	80	2
Debulk tumor	3.2	90	2

VII

ENDOSCOPY & PROCEDURES

7.01 ANTICOAGULATION & ANTI-INFLAMMATORY MANAGEMENT FOR ENDOSCOPY

(Gastrointest Endosc 2005;61:189-194)

WARFARIN THERAPY	HIGH-RISK PATIENTS: Afib associated with valvular disease Mechanical valve in the mitral position Mechanical valve and prior thromboembolic event	LOW-RISK PATIENTS: DVT Uncomplicated or paroxysmal Afib Bioprosthetic valve Mechanical valve in aortic position
HIGH-RISK PROCEDURES: Polypectomy Biliary Sphincterotomy Pneumatic or Bougie dilation PEG ERCP/EUS with FNA Laser ablation and coagulation Treatment of varices	Stop warfarin 3-5 days before; Consider heparin while INR below therapeutic	Stop warfarin 3-5 days before Restart warfarin after procedure
LOW RISK PROCEDURES: Diagnostic: EGD/Cscope/Flex Sig ± Biopsy ERCP without Sphincterotomy Biliary/Pancreatic stent without endoscopic sphincterotomy EUS without FNA Enteroscopy	No change in anticoagulation; Elective procedures should be delayed while INR is supratherapeutic	

OTHER MEDICATIONS

- ASA and NSAIDs
  - In the absence of pre-existing bleeding disorder, all endoscopic procedures can be performed in patients taking Aspirin and NSAIDs

- Dipyridamole: Similar to ASA/NSAIDs

- Plavix: There are no published studies
  - If Acute GI bleed, stop Plavix; Decision to reverse antiplatelet effect is individualized based on the risk-benefit assessment
  - For High Risk elective procedures: There's no guidelines available
    - If discontinued, hold it for 7-10 days prior to the procedure
    - If taking Plavix and ASA, consider switching to single agent such as ASA

- Glycoprotein IIb/IIIa receptors: There are no published studies
  - This is usually encountered during emergency endoscopy since this medication is given IV and should be discontinued in this setting
  - Duration of the antiplatelet effect of the drug:
    - Eptifibatide/Tirofiban - 4 hours
    - Abciximab-up to 24 hours

- LMWH: There are no published studies
  - Acute GI bleeding: The decision to stop or reverse LMWH is individualized based on the risk-benefit assessment
    - The anticoagulant effect of LMWH is reversed within 8 hours of last dose
  - Elective Procedures:
    - For low risk procedures-no adjustment is needed
    - For high risk procedures, discontinue for 8 hours; Time to restart therapy is individualized

NOTES

7.02 BALLOON TAMPONADE

Minnesota Tube (4 lumen) is current standard for use; Lumens include:
- Gastric suction
- Esophageal suction
- Gastric balloon and pressure monitoring
- Esophageal balloon and pressure monitoring

Sengstaken-Blakemore Tube (3 lumen): older style that did not include separate esophageal suction lumen

INDICATIONS:
- Acute bleeding from esophageal or gastric varices unresponsive to medical therapy (lavage, correction of clotting abnormalities, intravenous octreotide) and endoscopic therapy (band ligation and/or sclerotherapy)
  - Greatest role is temporarily stabilizing active bleeding while awaiting emergent TIPS
- Alternative: Angiography and/or TIPS for uncontrollable bleeding
- Efficacy: 50-92%
  - Worse outcome if patient has ascites, jaundice, encephalopathy
  - Long term efficacy depends in part on patients underlying liver disease

METHODS (IN GENERAL):
Pre-procedure
- Intubate patient to protect airway
- Always read a particular manufactures instructions
- EGD to confirm source of bleeding and attempt band ligation or sclerotherapy; Start Octreotide drip
- Test balloons by insufflating with air and examine for leaks under water
  - Gastric: inflate with 100 cc of air and record manometric pressures; Repeat to a total of 500 cc of air in 100 cc increments
- Deflate completely after testing and clamp with hemostats
- Lubricate tube, pass along the patient's mouth until the 45-50 cm mark is at teeth
  - Only use nares if oral fails (due to increased risk of necrosis of nasal septum)
- Apply suction to both gastric and esophageal ports to clear fluids
- Confirm position of tube fluoroscopically (Tip must be below diaphragm)
- Gastric balloon: inflate with 100 cc of air at a time to 450-500 cc total and check manometric readings for correlation with pre-insertion
  - If more than 15 mmHg greater than pre-insertion values, deflate as balloon may be located in esophagus
- Clamp the tube and pull back gently until resistance is felt against the GEJ
- Apply traction with weight of 500-1500 grams (a 500 ml bag of saline weighs 500 gm)

Esophageal Balloon
- Some recommend inflation if bleeding does not appear to be controlled after 4 hours and some recommend inflation in all patients
- If used, balloon should not exceed 25-45 mmHg (use lowest pressure needed to stop bleeding)
- Check esophageal balloon pressure with manometer every 3 hours
- Some recommend inflation deflating for 5-10 minutes every 6-8 hours to avoid necrosis

Post-procedure
- Verify tube position with portable X-ray
- Reduce pressure in esophageal balloon as soon as possible
- Manually check tube tension every 3 hours
- Medications can be given via gastric port if necessary
- Flush esophageal and gastric ports every 2 hours to prevent clogging
- If emergently needs to be removed, transect the tube with scissors and pull out
- If hemostasis after 24 hours: deflate esophageal balloon; If no recurrence of bleeding over next 6-12 hours, deflate the gastric balloon
  - Leave tube in place and if bleeding reoccurs the balloons can be re-inflated for another 24 hours
  - If no further bleeding after initial 24 hours, remove tube

COMPLICATIONS/RISK:
- Absolute contraindications, considerations include:
  - Cessation of variceal bleeding; Recent surgery of GEJ
- Relative contraindications:
  - Large hiatal hernias
  - Inability to demonstrate variceal source of bleeding;
  - Esophageal ulceration or stricture (do not use esophageal balloon)
  - Suspect perforation
  - Uncooperative
  - Irreversible coagulopathy
  - Lack of informed consent
- Complications
  - Aspiration (airway protection with intubation should be done), Pulmonary edema
  - Pressure effects:
    - Rupture of esophagus (especially with history of sclerotherapy in the past)
    - Laceration/ulceration of stomach
    - Pressure necrosis of hypopharynx with prolonged balloon inflation

7.03 CAPSULE ENDOSCOPY

INDICATIONS:
- Obscure GI bleeding
  - Signs of GI bleeding: Melena, Hematochezia, Iron deficient anemia
- Abnormal GI X-ray
- Crohn's disease
- Unexplained abdominal pain

AdvanCE: Endoscopic device to deliver the capsule to the stomach or duodenum
- Useful for patients with oropharyngeal or mechanical dysphagia, gastroparesis, and known or suspected anatomical abnormalities
- Helps minimize loss of battery life spent in the esophagus or stomach

PATENCY CAPSULE: A capsule that degrades within 30 hours of being in the gut; Given prior to real capsule in some patients to rule out obstruction
- KUB is taken at 24 hrs after administration and if still in the small bowel the Pillcam is not administered due to high risk of not passing/obstructing

COMPLICATIONS/RISK:
- Caution but not contraindicated
  - Dysphagia or Zenker's diverticulum-can use AdvanCE
  - Surgery of abdomen, bowel or pelvis in the preceding 12 months due to risk of obstruction due to adhesions
  - Crohn's due to risk of obstruction-can use Patency capsule first
  - Abdominal radiation due to risk of obstruction-can use Patency capsule first
  - Mentally or developmentally uncooperative-can use AdvanCE
  - Use of iron supplements: light from capsule is absorbed rendering poor quality images
  - Diabetics or chronic narcotic use have poor gastric emptying and capsule may stay in stomach - can use AdvanCE
  - If performing EGD and Biopsy, there can be a confused bleeding source
- Relative contraindications
  - Electromedical device (i.e. pacemaker or defibrillators): Not FDA approved, but substantial evidence suggest there is no deviation of function with an implanted device and concurrent capsule use; Some centers have done >150 studies without any problems
  - Pregnancy: has not been studied but has occurred unknowingly without problems
  - Suspected bowel obstruction-Patency capsule prior
- Repeating a second study
  - There is no limit to the number of capsule procedures a patient can have within a year
  - Some published data suggest there is a greater than 70% chance of significant findings found on a second capsule

PROCEDURE:
- Document Risk/Benefit/Alternatives in chart (including not FDA approved in those with electromedical devices)
- Take a history-any of the following?
  - dysphagia, diabetes, gastroparesis, abdominal surgery, abdominal radiation, Crohn's disease
  - signs/symptoms of obstruction, pregnant, electromedical device
  - Medications:
    - ASA/NSAIDS, Anti-coagulation, Iron supplements, PPI, Narcotics, Immunosuppressants

Before capsule administration
- Stop iron supplements at least 3-5 days prior to capsule
- Diet before morning of administration:
  - Clear liquids starting at noon the day prior (at least 12 hours)
  - NPO after midnight the day prior (adjust diabetic medication as necessary)
  - Any morning medications the day of the exam should be taken prior to 7 am
  - No carafate, antacids, barium for 4-6 hours prior to exam; Anticoagulants do not need to be stopped prior to exam
- Male abdominal wall should be shaved 4 inches above and below the waistline for lead placement

CHAPTER 7.03 CAPSULE ENDOSCOPY

During capsule
- Study time is 8 hours–may be extended if on narcotics
- Patient may drink clear liquids (water, soda, apple juice, coffee/tea or broth) 2 hours after swallowing the capsule
- Patients may resume their prior diet 8 hours after capsule administered (if high suspicion of bleeding, may want to keep NPO)
- Patient may ambulate during the study
- Patients may loosen the recording belt to go to restroom, but should not remove the belt
- Avoid going near MRI machines or radio transmitters
- The use of a computer, radio, cell phone or microwave is permitted

After capsule administration
- Pain and nausea are uncommon following a capsule endoscopy
- Patient may resume any prior activity and diet
- Patient may resume all medications immediately after study (do not make up for doses missed)
- The capsule naturally passes in a bowel movement typically within 24 hours (most likely patient will be unaware of passage)
  - Can be safely flushed down toilet (occasionally the light will still be flashing)
- MRI should be avoided until capsule passes (if unclear an abdominal X-ray can be obtained)

7.04 COLONOSCOPY

(Gastrointest Endosc 2003;57:441-5)

INDICATIONS:
Diagnostic:
- Screening for colon polyps/cancer; including preoperative evaluation of patients with known colon cancer
- Symptom evaluation: bleeding (occult or gross) or Abnormal X-ray findings (i.e. barium enema)
- Screening/Surveillance for neoplasia: IBD patients, familial polyposis

Therapeutic:
- Polypectomy, hemostasis of bleeding lesions, foreign body removal, decompression (Volvulus or Ogilvie's syndrome)

COMPLICATIONS/RISK:
- No absolute contraindications, considerations include:
  - Risk > Benefit; Risks are related to severity of underlying disease, comorbid disease, emergency/therapeutic procedures, elderly
  - Suspect perforation, acute diverticulitis, fulminant colitis, recent MI (risk may be greater than benefit)
  - Uncooperative
  - Irreversible coagulopathy, poor bowel preparation
  - Lack of informed consent
- Prep related complications (depends upon type of preparation used-see below)
  - PEG solutions:
    - 5-15% intolerance
  - Sodium phosphate or Magnesium citrate:
    - Fluid or electrolyte shifts
    - Increase in phosphate or magnesium, especially with chronic renal failure
    - Phosphate nephropathy
    - Mucosal changes: aphthoid like ulcers that can mimic IBD
  - Mannitol or lactulose:
    - Explosive gases
- Generally safe:
  - Complications include bleeding, perforation, myocardial infarction, and cerebral accidents
    - Cardiopulmonary complications related to sedation are most common
  - 0.35% overall complication rate, primarily bleeding and perforation (1 in 300)
  - 0.09% bleeding with diagnostic, 1-3% with polypectomy (can be immediate or delayed occurring on average in 1-12 days)
  - 0.14-0.26% perforation with diagnostic, 0.11-0.42% with polypectomy; need early diagnosis and surgery (1-2 in 1000)
  - 0.06% mortality related to colonoscopy (with or without polypectomy) (1 in 5000)
  - 4-5% bacteremia complication
- Most common complication: cardiopulmonary (40-45% of complications)
  - Minor change in vital signs or O_2 sats occur in 70%
  - Hypoxia related to: difficult intubation, age >65, obesity, higher dose of sedation, underlying CV or pulmonary disease, pre-existing cardiac disease
- Post-polypectomy coagulation syndrome:
  - Transmural burn resulting in inflammatory response of the serosa; Pain/fever/leukocytosis ~2 days post procedure (range 6 hr - 5 days)
  - Typically no free air and surgery not needed unless perforation (~0.3%)
  - Hospitalize for antibiotics and bowel rest

BEFORE PROCEDURE:
- Document Risk/Benefit/Alternatives in chart
- Labs: PT/PTT, Platelets
- Stop Warfarin × 3 days, Clopidogrel × 7 days, Ask about bleeding disorders
- Implantable devices & Electrical Therapy: Pacemakers (Endoscopic therapy current can change settings/deactivate); ICD (Endoscopic therapy current can cause benign/lethal arrhythmia)

Preparation (Gastrointest Endosc 2006;63:894–909)
- General
  - 5 days prior: No bulk-forming agents (i.e. Metamucil, Citrucel); No iron supplements, No NSAIDs
  - 3 days prior: No popcorn, seeds, nuts, multigrain bread, salad, cheese, high-fiber foods
  - 1 day prior: No solid foods, drink 8 oz of clear liquids every hour to avoid dehydration (avoid ETOH)

  Clear liquids: water, apple/white grape juice, broth, coffee/tee, clear carbonated beverages, sports drinks/jell-O/popsicles (not red color!)
  - Warn patients that with the preparation they may feel: bloating, nausea, and occasional vomiting may occur
    - Waiting 30 minutes or light activity or a few soda crackers and then resuming may help
- Polyethylene Glycol (GoLytely/NuLytely):
  - At 6 pm the evening prior to procedure: drink 8 oz of GoLytely/NuLytely every 10 minutes until the solution is finished (around 8 pm)
    - Continue to drink at least 8 oz of clear liquids every hour until bed time
  - Morning of procedure: continue to drink 8 oz of clear liquids every hour until two hours before the test
- Fleets Phospha-Soda:
  - *Do NOT use with patients who have kidney, liver or heart problems—use Polyethylene Glycol*
  - At 6 pm, mix 1.5 oz (3 tablespoons) of Fleets with 4 oz of clear liquids and drink followed by at least three more 8 oz of clear liquids
    - Continue to drink at least 8 oz of clear liquids every hour until bed time
  - At 8 pm, mix 1.5 oz (3 tablespoons) of Fleets with 4 oz of clear liquids and drink followed by at least three more 8 oz of clear liquids
  - Day of procedure: continue to drink 8 oz of clear liquids every hour until two hours before the test

7.05 ESOPHAGOGASTRODUO-DENOSCOPY (EGD)

(Gastrointest Endosc 2002;55:784-93 & 2000;52:831-837)

INDICATIONS:
Diagnostic:
- Upper GI symptoms that are persistent or worrisome: dysphagia/odynophagia; abdominal pain; gastric outlet obstruction; chest pain after cardiac evaluation, iron deficient anemia, document healing of ulcers; GERD; vomiting; evaluate toxic or caustic ingestion

Therapeutic:
- GI bleeding; Portal HTN
- Foreign bodies; Disintegration of bezoars
- Esophageal, gastric, duodenal polypectomy (including Familial polyposis)
- Esophageal dilation
- PEG placement
- Evaluate abnormal X-ray findings

COMPLICATIONS/RISK:
- No absolute contraindications, considerations include:
  - Risk > Benefit; Risks are related to severity of underlying disease, comorbid disease, emergency/therapeutic procedures, elderly
    - Shock and acute MI (risk may be greater than benefit)
  - Suspect perforation
  - Uncooperative
  - Irreversible coagulopathy
  - Lack of informed consent

- Generally safe:
  - Complications include bleeding, perforation, myocardial infarction, and cerebral accidents
    - Cardiopulmonary complications related to sedation are most common
  - 0.1-0.2% overall complication rate (1 in 500)
  - 0.03% perforation rate (however there is a 25% chance of mortality when they do rarely occur): need early diagnosis and surgery
  - 0.004-0.009% mortality related to EGD (1 in 10,000)
  - 4-8% bacteremia complication (up to 30% with dilation or sclerotherapy); 1% aspiration pneumonia
  - 0.05% bleeding related to low platelets or coagulopathy

- Most common complication: cardiopulmonary (40-45% of complications)
  - Minor change in vital signs or O_2 sats occur in 70%
  - Hypoxia related to: difficult intubation, age >65, obesity, higher dose of sedation, underlying CV or pulmonary disease, pre-existing cardiac disease

BEFORE PROCEDURE:
- Document Risk/Benefit/Alternatives in chart
- Labs: PT/PTT, Platelets
- Stop Warfarin × 3 days, Clopidogrel × 7 days

NOTES

7.06 ENDOSCOPIC RETROGRADE CHOLANGIOPANCREATOGRAPHY (ERCP)

(Gastrointest Endosc 2005;62:1-8 & 2003;57:633-38)

INDICATIONS:
- Biliary
  - Diagnosis and extraction of common bile duct stones (if high suspicion)
  - Diagnosis of primary sclerosing cholangitis
  - Investigation, brushing and therapy of bile duct strictures
  - Staging of bile duct cancer
  - Diagnosis of bile duct anomalies
  - Palliation of biliary obstruction from bile duct, ampullary, or pancreas cancer
  - Imaging of bile and pancreatic ducts prior to ampullectomy

  Questions to ask about a stricture:
  Long or short? Symmetric or asymmetric? What is above/below the stricture?

- Pancreatic
  - Acute recurrent pancreatitis (to rule out obstructive cause or sphincter dysfunction–should not be performed during acute episode)
  - Type I and II Sphincter of Oddi dysfunction (manometry and biliary/pancreatic sphincterotomy)
  - Therapy of chronic pancreatitis (pancreatic sphincterotomy, stone extraction, stent placement)
  - Transpapillary or transmural pseudocyst drainage
  - Diagnosis and presurgical staging of intraductal papillary mucinous neoplasm
  - Minor papillotomy for pancreas divisum

COMPLICATIONS/RISK:
- No absolute contraindications
- Prefer non-invasive tests (MRCP or EUS) for purely diagnostic purposes or if therapeutic potential is low
- Pancreatitis rate:
  - 5-10% for biliary procedures
  - 10-20% for pancreatic procedures
  - Up to 30% for evaluation of sphincter hypertension in young women
  - Most common predictor is prior post-ERCP pancreatitis (5-fold ↑), biliary sphincter dilation (4.5-fold ↑), difficult cannulation (3.5-fold ↑), Pancreatic sphincterotomy (3-fold ↑), More than 1 pancreatic injection (2.7-fold ↑)
- Bleeding in 2% after sphincterotomy
  - Increased risk with: coagulopathy before ERCP, Anticoagulation within 72 hours, Cholangitis before ERCP, Non-experience
- Periampullary perforation in 0.3-0.5%
- Cholangitis in up to 6%, particularly if there is failed stone extraction and no stenting
- Death in 0.4% (1 in 200)

BEFORE PROCEDURE:
- Document Risk/Benefit/Alternatives in chart
- Labs: PT/PTT, Platelets
- Stop Warfarin × 3 days, Clopidogrel × 7 days

NOTES

7.07 ENDOSCOPIC ULTRASOUND (EUS)

(Gastrointest Endosc 2005;61:8-12)

INDICATIONS:
- Esophagus
  - Esophageal carcinoma T and N staging
  - Submucosal nodules and extrinsic compression
- Stomach and Duodenum
  - Gastric cancer staging
  - Submucosal nodules and extrinsic compression
  - Prominent gastric folds
  - Gastric lymphoma staging
- Pancreas
  - Investigation of acute recurrent pancreatitis (rule out bile duct stones, pancreatic obstruction and chronic pancreatitis)
  - Diagnosis of chronic pancreatitis (parenchymal and ductal criteria)
  - Pancreas cancer (local staging and biopsy)
  - Screening for biochemically-proven neuroendocrine tumors
  - Pancreatic cysts (aspiration of cyst contents)
  - Celiac plexus blockade or neurolysis for pancreatic pain
  - Pseudocyst drainage
  - Pancreas divisum (?)
  - Familial pancreatic cancer screening (?)
- Biliary
  - Bile duct stones (good alternative to ERCP if suspicion of stones is low or moderate, or if stones may have passed)
  - Investigation of obstructive jaundice
  - Staging of ampullary neoplasms
- Rectum
  - Rectal cancer staging
  - Evaluation of fecal incontinence
- Miscellaneous
  - Biopsy of mediastinal masses or lymph nodes
  - Lung cancer lymph node staging
  - Biopsy of accessible liver masses
  - Assessment of portal hypertension (varices, splenic vein patency)

METHODS (IN GENERAL):
- Higher frequencies (12-20 Mhz) allow higher resolution imaging of lesions closer to the endoscope (↑ detail, ↓ depth of penetration)
- Lower frequencies (5 Mhz) allow increased penetration of tissue and imaging of distant lesions (↓ detail, ↑ depth of penetration)
- Radial: can image 360 degrees in a plane perpendicular to the endoscope
- Linear: in a plane roughly 180 degrees parallel with the endoscope (most commonly used for FNA)

Terms for brightness and texture with examples:

	Brightness:	**Hypoechoic (Dark)**	**Isoechoic (Neutral)**	**Hyperechoic (Bright)**
Texture:	**Homogenous (smooth)**	Cysts	Low-grade malig	Lipoma
	Heterogenous (rough)	Malignancy	Rare tumors	Fat necrosis

- Patterns of echogenicity (surface epithelium to deep structures):
  - Bright: superficial mucosa
  - Dark: Lamina propria & Muscularis mucosa
    Mucosa is comprised of superficial mucosa (epithelium), lamina propria and muscularis mucosa
  - Bright: Submucosa
  - Dark: Muscularis Propria (longitudinal and transverse muscles)

COMPLICATIONS/RISK:
- No absolute contraindications, considerations include (similar to EGD):
  - Risk > Benefit; Risks are related to severity of underlying disease, comorbid disease, therapeutic procedures, elderly
    - Shock and acute MI (risk may be greater than benefit)
  - Suspect perforation, Esophageal stricture, Duodenal obstruction, Zenker's diverticulum
  - Irreversible coagulopathy
  - Uncooperative, Lack of informed consent
- Generally safe:
  - 0.05% risk of major complications with diagnostic EUS (bleeding, perforation)
  - 0.003% 30-day mortality
  - Bleeding rate with FNA ~1–2%, usually self-limited
  - Pancreatitis rate with pancreatic FNA ~1%

BEFORE PROCEDURE (if FNA, pseudocyst drainage, or celiac plexus blockade planned):
- Document Risk/Benefit/Alternatives in chart
- Labs: PT/PTT, Platelets
- Stop Warfarin × 3 days, Clopidogrel × 7 days

7.08 FOREIGN BODIES

(Gastrointest Endosc 2002;55:802-06)

DEFINITION:
- Ingestion of a foreign substance

EPIDEMIOLOGY:
- Approximately 1500-3000 people die every year due to foreign body ingestion
- Only 10-20% of foreign bodies require removal through some form of therapeutic intervention; the rest pass via the GI tract without incident
- At risk:
  - 80% of ingestions are children (coins)
  - Adults: most common is food in pre-existing esophageal stricture/ring; almost all foreign bodies inserted into the rectum are in adults
  - Others: psychiatric patients, inmates, smugglers, alcoholics, elderly (dementia, poorly fitting dentures, dysphagia post-stroke)

PATHOPHYSIOLOGY:
- Several areas of anatomic or physiologic narrowing exist along the GI lumen and may compromise the spontaneous passage
  - Esophagus compression from aortic arch, LES, pylorus, ileocecal valve, anal sphincters
- Pathologic abnormalities can cause narrowing along the GI lumen
  - Strictures, tumors

Site	Anatomic Defect	Functional Defect
Esophagus	Stenosis, atresia, rings/webs, Zenker's(tics), vascular anomalies	Scleroderma, Achalasia, Chagas
Stomach	Pyloric stenosis (congenital, malignancy, post-op, ulcer)	Gastroparesis (diabetes, uremia, thyroid)
Intestine	Malignancy, Adhesions, Meckel's, Strictures (ischemic, surgical, IBD)	Idiopathic intestinal pseudoobstruction, Scleroderma
Colon	Strictures (ischemic, surgical, IBD, trauma, infection), Diverticula	Constipation, Megacolon, Pseudoobstruction
Anus	Stenosis (surgical, IBD, trauma, infection, radiation)	Hirschsprung's disease

Reprinted with permission from McNally P: GI/Liver Secrets 3rd ed. Elsevier/Mosby, 2006:529.

- Sharp objects (pins, needles, nails, toothpicks): may perforate the intestine, but in 70-90% they pass through without complications
  - Foreign bodies pass with axial flow down the lumen
  - Reflex relaxation and slowing of peristalsis causes sharp objects to turn around so sharp end trails down intestine
  - In colon, foreign objects are centered in the fecal bolus, which further protects bowel wall

CLINICAL MANIFESTATIONS/PHYSICAL EXAM:
- Adults correlate onset of symptoms to ingestion of specific meal or foreign body
  - Acute dysphagia (92%), Neck tenderness (60%), Inability to swallow oral secretions (indicates complete obstruction)
- Mentally retarded/psychiatric/children may remain asymptomatic for months after ingestion or may not volunteer information
- Respiratory compromise:
  - Wheezing, stridor, cough, or dyspnea associated may have entrapment in hypopharynx, trachea, pyriform sinus, Zenker's

DIAGNOSTIC STUDIES:
- X-ray: neck, chest, abdomen
- Never order a barium swallow

TREATMENTS:
- Identify the type of foreign body: Although most traverse the GI tract without complications, specific exceptions require immediate removal
    - Button alkaline batteries may cause coagulation necrosis in esophagus (in stomach, gastric acid neutralizes risk)
    - Objects longer than 6cm may become lodged in the C-loop of the duodenum and need removal with overtube
        - Blunt objects in stomach and <2.5 cm (adults) can be managed conservatively with weekly radiographs
    - Sharp objects carrying high risk of perforation should be removed before it passes to the level that is beyond reach of scope
        - Use overtube, keep sharp end facing down when removing
    - Any object lodged in esophagus that compromises ability to handle oral secretions and risk aspiration need immediate removal
- Surgical consultation: if perforation or other major complications are probable

Proposed algorithm
- Plain film of neck/chest/abdomen »
    - Free air: surgery
    - Asymptomatic/Negative X-rays: no treatment
    - Symptomatic/History of sharp objects or batteries/Negative perforation on X-rays: Urgent EGD
        - Coins: rat tooth, snare, roth net used to remove
        - Button batteries: roth net used to remove
        - Sharp objects: place overtube and use rat-tooth forceps to remove
        - Food bolus:
            - Distal visualization: push-through GEJ
            - Complete obstruction: snare, tripod, roth net; consider using overtube
            - Stricture/Ring: Peptic/Schatzki dilation

COMPLICATIONS:
- Bowel perforation, Mediastinitis, Hemorrhage, Death (overall very low)

7.09 GASTROINTESTINAL SURGERIES

BILLROTH TYPE-I PARTIAL GASTRECTOMY

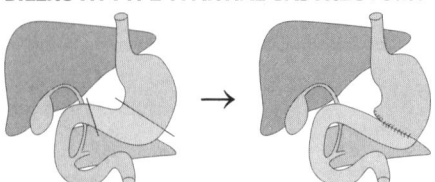

This operation removes part of the stomach. The top half of the stomach is reconnected with the duodenum.

Reprinted with permission from CancerHelp UK patient information website, cancerhelp.org.uk.

BILLROTH TYPE-II PARTIAL GASTRECTOMY

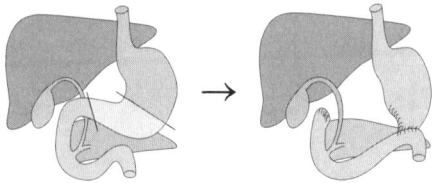

This operation removes part of the stomach. The top half of the stomach is reconnected more distally with the small bowel. The proximal end of the duodenum is sewn up to reestablish bile flow.

Reprinted with permission from CancerHelp UK patient information website, cancerhelp.org.uk.

ROUX-EN-Y TOTAL GASTRECTOMY

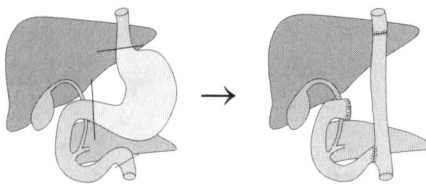

This operation removes all of the stomach, but allows the bile duct and pancreatic duct to continue to drain into the duodenum. The esophagus is reconnected directly to small bowel. The proximal end of the duodenum is sewn up, while the distal duodenum is reconnected to small bowel.

Reprinted with permission from CancerHelp UK patient information website, cancerhelp.org.uk.

WHIPPLE'S (PANCREATODUODENECTOMY)

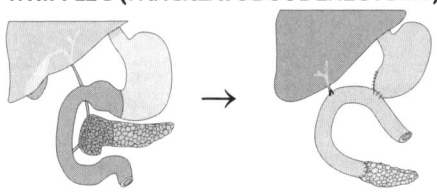

This operation removes the head of the pancreas, pylorus, duodenum, gallbladder, and part of the bile duct. Hepaticojujenostomy (re-establishes bile flow), pancreaticojujenostomy (re-establishes pancreatic flow). A pylorus preserving pancreaticoduodenectomy is often performed.

Reprinted with permission from CancerHelp UK patient information website, cancerhelp.org.uk.

PUESTOW (LONGITUDINAL PANCREATICOJEJUNOSTOMY)

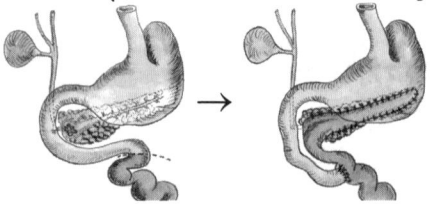

This operation, used for chronic pancreatitis, includes clearing the dilated pancreatic duct that causes blockage and pain. During the procedure, the duct is cleared and attached lengthwise to the small intestine. This increases the amount of pancreatic enzymes secreted into the small intestines.

Reprinted with permission from Medical University of South Carolina, www.ddc.musc.edu.

NOTES

7.10 INFECTIOUS ENDOCARDITIS PROPHYLAXIS FOR ENDOSCOPY

(Gastrointest Endosc 2003;58:475-82)
Note: Changes to these guidelines are likely forthcoming as GI societies adopt recent new recommendations, published (April 2007) in *Circulation: Journal of the American Heart Association,* that are based on a growing body of scientific evidence that shows that, for most people, the risks of taking prophylaxis antibiotics for certain procedures outweigh the benefits.

NEGLIGIBLE-RISK PATIENTS:
MVP without murmur/regurgitation
Physiologic murmurs
Secundum ASD
Surgical repair: ASD, VSD, PDA
Cardiac pacers, defibrillators
History of Rheumatic Fever without valve dysfunction
History of Kawasaki without valve dysfunction
CABG
Prosthetic joints

MODERATE-RISK PATIENTS:
MVP with regurgitation
HCM/IHSS
Acquired valve disease: stenosis/regurgitation/rheumatic
Ostium primum ASD
VSD, PDA
Bicuspid aortic valve
coarctation of aorta

HIGH-RISK PATIENTS:
Prosthetic heart valves
Previous infectious endocarditis
Complex cyanotic congenital heart disease
Surgical pulmonary shunts
Cirrhosis

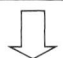

No Prophylaxis recommended
For all routine procedures with or without biopsy

Exception
Everyone gets prophylaxis with:
ERCP
EUS-FNA
Cirrhotics with GI bleed

IE Prophylaxis *Optional* for the following procedures
Sclerotherapy for esophageal varices
Esophageal stricture dilation
Any surgery to intestinal mucosa
PEG tubes

No Prophylaxis recommended
For all routine procedures with or without biopsies

IE Prophylaxis *Definitely* recommended for the following procedures
Sclerotherapy for esophageal varices
Esophageal stricture dilation
ERCP or biliary surgery
EUS-FNA
Any surgery to intestinal mucosa
PEG tubes

Optional Prophylaxis
For routine endoscopy (with or without biopsy) or EBL or TEE

GI Procedure Antibiotic Regimes

GI Procedure Antibiotic Regimes

Adults with GI procedures (except esophageal)

Amoxicillin, 2 g po 1 hr prior
 or
Ampicillin, 2 g IM/IV 30 min prior

If penicillin allergy:
Vancomycin, 1 g IV 30 min prior

Adults with GI procedures (except esophageal)

Ampicillin, 2 g IM/IV prior *with* Gentamycin, 1.5 mg/kg IV prior (<120 mg total)
 And a post procedure dose:
 Ampicillin 1 g IM/IV 6 hr after
  or
 Amoxicillin 1 g po 6 hr after

If penicillin allergy:
Vancomycin, 1 g IV prior
 And
Gentamycin, 1.5 mg/kg IV prior (<120 mg total)

Esophageal Procedure Antibiotic Regimes

Esophageal Procedure Antibiotic Regimes

Esophageal Procedures

Amoxicillin 2 g po 1 hr prior
 or
Ampicillin 2 g IV/IM 30 min prior

If penicillin allergy:
Clindamycin 600 po 1 hr prior
 or
Cephalexin 2 gm po 1 hr prior
 or
Azithromycin 500 po 1 hr prior

If penicillin allergy and NPO:
Clindamycin: 600 mg IV 30 min prior
 or
Cefazolin 1 gm IV/IM 30 min prior

Esophageal Procedures

Amoxicillin 2 g po 1 hr prior
 or
Ampicillin 2 g IV/IM 30 min prior

If penicillin allergy:
Clindamycin 600 po 1 hr prior
 or
Cephalexin 2 gm po 1 hr prior
 or
Azithromycin 500 po 1 hr prior

If penicillin allergy and NPO:
Clindamycin: 600 mg IV 30 min prior
 or
Cefazolin 1 gm IV/IM 30 min prior

Index

Pages followed by t indicate tables and f indicate figures.

A

Abciximab, for endoscopy, 296
Abdominal aneurysm, ruptured, 72
Abdominal pain, 70-71
    acute, 72-73
    chronic, 74-75
    general, 70-71
    referred, 70
    somatoparietal, 70
    visceral, 70
Abscess, liver, 160-161, 225
Abuse, alcohol, 166
Acetaminophen, liver disease from, 190-191
Acetylcholine, on gastric function, 66
Acetylcysteine, for trichobezoars, 67
Achalasia, 2-3, 45, 45f
Acid suppression, ICU indications, 34
Acini, hepatic, 216
Acute alcohol toxicity, 166
Acute fatty liver of pregnancy, 234
Acute liver failure, 162-165
    clinical manifestations of, 163
    definition of, 162
    epidemiology of, 162
    etiologies of, 162
    laboratory and diagnostic studies of, 163
    pathophysiology of, 162
    prognosis with, 165
    treatment of, 164
Acyclovir
    for EBV esophageal infection, 22
    for HSV infection, 22, 236
Adalimumab, for Crohn's and ulcerative colitis, 149
Adefovir, for hepatitis B, 202
Adenocarcinoma
    colorectal, 90
    esophageal, 20
    gastric, 24
    pancreatic, 266-268
    small bowel, 136-137
Adenoma
    Brunner's gland, 137
    liver cell, 219
    small bowel, 136-137
    sporadic, 154
Adenoma-like mass (ALM), 154
Adenomatous polyposis coli, small bowel tumors with, 136
Aeromonas diarrhea, 103
African iron overload, 194
Albendazole, for hydatid cyst disease, 209
Albumin, in liver function tests, 220
Albumin replacement
    for ascites and portal hypertension, 170-173
    for hepatorenal syndrome, 215
Alcohol abuse, 166
Alcohol dependency, 166
Alcoholic cirrhosis, 217
Alcoholic hepatitis, 166-167, 217
Alcoholic liver disease, 166-168, 217
Alcohol toxicity, acute, 166
Aldactone, for ascites and portal hypertension, 171
Alkaline phosphatase, abnormal, 220
Alosetron, for irritable bowel syndrome, 116
α-1-antitrypsin deficiency, 158-159, 219
Alprazolam, for nausea and vomiting, 49
ALT, abnormal, 220
AMA-negative primary biliary cirrhosis, 230
Amanita phalloides, liver disease from, 192
Amebic abscess of liver, 160-161
Aminoglycosides. *See also specific agents*
    for *H. Pylori* esophageal infection, 22
    for pyogenic liver abscess, 161
5-Amino salicylic acid (5-ASA). *See also specific agents*
    for Crohn's and ulcerative colitis, 148
    for endoscopy, 296
    for radiation colitis, 147
Aminotransferases, abnormal, 220
Amiodarone, liver disease from, 193
Amitriptyline
    for esophageal spasm, 62
    for irritable bowel syndrome, 116
Amoxicillin
    for *H. Pylori* peptic ulcer disease, 60
    liver disease from, 192
Amphotericin B, for *Candida* esophageal infection, 22
Ampicillin
    for diverticulitis, 107
    for pyogenic liver abscess, 161
Ampicillin/sulbactam, for cholecystitis and cholangitis, 256
Amylase, 280
Anal fissures, 77
Anal foreign bodies, 310-311
Anesthetic agents, liver disease from, 192
Anorectal diseases, 76-77
Anorexia, 48, 67
Antacids
    for esophagitis, 38
    for gastroesophageal reflux disease, 38
    for peptic ulcer disease, 60
Antiarthritics, liver disease from, 193
Anticholinergics. *See also specific agents*
    for nausea and vomiting, 49
Anticoagulants. *See also specific agents*
    for endoscopy, 296

INDEX

Antidepressants. *See also specific agents*
    for esophageal spasm, 63
    for sphincter of Oddi dysfunction, 279
    tricyclic, for esophageal spasm, 63
Antispasmodics, for sphincter of Oddi dysfunction, 279
Antral gastritis, chronic, 35
Appendicitis, 72, 78-79
Argon plasma coagulation (APC) therapy, 294
Ascites, portal hypertension and, 170-172
Ascites fluid total protein (AFTP), 171
Aspirin, for Barrett's esophagus, 5
AST, abnormal, 220
Attenuated adenomatous polyposis coli (AAPC), 90
Augmentin, for bacterial overgrowth, 81
Autoimmune cholangitis, 230
Autoimmune hepatitis (AIH), 174-177, 234
Azathioprine (6-MP)
    for autoimmune hepatitis, 176, 234
    for Crohn's and ulcerative colitis, 149, 150
    for microscopic colitis, 146
    in pregnancy, 234
    for transplant immunosuppression, 242

B

Backwash ileitis, 152
Baclofen, for hiccups, 67
Bacterial infection. *See also specific infections*
    esophageal, 22
Bacterial overgrowth, GI tract, 80-81
Bacterial peritonitis, 178-179
Bactrim
    for bacterial overgrowth, 81
    for bacterial peritonitis prophylaxis, 178
Balloon tamponade, 298-299
Balsalazide, for Crohn's and ulcerative colitis, 148
Bantu hemosiderosis, 194
Barrett's esophagus, 4-6
Battery ingestion, 311
Batts & Ludwig system, 217-218
Beta-blockers. *See also specific agents*
    for variceal bleeding, 292-293
Beta-lactam antibiotics. *See also specific agents*
    for *H. Pylori* esophageal infection, 22
Bethanechol, for gastroparesis, 31
Bezoars, 67
Bile duct cancers, 252-255. *See also* Cholangiocarcinoma
Bile duct cysts, 208, 208f
Bile duct disorders, 218
Bile salt diarrhea, 156
Biliary cirrhosis, primary, 218, 230-231
Biliary dyskinesia, 278
Bilirubin, in liver function tests, 220
Billroth type-I partial gastrectomy, 312, 312f
Billroth type-II partial gastrectomy, 312, 312f
Biopsy, liver, 222
Biotin, 125
Bisacodyl, for constipation, 96
Bismuth subsalicylate
    for diarrhea, 101
    for microscopic colitis, 146

Bleeding, gastrointestinal, 282-294
    acute, 282
    argon plasma coagulation therapy for, 294
    diverticular, 284
    endoscopy-related, 282
    lower, 288-291
    occult and obscure, 286-287
    upper, 288-291
    variceal, 292-293
Bloating
    differential diagnosis of, 114
    with IBS, 115
Blood sugar management, in TPN, 130
Body mass index (BMI), 124, 129
Body weight, ideal, 129
Bosentan, for portopulmonary hypertension, 240
Botulinum toxin, for esophageal spasm, 63
Bridging fibrosis, in liver, 216
Brunner's gland adenoma, 137
Budd-Chiari syndrome, 185, 235
Budesonide
    for Crohn's and ulcerative colitis, 148
    for microscopic colitis, 146
Bulimia, 67
Button alkaline battery ingestion, 311

C

Calcium, 125
Calcium-channel blockers. *See also specific agents*
    for esophageal spasm, 63
Calcium oxalate stones, in inflammatory bowel disease, 156
Campylobacter diarrhea, 103
Cancer. *See also specific types*
    bile duct, 252-255
    colorectal, 90-93, 154 (*See also* Colorectal cancer)
    esophageal, 20-21
    gastric, 24-26
    liver, 219
Candida albicans esophageal infection, 22
Capsule endoscopy, 300-301
Captopril, liver disease from, 193
Carcinoid syndrome, treatment of, 85
Carcinoid tumors (carcinoids)
    classification of, 84
    complications of chronic gastritis, 35
    mid-gut, 84-85
    small bowel, 136-137
Caroli's disease, 209
Caroli's syndrome, 209
Castor oil, for constipation, 96
Cathartics, for constipation, 96
Caustic agents, esophageal injury from, 40-41
Cavernous hemangiomas, 224
Cefotaxime, for bacterial peritonitis, 178
Cefotetan, for diverticulitis, 107
Ceftriaxone
    for bacterial peritonitis, 178
    for Whipple's disease, 139
Celiac sprue, 86-87
Cephalexin, for diverticulitis, 107

INDEX

Cephalosporin, for pyogenic liver abscess, 161
Cephalosporin, third-generation
   for bacterial peritonitis, 178
   for cholecystitis and cholangitis, 256
   for variceal bleeding, acute, 293
   for Whipple's disease, 139
Chaparral leaf, liver disease from, 193
Charcot's triad, 78, 257
Chest pain, noncardiac, 52-53
Chief cells, 66
Chlordiazepoxide, for irritable bowel syndrome, 116
Chlorzoxazone, liver disease from, 193
Cholangiocarcinoma, 225, 252-255
   clinical manifestations of, 253
   definition and classification of, 252
   diagnostic studies of, 253-254
   epidemiology of, 252
   etiology of, 252-253
   laboratory studies of, 253
   pathophysiology of, 253
   prognosis in, 255
   treatment of, 254-255
Cholangitis, 230, 256-257
Cholecystitis, 72, 256
Choledochal cyst, 208, 208f
Choledochal dilation, segmental, 208, 208f
Choledochocele, 208, 208f
Choledocholithiasis, 260
Cholelithiasis, 258-260
Cholestasis, 218
   intrahepatic, of pregnancy, 235
   on liver function tests, 220, 221
Cholestyramine
   for *C. Difficile* diarrhea, 83
   for carcinoid syndrome, 85
   for diarrhea, 101
   for fecal incontinence, 109
   for intrahepatic cholestasis of pregnancy, 235
   for microscopic colitis, 146
   for primary biliary cirrhosis, 231
   for primary sclerosing cholangitis, 233
   for short bowel syndrome, 134
Chromium, 125
Ciprofloxacin
   for bacterial overgrowth, 81
   for bacterial peritonitis prophylaxis, 178
   for Crohn's and ulcerative colitis, 148
   for diverticulitis, 107
Cirrhosis
   alcoholic, 217
   ascites and portal hypertension from, 170
   encephalopathy and, 180-182
   histopathology of, 216
   primary biliary, 218, 230-231
Cisapride
   for constipation, 96
   for gastroparesis, 31
Clarithromycin, for *H. Pylori* peptic ulcer disease, 60
Clavulanic acid, liver disease from, 192
Clidinium, for irritable bowel syndrome, 116
Clindamycin
   for cholecystitis and cholangitis, 256
   for pyogenic liver abscess, 161

Clonidine, for diarrhea, 101
Clopidogrel, for endoscopy, 296
Clostridium Difficile diarrhea, 82-83, 103
Clots, from liver disease, 184-187
Cobalamin, 125
Cocaine, liver disease from, 191-192
Codeine
   for diarrhea, 101
   for fecal incontinence, 109
Colchicine, for primary biliary cirrhosis, 231
Colitis
   collagenous, 146-147
   Crohn's disease, 142-144, 148-151
   intermediate, 152
   ischemic, 118-119
   lymphocytic, 146-147
   microscopic, 146-147
   pseudomembranous, from *C. Difficile* diarrhea, 82
   radiation, 147
   ulcerative, 152-155
      treatment of, 148-151
Collagenous colitis, 146-147
Colon foreign bodies, 310-311
Colonoscopy, 302-303
Colorectal cancer, 90-93
   clinical manifestations and physical exam for, 91
   definition of, 90
   diagnostic studies of, 91
   epidemiology of, 90
   etiologies of, 90
   from inflammatory bowel disease, 154
   laboratory studies of, 91
   pathophysiology of, 91
   postoperative surveillance after resection in, 93
   prognosis in, 93
   screening for, 92
   surveillance post-polypectomy in, 92
   treatments for, 93
Comfrey, liver disease from, 193
Congenital hepatic fibrosis, 188
Constipation, 94-96
Copper, 125
Corrosive injury, of esophagus, 40-41
Corticosteroids. *See also specific agents*
   for Crohn's and ulcerative colitis, 148
   for eosinophilic esophagitis, 17
   for nausea and vomiting, 49
Costochondritis, noncardiac chest pain from, 52
Courvoisier's sign, 266
Crohn's disease, 142-144
   small bowel tumors with, 136
   treatment of, 148-151
Cromolyn
   for eosinophilic esophagitis, 17
   for eosinophilic gastroenteritis, 19
Cuffitis, 155
Cyanoacrylate injection, for variceal bleeding, 293
Cyclosporine
   for Crohn's and ulcerative colitis, 149, 151
   for transplant immunosuppression, 242
Cylindrical duct dilation, 208, 208f

INDEX

Cyst
    bile duct, 208, 208f
    choledochal, 208, 208f
    hepatic, 225
    hepatic, simple, 209
    in hydatid cyst disease, 209
    intrahepatic duct, 208, 208f
    pancreatic, 262–264
Cystic disease of the pancreas, 262–264
Cystic neoplasms, pancreatic, 262–264
Cytomegalovirus (CMV) infection, esophageal, 22

D

Deferoxamine, for hemochromatosis and iron overload, 196
Dependency, alcohol, 166
Dexamethasone, for nausea and vomiting, 49
Diarrhea, 98–101
    antibiotic associated, 82
    bile salt, 156
    Clostridium Difficile, 82–83
    definition of, 98
    fatty acid, 156
    fatty (malassimilation), 99
    infectious, 98
    inflammatory, 98
    motility/functional, 99
    traveler's, 104
    treatment of, 101
    watery, 98–99
    workup for
        acute, 99
        chronic, 100
Diarrheal infections, 98, 102–104
    acute, 102–103
    chronic, 104
    food poisoning, 104
    oral solutions for, 104
    traveler's, 104
    treatment of, 104
Diazoxide, for insulinoma, 111
Diclofenac, liver disease from, 193
Dicyclomine, for irritable bowel syndrome, 116
Diffuse duct dilation, 208, 208f
Diffuse esophageal spasm, esophageal manometry for, 46, 46f
Dilation, esophageal, 14, 62
Diltiazem, for esophageal spasm, 63
Dimenhydrinate, for nausea and vomiting, 49
Diphenhydramine
    for nausea and vomiting, 49
    for primary biliary cirrhosis, 231
    for primary sclerosing cholangitis, 233
Diphenoxylate, for diarrhea, 101
Dipyridamole, for endoscopy, 296
Diuretics. *See also specific agents*
    for ascites and portal hypertension, 171
    for Budd-Chiari syndrome, 185
Diverticula
    of esophagus, 8
    extrahepatic duct, 208, 208f

Diverticular bleeding, 284
Diverticulitis, 72, 106–107
Diverticulosis, 106
Docusate sodium, for constipation, 96
Dolasetron, for nausea and vomiting, 49
Domperidone
    for gastroparesis, 31
    for nausea and vomiting, 49
Dopamine antagonists. *See also specific agents*
    for nausea and vomiting, 49
Doxycycline, for bacterial overgrowth, 81
Drug-induced liver disease, 190–193, 218. *See also specific drugs*
Dumping syndrome, 32
Dyspepsia, 10–11
Dysphagia, 12–14
Dysphagia lusoria, 12
Dysplasia-associated lesion/mass (DALM), 154

E

Eating disorders, 67
Eclampsia, liver function in, 235–236
Ecstasy, liver disease from, 192
Ectopic pregnancy, ruptured, abdominal pain in, 72
Electrolytes, in TPN, 130
Enalapril, liver disease from, 193
Encephalopathy
    cirrhosis and, 180–182
    hepatic, 180–182
Endocarditis prophylaxis, for endoscopy, 314–315
Endocrine tumors, GI, 110–113
Endoscopic retrograde cholangiopancreatography (ERCP), 306
Endoscopic ultrasound (EUS), 308–309
Endoscopy
    anticoagulation and anti-inflammatory agents for, 296
    capsule, 300–301
    endocarditis prophylaxis for, 314–315
Endothelin receptor antagonists. *See also specific drugs*
    for portopulmonary hypertension, 240
Enemas, for constipation, 96
Energy requirements, 129
Enflurane, liver disease from, 192
Entecavir, for hepatitis B, 202
Enterohemorrhagic *E. coli* O157:H7 (EHEC) diarrhea, 103
Enteroinvasive *E. coli* (EIEC) diarrhea, 103
Enteropathogenic *E. coli* (ETEC) diarrhea, 102
Enterotoxicogenic *E. coli* (ETEC) diarrhea, 102
Eosinophilic esophagitis, 16–17
Eosinophilic gastroenteritis, 18–19
Epiphrenic diverticula, 8
Epoprostenol, for portopulmonary hypertension, 240
Epstein-Barr virus (EBV) infection, esophageal, 22
Eptifibatide, for endoscopy, 296
Erythromycin
    for gastroparesis, 31
    for nausea and vomiting, 49

INDEX

Erythromycin estolate, liver disease from, 192
Esomeprazole
  for esophagitis, 38
  for gastroesophageal reflux disease, 38
Esophageal cancer, 20-21
Esophageal disorders, 2-22
  achalasia, 2-3
  Barrett's esophagus, 4-6
  cancer, 20-21
  diverticula of esophagus, 8
  dyspepsia (indigestion), 10-11
  dysphagia/odynophagia, 12-14
  eosinophilic esophagitis, 16-17
  eosinophilic gastroenteritis, 18-19
  esophageal intramural pseudodiverticulosis, 8
  esophagitis and reflux esophagitis, 36-39
  gastroesophageal reflux disease, 36-39
  infections, 22
  lichen planus, 67
  manometry for, 44-47
  noncardiac chest pain, 52-53
  nonerosive reflux disease, 36-39
  Schatzki's ring, 62
  spasms, 62-63
Esophageal dysmotility, noncardiac chest pain from, 52
Esophageal dysphagia, 12-14
Esophageal foreign bodies, 310-311
Esophageal infections, 22
Esophageal injury
  corrosive, 40-41
  pill-induced, 42
Esophageal intramural pseudodiverticulosis, 8
Esophageal lichen planus, 67
Esophageal manometry, 44-47
Esophageal motility abnormalities, 44, 62-63
Esophageal spasm, diffuse, manometry for, 46, 46f
Esophageal spasms, 62-63
Esophagitis
  eosinophilic, 16-17
  erosive, 36-39
Esophagogastroduodenoscopy (EGD), 304
Estrogen, for fecal incontinence, 109
Extrahepatic duct diverticula, 208, 208f

F

Familial adenomatous polyposis (FAP), 90. *See also* Colorectal cancer
Familial colon cancer syndromes, 90
Famotidine
  for esophagitis, 38
  for gastroesophageal reflux disease, 38
Fat, fecal, 140
Fatty acid diarrhea, 156
Fatty change, in liver, 217
Fatty infiltration, of liver, 225
Fatty liver disease, non-alcoholic, 228-229
Fatty liver of pregnancy, 234
Fecal fat, 140
Fecal incontinence, 108-109

Fiber
  for constipation, 95
  for irritable bowel syndrome, 116
Fibrolamellar carcinoma, 210
Fibrosis, congenital hepatic, 188
FK506, for transplant immunosuppression, 242
Fluconazole, for *Candida* esophageal infection, 22
Fluoride, 125
Fluticasone, for eosinophilic esophagitis, 17
Focal nodular hyperplasia (FNH), hepatic, 219, 224
Folic acid, 125
  for tropical sprue, 88
Food allergy, 18
Food poisoning, diarrhea from, 104
Foreign bodies, 310-311
Fulminant hepatic failure, 162-165. *See also* Acute liver failure
Functional dyspepsia, 10
Fundal gastritis, chronic, 35
Fungal infections, esophageal, 22

G

Gallbladder polyps, 280
Gallstones
  noncardiac chest pain from, 52
  in pregnancy, 235
Ganciclovir, for CMV esophageal infection, 22
Gastrectomy
  partial, Billroth type-I, 312, 312f
  partial, Billroth type-II, 312, 312f
  total, roux-en-Y, 312, 312f
Gastric cancer, 24-26
Gastric carcinoid, 24
Gastric disorders, 24-70
  chronic antral gastritis, 35
  chronic fundal gastritis, 35
  dumping syndrome, 32
  gastric cancer, 24-26
  gastroesophageal reflux disease, 36-39
  gastroparesis, 30-32
  gastropathy, 34-35
  nausea and vomiting, 48-50
  noncardiac chest pain, 52-53
  nonerosive reflux disease, 36-39
  peptic ulcer disease, 58-61
  percutaneous endoscopic gastrostomy tubes for, 54-57
  polyps and thickened folds, 28-29
  Zollinger-Ellison syndrome (gastrinoma), 64-65
Gastric folds, thickened, 28-29
Gastric foreign bodies, 310-311
Gastric juice, 66
Gastric lymphoma, 24
Gastric physiology, 66
Gastric polyps, 28-29
Gastric variceal bleeding, 292-293
Gastrin, 66
Gastrinoma, 64-65
Gastritis, chronic antral, 35

Gastritis, chronic fundal, 35
Gastroenteritis
　abdominal pain in, 72
　eosinophilic, 18–19
　viral, diarrhea from, 102
Gastroesophageal reflux disease (GERD), 36–39, 52
Gastrointestinal bleed, 282–294
　acute, 282
　argon plasma coagulation therapy for, 294
　diverticular, 284
　endoscopy-related, 282
　lower, 288–291
　occult and obscure, 286–287
　upper, 288–291
　variceal, 292–293
Gastrointestinal endocrine tumors, 110–113. See also Carcinoid tumors (carcinoids); Zollinger-Ellison syndrome
　general information on, 110
　glucagonoma, 112
　insulinoma, 110–111
　somatostatinoma, 112–113
　VIPoma, 111
Gastrointestinal foreign bodies, 310–311
Gastrointestinal stromal tumors (GISTs), 24, 136–137
Gastrointestinal surgeries, 312, 312f
Gastroparesis, 30–32
Gastropathy, 34–35
Gastrostomy tubes, percutaneous endoscopic, 54–57
G cells, 66
Gemcitabine, for pancreatic carcinoma, 267
Gentamicin, for diverticulitis, 107
Globus (hystericus), 12
Glucagonoma, 112
Gluten-free diet, for celiac sprue, 87
Graft vs. host disease (GVHD), after liver transplantation, 219
Granuloma, 218
Granulomatous inflammation, hepatic, 218

H

Haloperidol, for nausea and vomiting, 49
Halothane, liver disease from, 192
Hamartomatous polyp syndromes, 90
H2 blockers. See also specific agents
　for esophagitis, 38
　for gastritis, chronic, 35
　for gastroesophageal reflux disease, 38
Helicobacter Pylori infection
　esophageal, 22
　peptic ulcer disease from, 58–61
HELLP syndrome, liver function in, 235–236
Hematemesis, 288
Hematochezia, 288
Hemochromatosis, 194–197, 219
　clinical manifestations of, 195
　complications of, 196–197
　definitions in, 194
　diagnostic studies of, 196

epidemiology and etiologies of, 194
laboratory studies of, 195–196
liver in, 219
pathophysiology of, 194–195
prognosis in, 197
treatment of, 196
Hemorrhage. See Bleeding; Gastrointestinal bleed
Hemorrhoids, 76
Hemosiderosis, Bantu, 194
Hemosuccus pancreaticus, 262
Heparin, for Budd-Chiari syndrome, 185
Hepatic acini, 216
Hepatic artery thrombosis, 187
Hepatic cysts, 225
　simple, 209
Hepatic encephalopathy, 180–182
Hepatic failure, fulminant, 162–165. See also Acute liver failure
Hepatic fibrosis, congenital, 188
Hepatic function tests, 220
Hepatic lymphoma, 225
Hepatic Venous Wedge Pressure Gradient (HVWPG), 171
Hepatitis
　alcoholic, 166–167, 217
　autoimmune, 174–177, 234
　in pregnancy, 234, 236
　viral, 217, 236 (See also *specific types*)
Hepatitis A, 198, 217, 236
Hepatitis A immune globulin (HAIG), in pregnancy, 236
Hepatitis A vaccine, in pregnancy, 236
Hepatitis B, 200–203, 217
　clinical manifestations of, 200
　complications of, 203
　definition of, 200
　diagnostic studies of, 201, 201t
　epidemiology and etiologies of, 200
　laboratory studies of, 200–201, 201f
　pathophysiology of, 200
　in pregnancy, 236
　prognosis in, 203
　treatment of, 202–203
Hepatitis B immune globulin (HBIG)
　for hepatitis B treatment, 202
　as hepatitis B vaccine, 203
　in pregnancy, 236
Hepatitis C, 204–207, 217, 236
Hepatitis D (delta), 198–199
Hepatitis E, 199, 236
Hepatobiliary cystic disease, 208–209
Hepatocellular carcinoma (HCC), 210–212
　differential diagnosis of, 225
　histopathology of, 219
　screening for, 226
Hepatocellular injury, on liver function tests, 220
Hepatocytes, 216
Hepatoma, 210–212
Hepatopulmonary syndrome, 238–239
Hepatorenal syndrome, 214–215
Herbs, liver disease from, 193
Hereditary hemochromatosis, 194–197

INDEX

Hereditary nonpolyposis colorectal cancer (HNPCC), 90, 136
Herpes simplex virus (HSV) infection
  esophageal, 22
  in pregnancy, 236
Hiccups, 66-67
Hirschsprung's, 122
H2RA, for peptic ulcer disease, 60
H2R antagonists, 66
5-HT3 agonist, for irritable bowel syndrome, 116
5-HT4 agonist, for constipation, 96
5-HT3 antagonist. *See also specific agents*
  for irritable bowel syndrome, 116
  for nausea and vomiting, 49
Human papilloma virus (HPV) infection, esophageal, 22
Hydatid cyst disease, 209
Hydralazine, liver disease from, 193
Hydrocortisone, for Crohn's and ulcerative colitis, 148
Hydroxyzine, for intrahepatic cholestasis of pregnancy, 235
Hyoscyamine sulfate, for irritable bowel syndrome, 116
Hyperbilirubinemia, isolated, on liver function tests, 220, 221
Hypertension, portal, ascites and, 170-172
Hypertensive lower esophageal sphincter, isolated, manometry for, 47
Hypertensive peristalsis, manometry for, 47
Hypoalbuminemic malnutrition, 124

I

Ibuprofen, liver disease from, 193
Ileitis, backwash, 152
Imidazoles, oral. *See also specific agents*
  for *Candida* esophageal infection, 22
Imipenem
  for cholecystitis and cholangitis, 256
  for pancreatitis, acute necrotizing, 272
Imipramine
  for esophageal spasm, 63
  for irritable bowel syndrome, 116
Immunomodulators. *See also specific agents*
  for Crohn's and ulcerative colitis, 149
Immunosuppression, after liver transplant, 242-243
Incontinence, fecal, 108-109
Indigestion, 10-11
Ineffective esophageal motility, manometry for, 47, 47f
Infections. *See also specific infections*
  diarrheal, 98, 102-104 (*See also* Diarrheal infections)
  esophageal, 22
Infiltrative pattern, on liver function tests, 221
Inflammatory bowel disease (IBD), 141-156
  Crohn's disease, 142-144
    small bowel tumors with, 136
    treatment of, 148-151
  kidney stones in, 156
  microscopic colitis, 146-147

mimickers of, 156
pearls on, 156
in pregnancy, 151
radiation colitis, 147
small bowel resection and malabsorption in, 156
ulcerative colitis, 152-155
treatment of, 148-151
Infliximab, for Crohn's and ulcerative colitis, 149, 150-151
Inherited colon cancer syndromes, 90
Inherited liver disease, 219
Insulinoma, 110-111
Interferon-α, for carcinoid syndrome, 85
Interferon-α-2a, PEG (PEG-IFN-α-2a), for hepatitis B, 202
Interferon-α-2b (PEG-IFN-α-2b), for hepatitis C, 205-206
Intermediate colitis, 152
Intestinal failure, 132
Intestinal foreign bodies, 310-311
Intraductal papillary mucinous neoplasm (IPMN), pancreatic, 262-264
Intrahepatic cholestasis of pregnancy, 235
Intrahepatic duct cysts, 208, 208f
Iodine, 125
Iron, 125
Iron overload, 194-197
  clinical manifestations of, 195
  complications of, 196-197
  definitions in, 194
  diagnostic studies of, 196
  epidemiology and etiologies of, 194
  laboratory studies of, 195-196
  pathophysiology of, 194-195
  prognosis in, 197
  treatment of, 196
Irritable bowel syndrome (IBS), 114-117
  clinical manifestations of, 115
  definition of, 114
  epidemiology of, 114
  etiology of, 114
  laboratory and diagnostic studies of, 115
  pathophysiology of, 114
  treatment of, 116-117
Ischemic colitis, 118-119
Ischemic small bowel, 120-121
Isoflurane, liver disease from, 192
Isolated hypertensive lower esophageal sphincter, manometry for, 47
Isoniazid (INH), liver disease from, 192

J

Jaundice, on liver function tests, 220, 221
Juvenile polyposis, 90

K

Ketoconazole, liver disease from, 192
Kidney stones, in inflammatory bowel disease, 156
Kilocalorie requirements, 129

INDEX

King's College criteria, 165
Kupffer cells, 216

L

Lactulose
    for acute liver failure, 164
    for constipation, 96
Lamivudine, for hepatitis B, 202
Lansoprazole
    for esophagitis, 38
    for gastroesophageal reflux disease, 38
Laryngopharyngeal reflux, 37
Laxatives
    for constipation, 96
    for irritable bowel syndrome, 116
Lichen planus, 67
Lipase, 280
Liver
    injury patterns of, 216
    microanatomy of, 216
    vascular anatomy of, 184, 184f
Liver abscess, 225
Liver biopsy, 222
Liver cancer, primary, 219
Liver disease, 157-250
    abscess, 160-161
    from acetaminophen, 190-191
    acute liver failure, 162-165 (*See also* Acute liver failure)
    alcoholic, 166-168, 217
    α-1-antitrypsin deficiency, 158-159, 219
    ascites and portal hypertension, 170-172
    autoimmune hepatitis, 174-177
    bacterial peritonitis, 178-179
    bile duct cysts, 208, 208f
    Caroli's disease, 209
    cirrhosis and encephalopathy, 180-182
    clots, 184-187
    from cocaine, 191-192
    congenital hepatic fibrosis, 188
    drug and toxin induced, 190-193, 218 (*See also specific drugs and toxins*)
    from ecstasy, 192
    fulminant hepatic failure, 162-165 (*See also* Acute liver failure)
    hemochromatosis, 194-197, 219
    hepatitis A, 198, 217
    hepatitis B, 200-203, 217 (*See also* Hepatitis B)
    hepatitis C, 204-207, 217
    hepatitis D (delta), 198-199
    hepatitis E, 199
    hepatobiliary cystic disease, 208-209
    hepatocellular carcinoma, 210-212
    hepatorenal syndrome, 214-215
    hydatid cyst disease, 209
    inherited, 219
    iron overload, 194-197
    liver cell injury in, 216
    liver mass evaluation in, 224-228 (*See also* Liver mass evaluation)
    metastatic neoplasms, 219
    from mushrooms, 192
    neoplasms, 219
    non-alcoholic fatty liver disease, 228-229
    polycystic liver disease, 209
    primary biliary cirrhosis, 230-231
    pulmonary complications of, 238-240
        hepatopulmonary syndrome, 238-239
        portopulmonary hypertension, 239-240
    simple hepatic cysts, 209
    transplantation for, 244-246
        immunosuppression after, 242-243
    Wilson's disease, 219, 248-250
Liver disease in pregnancy, 234-237
    acute fatty liver of pregnancy, 234
    autoimmune hepatitis, 234
    Budd-Chiari syndrome, 235
    gallstones, 235
    herpes simplex virus, 236
    intrahepatic cholestasis of pregnancy, 235
    in pre-eclampsia, eclampsia, HELLP syndrome, 235-236
    viral hepatitis, 236
    Wilson's disease, 236
Liver failure, acute, 162-165. *See also* Acute liver failure
Liver function, in pregnancy, 234
Liver function tests, 220-222
    abnormal, 220
    algorithms in, 221-222
    for hepatic function, 220
    patterns of liver injury in, 220-221
Liver granulomas, 218
Liver histology, in pregnancy, 234
Liver histopathology, 216-219
    alcoholic cirrhosis, 217
    α-1-antitrypsin deficiency, 219
    Batts & Ludwig system for, 217-218
    bile duct disorders, 218
    cholestasis, 218
    drug injury, 190-193, 218
    fatty change and steatohepatitis, 217
    granulomatous inflammation, 218
    hemochromatosis, 219
    hepatitis, alcoholic, 217
    hepatitis, viral, 217
    inherited liver disease, 219
    liver cell injury in, 216
    metastatic neoplasms, 219
    neoplasms, 219
    non-alcoholic fatty liver disease, 217
    primary tumors, 219
    steatosis, macrovesicular, 217
    steatosis, microvesicular, 217
    transplantation, 219
    Wilson's disease, 219
Liver injury, on liver function tests, 220-221
Liver mass evaluation, 224-228
    clinical manifestations in, 225
    definition of, 224
    diagnostic studies in, 226-227
    etiologies and differential diagnosis of, 224-225
    laboratory studies in, 226
    treatment in, 227
Liver transplantation, 242-243. *See also specific indications*

INDEX

Liver transplantation, immunosuppression after, 244–246
Lomotil, for fecal incontinence, 109
Longitudinal pancreaticojejunostomy, 312, 312f
Loperamide
    for diarrhea, 101
    for diarrhea from eosinophilic gastroenteritis, 19
    for fecal incontinence, 109
    for irritable bowel syndrome, 116
    for microscopic colitis, 146
Lorazepam, for nausea and vomiting, 49
Lower gastrointestinal bleeding, 288–291
Low-molecular-weight heparin, for endoscopy, 296
Lubiprostone
    for constipation, 96
    for diarrhea, 101
Lymphocytic colitis, 146–147
Lymphoma, hepatic, 225
Lynch II syndrome, small bowel tumors with, 136

M

Macrovesicular steatosis, 217
Maddrey Discriminate Function, 167
Magnesium, 125
Magnesium citrate, for constipation, 96
Magnesium sulfate, for constipation, 96
Malabsorption
    in short bowel syndrome, 132–134, 156
    from small bowel enteropathy vs. pancreatic insufficiency, 140
Malassimilation, 99
Malnutrition, 124–126
Manganese, 125
Mannitol, for acute liver failure, 164
Manometry, esophageal, 44–47
Marasmus, 124
Marseilles-Rome/Sarles classification, of chronic pancreatitis, 274
McBurney's point, 78
Meckel's diverticulum, 78–79
Meclizine, for nausea and vomiting, 49
Megacolon, 122–123
MELD (Model for End Stage Liver Disease), 182, 244
Melena, 288
Menetrier's disease, thickened gastric folds from, 29
Meperidine, for pancreatitis, acute, 272
Mercaptopurine (6MP), for Crohn's and ulcerative colitis, 149, 150
Meropenem
    for acute necrotizing pancreatitis, 272
Mesalamine, for Crohn's and ulcerative colitis, 148
Mesenteric ischemia, abdominal pain in, 72
Metastases, to liver, 219, 225
Metformin, for non-alcoholic fatty liver disease, 229
Methimazole, liver disease from, 192
Methotrexate (MTX)
    for Crohn's disease, 149
    liver disease from, 193
    for primary biliary cirrhosis, 231
Methoxyflurane, liver disease from, 192
Methylcellulose, for constipation, 95
Methyldopa, liver disease from, 193
Methylprednisolone, for Crohn's and ulcerative colitis, 148
Metoclopramide
    for constipation, 96
    for esophagitis, 38
    for gastroparesis, 31
    for nausea and vomiting, 49
Metronidazole
    for acute liver failure, 164
    for amebic liver abscess, 161
    for bacterial overgrowth, 81
    for *C. Difficile* diarrhea, 83
    for Crohn's and ulcerative colitis, 148
    for diverticulitis, 107
    for *H. Pylori* peptic ulcer disease, 60
    for pyogenic liver abscess, 161
Micronutrients, 125
Microscopic colitis, 146–147
Microvesicular steatosis, 217
Midodrine, for hepatorenal syndrome, 215
Milk of magnesia, for constipation, 96
Milk thistle, liver disease from, 193
Mineral oil, for constipation, 96
Minerals, 125
    in TPN, 129, 130
Misoprostol, 66
    for peptic ulcer disease, 60
Model for End Stage Liver Disease (MELD), 182, 244
Molybdenum, 125
Montelukast
    for eosinophilic esophagitis, 17
    for eosinophilic gastroenteritis, 19
Morphine, for diarrhea, 101
Mucinous cystic neoplasm (MCN), pancreatic, 262–264
Mucosal associated lymphoid tumors (MALT) gastric, 24
    thickened gastric folds from, 29
Mucosal defense factors, 66
Muromonab-CD3, for transplant immunosuppression, 243
Murphy's sign, 256
Mushrooms, liver disease from, 192
Mycophenolate, for transplant immunosuppression, 242

N

Nadolol, for variceal bleeding, 292–293
Nausea, 48–50
Nefopam, for hiccups, 67
Neomycin
    for acute liver failure, 164
    for bacterial overgrowth, 81
Neostigmine, for Ogilvie's syndrome, 123
Neurofibromatosis type 1, small bowel tumors with, 136
Niacin, 125
    liver disease from, 192

INDEX

Nicotinic acid supplements, for carcinoid syndrome, 85
Nifedipine, liver disease from, 193
Nitrofurantoin, liver disease from, 192
Nitroglycerin, for variceal bleeding, acute, 293
Non-alcoholic fatty liver disease (NAFLD), 217, 228-229
Non-alcoholic fatty liver (NAFL), 228-229
Non-alcoholic steatohepatitis (NASH), 228-229
Nonerosive reflux disease (NERD), 36-39
Non-Hodgkin lymphoma, thickened gastric folds from, 28
Nonsteroidal antiinflammatory agents (NSAIDs). *See also specific agents*
    for Barrett's esophagus, 5
    for endoscopy, 296
    peptic ulcer disease from, 58-61
Noradrenaline, for hepatorenal syndrome, 215
Norfloxacin, for bacterial peritonitis prophylaxis, 178
Norwalk virus, diarrhea from, 102
Nutcracker esophagus, manometry for, 47
Nutrition
    general questions on, 128
    malnutrition, 124-126
    obesity, 124-126
    refeeding syndrome, 131
    total parenteral, 128-131
Nutritional status, 124
Nystatin, for *Candida* esophageal infection, 22

O

Obesity, 124-126
Obscure bleeding, 286
Occult bleeding, 286
Octreotide
    for carcinoid syndrome, 85
    for diarrhea, 101
    for dumping syndrome, 32
    for GI bleeding from peptic ulcer disease, 290
    for glucagonoma, 112
    for hepatorenal syndrome, 215
    for insulinoma, 111
    for nausea and vomiting, 49
    for short bowel syndrome, 134
    for variceal bleeding, acute, 293
    for VIPoma, 111
Odynophagia, 12-14
Ogilvie's syndrome, 122-123
Olsalazine, for Crohn's and ulcerative colitis, 148
Omeprazole
    for esophagitis, 38
    for gastroesophageal reflux disease, 38
Ondansetron, for nausea and vomiting, 49
Opioids, for diarrhea, 101
Opium, tincture of, for diarrhea, 101
Oropharyngeal dysphagia, 12-14
Overlap syndrome, in primary biliary cirrhosis, 230
Oxalate, dietary restrictions, 134

P

Pancreas
    anatomy and physiology of, 280
    cystic disease of the, 262-264
Pancreatic carcinoma, 266-268
Pancreatic cyst, true, 262, 263
Pancreatic cystic neoplasms, 262-264
Pancreatic fibrosis, 274-276
Pancreatic insufficiency, malabsorption from, 140
Pancreaticojejunostomy, longitudinal, 312, 312f
Pancreatic pseudocyst, 262-264
Pancreatitis
    abdominal pain in, 72
    acute, 270-273
    chronic, 274-276
Pancreatoduodenectomy, 312, 312f
Pancrelipase, for chronic pancreatitis, 274
Pantoprazole
    for esophagitis, 38
    for gastroesophageal reflux disease, 38
Pantothenic acid, 125
Papaverine, for ischemic small bowel, 121
Parietal cell, 66
Pediatric Model for End Stage Liver Disease (PELD), 245
PEG-interferon-α-2a (PEG-IFN-α-2a)
    for hepatitis B, 202
    for hepatitis C, 205-206
PELD (Pediatric Model for End Stage Liver Disease), 245
D-Penicillamine, for Wilson's disease, 236, 249
Penicillin
    liver disease from, 192
    for pyogenic liver abscess, 161
Penicillin G, for Whipple's disease, 139
Pentoxifylline, for alcoholic liver disease, 167
Pepsin, 66
Pepsinogen, 66
Peptic ulcer disease (PUD), 58-61, 72
Percutaneous endoscopic gastrostomy (PEG) tubes, 54-57
Peritonitis, bacterial, 178-179
Peutz-Jeghers syndrome, 90, 136
Phenytoin, liver disease from, 193
Phospha-soda, for colonoscopy prep, 303
Phosphate sulfates, for constipation, 96
Phosphodiesterase inhibitors. *See also specific drugs*
    for portopulmonary hypertension, 240
Phosphorus, 125
Phytobezoars, 67
Pill-induced esophageal injury, 42
Piperacillin/tazobactam
    for bacterial peritonitis, 178
    for cholecystitis and cholangitis, 256
Plesiomonas, diarrhea from, 103
Polycystic liver disease, 209
Polyethylene glycol
    for colonoscopy prep, 303
    for constipation, 96

INDEX

Polyps
  colon, 91
  gallbladder, 280
  gastric, 28–29
  in hamartomatous polyp syndromes, 90
Portal hypertension, ascites and, 170–172
Portal tracts, 216
Portal vein thrombosis (PVT), 186
Portopulmonary hypertension, 239–240
Pouchitis, 155
Prague classification for Barrett's esophagus, 5
Prednisolone
  for alcoholic liver disease, 167
  for autoimmune hepatitis, 176
Prednisone
  for alcoholic liver disease, 167
  for autoimmune hepatitis, 176
  for Crohn's and ulcerative colitis, 148
  for eosinophilic gastroenteritis, 19
  for microscopic colitis, 146
  for radiation colitis, 147
Pre-eclampsia, liver function in, 235–236
Pregnancy
  inflammatory bowel disease in, 151
  liver disease in, 234–237 (See also Liver disease in pregnancy)
  liver in, 234
  ruptured ectopic, 72
Primary biliary cirrhosis (PBC), 218, 230–231
Primary sclerosing cholangitis (PSC), 218, 232–233
Probiotics, for C. Difficile diarrhea, 83
Procainamide, liver disease from, 193
Prochlorperazine, for nausea and vomiting, 49
Prokinetics, for constipation, 96
Promethazine, for nausea and vomiting, 49
Propranolol, for variceal bleeding, 292–293
Propylthiouracil, liver disease from, 192
Prostacyclin, for portopulmonary hypertension, 240
Prostaglandin E analogs, 66
Prostanoids, for portopulmonary hypertension, 240
Proteases, 280
Protein requirements, 129
Prothrombin time, in liver function tests, 220
Proton pump, 66
Proton pump inhibitor (PPI). See also specific agents
  for Barrett's esophagus, 5
  for eosinophilic esophagitis, 17
  for esophageal intramural pseudodiverticulosis, 8
  for esophagitis, 38
  for gastritis, chronic, 35
  for gastroesophageal reflux disease, 38
  for gastropathy, 34
  for GI bleeding from peptic ulcer disease, 290
  for H. Pylori peptic ulcer disease, 60
  for noncardiac chest pain, 53
  for short bowel syndrome, 134
  for variceal bleeding, acute, 293
  for Zollinger-Ellison syndrome (gastrinomas), 65

Pruritus ani, 77
Pseudoachalasia, 2, 20
Pseudocyst, pancreatic, 262–264
Pseudomembranous colitis, from *Clostridium Difficile* diarrhea, 82
Psyllium, for constipation, 95
Puestow procedure, 312, 312f
Pulmonary complications of liver disease, 238–240
  hepatopulmonary syndrome, 238–239
  portopulmonary hypertension, 239–240
Pyogenic abscess of liver, 160–161
Pyridoxine, 125
  for Wilson's disease, 249
Pyrimethamine-sulfadoxine, liver disease from, 192

Q

Quinidine, liver disease from, 193

R

Rabeprazole
  for esophagitis, 38
  for gastroesophageal reflux disease, 38
Radiation colitis, 147
Ranitidine
  for esophagitis, 38
  for gastroesophageal reflux disease, 38
Refeeding syndrome, 131
Reflux esophagitis, 36–39
Regurgitation, 48
Retching, 48
Reynold's pentad, 257
Ribavirin, for hepatitis C, 205–206
Riboflavin, 125
Rifamixin
  for bacterial overgrowth, 81
  for Crohn's and ulcerative colitis, 148
Rifampin
  for primary biliary cirrhosis, 231
  for primary sclerosing cholangitis, 233
Right lower quadrant pain, 78
Rotavirus, diarrhea from, 102
Roux-en-Y total gastrectomy, 312, 312f
Rovsing's sign, 78
Rumination, 48, 50

S

Saccharomyces boulardii, for *C. Difficile* diarrhea, 83
Salmonella, diarrhea from, 103
Schatzki's ring, 62
Scleroderma, esophageal manometry for, 47, 47f
Scopolamine, for nausea and vomiting, 49
Screening, for colorectal cancer, 92
Segmental choledochal dilation, 208, 208f

INDEX

Selective serotonin reuptake inhibitors (SSRIs)
  for irritable bowel syndrome, 116
  for sphincter of Oddi dysfunction, 279
Selenium, 125
Senna, for constipation, 96
Serum-ascites albumin gradient (SAAG), 170–171
Shigella diarrhea, 103
Short bowel syndrome, 132–134, 156
Sildenafil, for portopulmonary hypertension, 240
Simple hepatic cysts, 209
Sinusoids, hepatic vascular, 216
Sirolimus, for transplant immunosuppression, 242
Sitophobia, 48
Small bowel enteropathy, malabsorption from, 140
Small bowel obstruction, abdominal pain in, 72
Small bowel resection, malabsorption with, 132–134, 156
Small bowel tumors, 136–137
Solitary rectal ulcer syndrome, 77
Somatostatinoma, 112–113
Sorbitol, for constipation, 95, 96
Spasms, esophageal, 62–63
Sphincter of Oddi, 278–279
Sphincter of Oddi dysfunction (SOD), 278–279
Sporadic adenoma, 154
Sprue
  celiac, 86–87
  tropical, 87–88
Statins, liver disease from, 192
Steatohepatitis, 217
Steatohepatitis, non-alcoholic, 228–229
Steatosis
  macrovesicular, 217
  microvesicular, 217
Steroids. *See also* Corticosteroids; *specific agents*
  for lichen planus, 67
  liver disease from, 192
  for transplant immunosuppression, 242
Stomach cancer, 24–26
Stomach foreign bodies, 310–311
Stomach physiology, 66
Streptokinase, for Budd-Chiari syndrome, 185
Streptomycin, for Whipple's disease, 139
Sucralfate
  for esophagitis, 38
  for gastroesophageal reflux disease, 38
  for peptic ulcer disease, 60
Sulfasalazine
  for Crohn's and ulcerative colitis, 148
  for microscopic colitis, 146
Sulfonamides, liver disease from, 192
Sulfonylureas, liver disease from, 192
Sulindac, liver disease from, 193
Surgeries, gastrointestinal, 312, 312f

T

Tacrolimus, for transplant immunosuppression, 242
Tegaserod
  for constipation, 96
  for gastroparesis, 31
  for irritable bowel syndrome, 116

Terlipressin, for hepatorenal syndrome, 215
Tetracycline
  liver disease from, 192
  for tropical sprue, 88
Thiamine, 125
  for acute pancreatitis, 272
Thickened gastric folds, 28–29
Thrombosis
  hepatic artery, 187
  portal vein, 186
Thumbprinting on X-ray, 119, 121
Tincture of opium, for diarrhea, 101
Tirofiban, for endoscopy, 296
Tissue plasminogen, for Budd-Chiari syndrome, 185
Tolazine, for ischemic small bowel, 121
Total parenteral nutrition (TPN), 128–131
  for short bowel syndrome, 133
Toxic megacolon, 122–123, 152
Toxin-induced liver disease, 190–193
Traction diverticula, 8
Transplantation, liver, 219, 244–246. *See also specific indications*
Transplant immunosuppression, 242–243
Traveler's diarrhea, 104
Trazodone, for esophageal spasm, 63
Trichobezoars, 67
Tricyclic antidepressants (TCAs), for irritable bowel syndrome, 116
Trientine, for Wilson's disease, 249
Trimethoprim-sulfamethoxazole, for diverticulitis, 107
Troglitazone, liver disease from, 192
Tropical sprue, 87–88
Trypsin, 280
Tylenol, with alcoholic liver disease, 168
Tylosis, 20

U

Ulcer, in solitary rectal ulcer syndrome, 77
Ulcerative colitis, 152–155
Ulcerative colitis treatment, 148–151
Ultrasound, endoscopic, 308–309
Upper gastrointestinal bleeding, 288–291
Ursodeoxycholic acid (UDCA)
  for non-alcoholic fatty liver disease, 229
  for primary biliary cirrhosis, 231
  for primary sclerosing cholangitis, 233
Ursodiol, for cholelithiasis, 259

V

Vancomycin, for *C. Difficile* diarrhea, 83
Variant syndrome, in primary biliary cirrhosis, 230
Variceal bleeding, 292–293
Varicella zoster virus (VSV) infection, esophageal, 22
Vascular anatomy, of liver, 184, 184f
Vascular sinusoids, hepatic, 216
Vasoconstrictors. *See also specific agents*
  for hepatorenal syndrome, 215
Vasopressin, for acute variceal bleeding, 293

INDEX

Veno-occlusive disease (VOD), 186–187
    after liver transplantation, 219
Verapamil, liver disease from, 193
Vibrio cholera, diarrhea from, 102
Vibrio parahemolyticus, diarrhea from, 103
VIPoma, 111
Viral gastroenteritis, diarrhea from, 102
Viral infection. *See also* Hepatitis; *specific infections*
    esophageal, 22
Vitamin A, 125
    for primary biliary cirrhosis, 231
    for primary sclerosing cholangitis, 233
Vitamin B1, 125
Vitamin B2, 125
Vitamin B3, 125
Vitamin B6, 125
    for Wilson's disease, 249
Vitamin B12, 125
    for gastritis, chronic fundal, 35
    low, differential diagnosis of, 35
    for short bowel syndrome, 134
    for tropical sprue, 88
Vitamin B12 injection, for fundal gastritis, 35
Vitamin C, 125
Vitamin D, 125
    for primary biliary cirrhosis, 231
    for primary sclerosing cholangitis, 233
Vitamin E, 125
    for primary biliary cirrhosis, 231
Vitamin K, 125
    for intrahepatic cholestasis of pregnancy, 235
    for primary biliary cirrhosis, 231
    for primary sclerosing cholangitis, 233
Volume calculations, in TPN, 129
Vomiting, 48–50

Von Recklinghausen's disease, small bowel tumors with, 136

W

Warfarin
    for Budd-Chiari syndrome, 185
    for endoscopy, 296
Weight, ideal body, 129
Weil's syndrome, 257
Wheat dextrin, for constipation, 95
Whipple's disease, 138–139
Whipple's surgery, 312, 312f
Wilson's disease, 248–250
    liver in, 219
    in pregnancy, 236

X

D-Xylose test, 140

Y

Yersinia, diarrhea from, 103

Z

Zenker's diverticula, 8
Zinc, 125
    for Wilson's disease, 236, 249
Zollinger-Ellison syndrome, 64–65